To Fred Ke

I thought t k.

might have use

Thanks for your excellen

Bob

Postcholecystectomy Syndromes

POSTCHOLECYSTECTOMY SYNDROMES • A Clinical Approach to Etiology, Diagnosis, and Management

CLARENCE J. SCHEIN, M.D.

PROFESSOR OF SURGERY, MONTEFIORE
HOSPITAL MEDICAL CENTER AND
ALBERT EINSTEIN COLLEGE OF MEDICINE,
BRONX, NEW YORK

MEDICAL DEPARTMENT
HARPER & ROW, PUBLISHERS
HAGERSTOWN, MARYLAND
NEW YORK, SAN FRANCISCO, LONDON

DRUG DOSAGE

The author and publisher have exerted every effort to ensure that drug selection and dosage set forth in this text are in accord with current recommendations and practice at the time of publication. However, in view of ongoing research, changes in government regulations, and the constant flow of information relating to drug therapy and drug reactions, the reader is urged to check the package insert for each drug for any change in indications and dosage and for added warnings and precautions. This is particularly important when the recommended agent is a new and/or infrequently employed drug.

78 79 80 81 82 83 10 9 8 7 6 5 4 3 2 1

Library of Congress Cataloging in Publication Data

Schein, Clarence J
Postcholecystectomy syndromes.

Bibliography: p.
Includes index.
1. Cholecystectomy—Complications and sequelae.
I. Title. [DNLM: 1. Cholecystectomy—Adverse effects.
2. Postoperative complications. WI750 S319p]
RD546.S3 617'.556 77-11662
ISBN 0-06-142337-8

On the principle that one acts best in advance
of the anticipated result, I dedicate
this to others who also see in
each biliary problem
an exciting and a somewhat
different anatomic physiologic
event.

CONTENTS

PART IV **SECONDARY BILIARY TRACT OPERATIONS**

PART V **CASE STUDIES**

PREFACE

The prevalence of cholelithiasis and its complications makes cholecystectomy and bile duct surgery the most frequently performed intraabdominal operation. The postoperative results are not always satisfactory.

The incidence of postcholecystectomy dissatisfaction is in the 10–30% range. In general, the tangential experience of optimistic, mechanically oriented surgeons has tended to regard the results of procedures for calculus disorders in a better light than the family doctor's day-to-day follow-up would support (218,628).

The historical perspective accentuates the dismay which attends operative failures, for virtually all of the techniques employing drainage, bypass and excisional procedures were well established by the first decade of this century, and monographically documented by Moynihan (432) in 1905 and Kehr (322) in 1910.

Disappointed patients turn to virtually every speciality oriented consultant for advice—family physician, internist, gastroenterologist, radiologist, psychiatrist and surgeon. The residual problem can be as obvious as the retained stone in the neurotic, or as problematic as being confronted with typical symptoms and no objective abnormalities. The aim of this monograph has been the comprehensive presentation of the problem from an etiologic and diagnostic viewpoint, combining an experienced tested attitude toward comprehensive management and a detailed consideration of the pertinent literature.

Because of the variety of physicians involved, I have directed the text to consider all of the concerned disciplines. The psychiatrist and internist have important roles in the selection and evaluation of patients. In the majority of instances radiologic techniques are required for specific diagnosis. The surgical techniques are detailed because there are no trivia. The advances in peroral endoscopic stone extraction are considered, but await a long-term evaluation. The magnitude of the problem justifies this monograph—which is the first comprehensive consideration of the entire spectrum of postcholecystectomy disorders.

The organization of the text proceeds from fundamental considerations to in-fact case studies. The orientation is pertinently practical at the clinical level.

The case material comprises two groups of patients. Those in the first group underwent a revisional procedure. No surgery was advised for the second group. The indication for reintervention after a prior surgical failure is the demonstration of an anatomic abnormality that can cause infection, pain or obstruction. The goal of the revisionary surgical procedure is to establish a free flow of bile through an unobstructed conduit.

I present the attitudes and the techniques that I have found useful, together with their limitations and complications. These are based on the Montefiore Hospital Medical Center (MHMC) experience with 250 cases that were managed for these problems. Other viewpoints are included as a sincere concession to the efficacy of alternative methods. In these problems there is much to be learned in the well documented experiences of the past.

The procedures, attitudes and techniques are presented in great detail because good results follow attention to minutiae. Each chapter is intended to be complete for its specific subject material; therefore, some of the data overlaps chapter headings. The stripped-down case presentations are a convenient way of illustrating the concepts elaborated in the text.

The lessons learned in the management of the previously operated patients have served to suggest certain prophylactic and precautionary measures that can then be routinely applied to the first procedure. That would significantly reduce the incidence of this disorder.

Applied retrospective experiences can make the first operation definitive. That aphorism also applies to biliary problems. "Those who have not learned the lessons of the past, will have to repeat its errors."

Scarsdale, New York 1978 C.J.S.

ACKNOWLEDGMENTS

This monograph is not a parthogenetic product. The twenty-five year exposure to biliary problems occurred in relation to other individuals at the Montefiore Hospital Medical Center. I am anxious to acknowledge the pleasures and rewards of those mutual experiences.

To Dr. Thomas C. Beneventano, I am indebted for his continuous and continuing cooperation in the study of radiologic and physiologic aspects of common bile duct disorders. I remember Dr. Hans Wildegans of Berlin, who taught me choledochoscopy. Stanley Waine, who has illustrated two of my previous monographs I thank again, for his excellent clear and uncluttered drawings which graphically clarify the thousands of words. George N. Tanis did a superb job in the reproduction of x-rays and the photographic aspects of the text. Without his cooperation the manuscript would have been considerably delayed. Mrs. Marjorie de Forest went beyond the chore of most librarians in making the reference material available. Mrs. Lilla Kumme is credited for the excellence of the intraoperative cholangiograms. Dr. George Berci's ebullience caused my concepts to surface into print. I acknowledge with thanks the financial support of the MHMC, and Mrs. Rose Miller.

The most arduous and difficult task of collating all the material into a suitable manuscript fell upon Carol Grossman. Again—no words and many thanks.

To the personnel and the not impersonal nature of the Montefiore Hospital Medical Center, I am grateful for the opportunity to acquire this experience.

This book could not have been completed without the ambience created by early breakfasts and by Ada, Aviva and Amy Schein.

C.J.S.

Postcholecystectomy Syndromes

1 Fundamental Considerations

1 Anatomy and Physiology of the Normal Postcholecystectomy State

DEFINITION OF TERMS–INCIDENCE

The term **postcholecystectomy syndrome** (PCS) refers to a state in time. It is applied to those who, having already undergone biliary surgery, still have symptoms referable to persistent or new anatomic–physiologic derangements in the extrahepatic bile ducts. In the vast majority of instances these problems are related to persisting calculus disorders. Patients whose initial surgery was for cancer of the gallbladder or extrahepatic ducts are not included. The term PCS should not be applied to a wide variety of nonspecific dyspeptic symptoms whose origin is not in the biliary tract as the function of this conduit is presently understood. Eructations, flatulence, and intolerance of fatty food are not symptoms of biliary dysfunction. The first may be air swallowing, the second a functional bowel disorder, and third is not specific to any particular organ.

A more precise diagnosis can be applied to individual instances: incomplete biliary tract surgery, retained stone, iatrogenic complications of cholecystectomy, extrabiliary complications of cholecystolithiasis, or cholangiomanometric derangements. However, the term PCS is an acceptable concession to popular usage and encompasses a definite clinical spectrum; any other designation might be more accurate but less useful and less widely understood. All things considered, this accommodation is necessary. An alternative title I had considered was "Reoperative Biliary Surgery: Indications and Techniques." The term covers the broad medical, radiologic, and surgical aspects of the problem that are encountered by the variety of clinicians who deal with it. The term excludes unrelated primary disease in the liver, pancreas, or bowel although it does encompass diseases in those organs that are secondary to obstruction, infection, or fistulization originating in the biliary tract.

When patients regarded as having PCS are found to have disease elsewhere, it is least often in the appendix or hiatus of the diaphragm. It is most often in the pyloroduodenal sweep or in the colon.

Immediate postoperative complications such as early postoperative biliary fistulas, bile duct strictures, and intraabdominal abscess have been excluded from the PCS designate.

The term biliary dyskinesia or one of its equivalents applies to a specific clinical complex. A variety of disturbances in the Vaterian segment can be defined only by specific cholangiomanometric and debimetric techniques.

There is a diagnostic gap between the demonstration of an abnormality and its adjudication as the cause of symptoms. Some people go through a lifetime with completely silent choledocholithiasis, significant choledochalectasia, and sizable gallbladder remnants. The roentgen findings have to be integrated into the total clinical syndrome. If the term PCS is to have clinical validity, its symptoms must be objectively definable in terms of an anatomic, pathologic, or functional derangement (56, 255, 584, 593).

Obviously PCS does not apply to the complex of residual biliary disease incidentally associated with carcinoma of the bowel, cirrhosis of the liver, tumors of the pancreas, or the broad variety of medical disorders in the hepatoenteric system. When the antecedent procedure has been a cholecystostomy, the surgeon anticipates that there may be subsequent problems. When the tube vent is withdrawn, the gallbladder and its ductal system is again liable to all the problems of its still diseased but previously unmolested state.

Incidence of PCS

The incidence in females is strikingly high, far more than can be accounted for by the respective incidence of cholelithiasis in males and females. Women constitute over 80% of most PCS series, especially in the 40–49 age group. This high ratio has been ascribed to endocrine influences.

The frequency of the PCS is also a function of the avidity with which the entity is investigated, the depth of the inquiry into symptoms, and the criteria for the diagnosis. Some of the most valuable data have come from the countries that have a national health service. In general terms, few reports give a figure lower than 5–8% or greater than 40%.

Glenn's (225) 1972 evaluation of gallbladder disease as a national problem indicates that 5% of biliary operations are secondary procedures. In the Rigshospitalet (Copenhagen) (190) experience, 77 patients with severe PCS were referred for surgical consideration. In 51 a basis for complaints was established, and 65% of these benefited from secondary surgery. In 53% of this group there had been no subjective improvement after the first operation, and their symptoms appeared immediately or within 2 months. The most common cause for symptoms, other than biliary, was a musculoskeletal problem (including the scar), urologic disease, or a psychiatric problem. In the latter group the disorders included character neurosis, hysteria, psychopathology and paranoia.

Even with careful screening of the PCS patients, in about 50% no anatomic treatable derangement is brought to light.

Another Scandinavian study (70) indicates that the longer patients are followed—5 or 6 years, rather than 2 years—the greater the frequency of postoperative complaints. In the Montefiore Hospital and Medical Center experience this is especially true in patients originally operated upon for cholesterolosis or noncalculus cholecystitis.

Some reports are those of a large personal experience. Thus, Kourias (335) reviewed 18 series of secondary biliary operations and found the overall incidence of postoperative disease to vary between 10% and 23%. Of these recurrences, 16% appeared early and 84% presented remotely. The recurrences were most often due to residual calculi (50.6%), stenosing papillitis (13.0%), or pancreatopathy (7.0%). As the techniques have become more refined, the frequency of PCS in Kourias' personal series has decreased from 5% to 1% (335).

Mallet-Guy (397) reports an 8.2% incidence of PCS in a series of 6000 personal cases. He emphasizes functional derangements and exhibits a greater sensitivity to these factors than is credited in the American and English literature.

Weitz (621), of Hamburg, reports on a 4–5% incidence in 3194 cases, in which 50% of the problems were due to persistent stone disease; papillary stenosis was the second most common problem.

The magnitude of the problem is staggering from the standpoint of incidence and economics. About 750,000 primary biliary operations are done in one year in this country. If one accepts not the "medical" dissatisfactions, but the fact that 5–8% of these require some type of secondary surgical management, the toll is considerable. Some of these secondary operations might have been avoided if the first procedure had anticipated the potential of a residual problem.

The problem is especially important in this country, where the incidence of biliary surgery is six times that in Western Europe and nine times as frequent in patients below age 35. The most significant etiologic factor is choledocholithiasis and its sequelae. The overall published figure places its general incidence at 7–8% of all cases of cholelithiasis. Yet in a survey of cases requiring reoperation it involves about 70% of cases. Therefore, adequate initial common duct surgery can avoid the retained stone and bypass the stasis factor responsible for the primary stasis stone.

The statistical survey of the incidence of the problem correlates directly with the fact that biliary disease becomes more complicated pathologically and technically the longer it is permitted to go uncorrected. Hence, the high incidence of the disorder in the older patient. It has also been observed that the secondary biliary tract operation performed on a separate admission carries a higher mortality than the primary procedure. Glenn and McSherry (226) report a mortality of 6.7% in 253 cases. For elective cholecystectomy, the mortality was under 2%.

PERTINENCE OF CERTAIN FACETS OF BILIARY ANATOMY

The terms **choledochus** and **common bile duct** are employed interchangeably to include the extrahepatic conduit extending from the confluence of the right and left hepatic ducts to the duodenal papilla. This obviates the issue of the site of cystic duct insertion in relation to the anatomic distinction between the common hepatic and common bile duct.

For the purpose of nomenclature, the common bile duct is segmentally named in relation to the duodenum. That portion superior to the duodenum in the hepatoduodenal ligament is termed **supraduodenal**—this is the usual arena for choledochal exploration. The segment behind the duodenum, termed **retroduodenal,** is the occasional target for duodenal ulcer penetration. The infraduodenal segment passes through the pancreas and is termed **transpancreatic;** in this position it is inaccessible to exploration, but is influenced by the pancreatic reaction. The terminal common duct passes through the duodenum as the transduodenal segment, to exit at the duodenal papilla. Hence the distal choledochus and the major proximal divisions are not ordinarily exposed. The entire adult choledochus is approximately 11.5 cm in length.

Certain purely anatomic aspects of the area have surgically pertinent implications for decision-making. Specifically important are the course of the right and left hepatic ducts, the relationship between the common bile duct and pancreatic duct at their termination, and the components of the choledochoduodenal junction mechanism.

There is a strong probability that the variety of individual responses to the same nociceptive factor in the biliary tree is based in part on anatomic differences. The pancreatic response is influenced by whether the pancreatic ducts course through the parenchyma, whether the individual is one of the 13% who have a sphincter of the pancreatic duct or of the ampulla, and how important the drainage is from the duct of Santorini.

Hepatic Ducts

The right hepatic duct is formed by the confluence of its dorsocaudal and ventrocranial tributaries. That junction is intrahepatic. The latter tributary is in direct line with the common duct while the former enters the bifurcation from a sharp curve. For this anatomic reason, calculi are far less common in the dorsocaudal than in the ventrocranial division except in those instances in which they have been forcibly flushed beyond the curve. However, the lobular incidence of focal liver abscess in association with choledocholithiasis is equal and possibly even greater in the area served by the dorsocaudal branch. This may be related to less direct drainage of the dorsocaudal division into the choledochus.

The left hepatic duct ordinarily has no major tributaries. It has a long extrahepatic segment that is not buttressed by hepatic substance. This permits its unopposed dilation in association with distal obstruction. Therefore, it is the usual reservoir for hepatic duct calculi. In 50 patients who underwent a second operation for stones retained in the hepatic ducts, about 80% of the calculi were in the left hepatic duct, and none were in the dorsocaudal division of the right hepatic duct (Fig. 1-1).

Hepatic Segments

The segmental nature of the liver's architecture is recognized in the fact that each area has an artery, vein, and bile duct (portal triad) draining into a central vein. The liver parenchyma is divided into anatomic segments on this basis. This concept has had less clinical significance than that of the regional segments in the lung. However, stone-linked, congenital, and neoplastic disorders may have a segmental distribution that determines drainage and patterns of resection. Thus, liver resection in this regard is segmental: right hepatic lobectomy, extended right hepatic lobectomy, left lateral segmentectomy, and left lobar hepatectomy. The plane from the gallbladder to the inferior vena cava is considered to separate the right lobe from the left. The falciform ligament divides the medial from the lateral segment of the left lobe. These segmental considerations are pertinent to suppurative disease, parasitic infections,

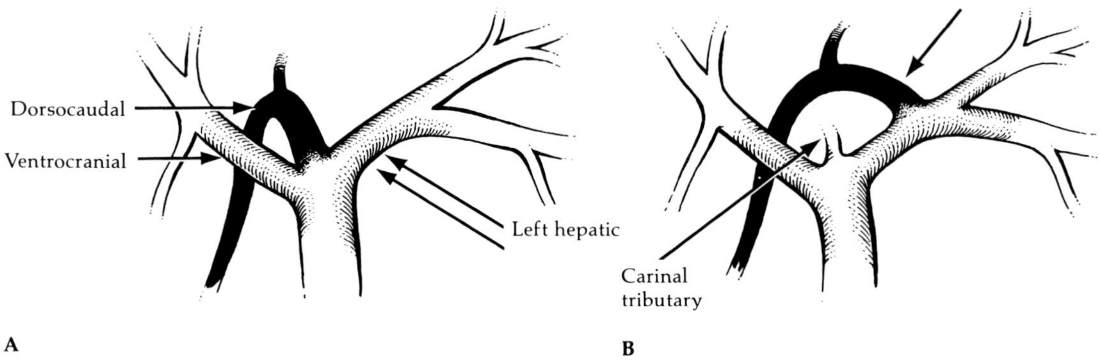

FIG. 1-1. Hepatic ducts. **A.** Ventrocranial division of right hepatic duct **(short arrow)** and dorsocaudal division of right hepatic duct **(long arrow)**; long extrahepatic segment of the left hepatic duct **(double arrow)**. The latter duct is anterior. **B.** An accessory duct drains into the carina **(long arrow)**. Origin of dorsocaudal division from the left hepatic duct is a variant **(short arrow)**. These illustrate the anatomic basis for the observation that the left hepatic duct is more sensitive to distal obstruction because of its longer anterior extrahepatic segment.

FIG. 1-2. Lateral of oblique cholangiogram, made at the time of operation and obtained via a T tube positioned more distally than usual. The left hepatic duct **(lhd)** is anterior and has a long segment free of tributaries. The right hepatic duct **(rhd)** is short and is directed posteriorly. Its ventrocranial **(vc)** tributary is in direct line. The dorsocaudal **(dc)** division is at right angles, directed posteriorly.

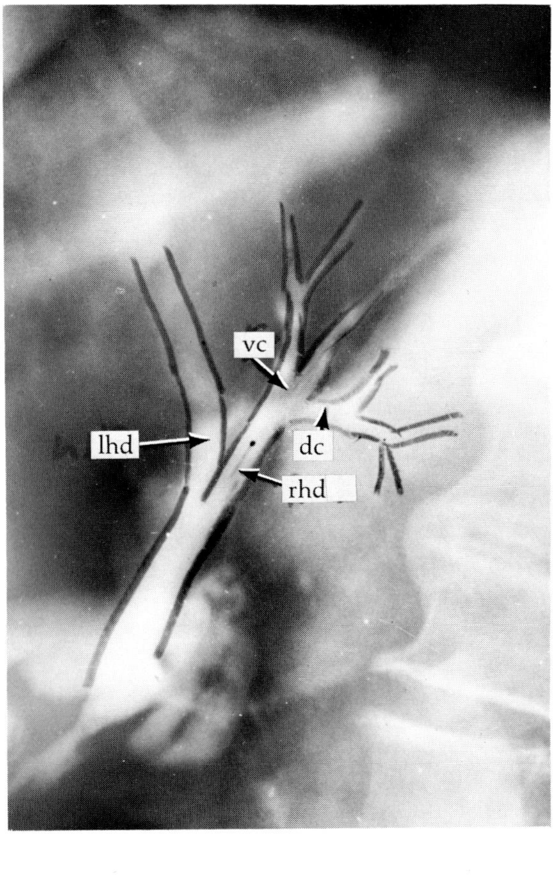

and tumors (83, 85, 86). Bile duct strictures, tumors, clots and impacted stones can produce a derangement in the liver that is patterned on this basis. The segmental nature of lobular hepatic duct disease can go unappreciated if there is no cholangiogram in the lateral or oblique projection (Fig. 1-2) (449, 573).

Common Bile Duct

The supraduodenal common bile duct disappears from view as it passes beneath the duodenum (retroduodenal segment), and goes through the pancreas (transpancreatic segment) until it enters the duodenal wall (intraduodenal). The contour of the duct has a gentle curve with the convex surface to the left. Normally, there are no angulations or areas of dilation. Any such change is abnormal. In about 10% of people, the course of the common bile duct is relatively vertical so that it opens into the third part of the duodenum. The first time that a surgeon frustratedly searches for the ampulla in the second portion of the duodenum and fails to find it, there is a searing initiation into the realities of biliary anomalies and variations (466, 486).

In pancreatitis associated with biliary disorders, there is an advantage to defining the course of the common duct by cholangiography before direct exploration. The manner of angulation and distortion of the common duct determines the technical facility with which stones can be extracted from this segment, as well as the wisdom of attempting to negotiate it.

The human common bile duct contains no muscle except at the choledochal sphincter (257, 374, 375, 386). The biliary epithelium rests on a loose stroma containing many elastic fibers. When the elastic tissue is attenuated by age or is functionally destroyed by infection or prolonged distention, the elastic recoil is also lost.

This distensibility of the duct is a function of the intraluminal pressure. When the perfusion pressure, as in unmonitored T-tube cholangiography, exceeds the passage pressure, the size of the duct on the film, as measured by the opacified contrast, will be related to the force with which the material is introduced. The flat duct seen at autopsy does not reflect this elasticity. For clinical purposes the size of the duct at residual pressure, as measured just above the cystic duct entrance, is the basic width. Perfusion pressure may increase the width by a factor of 2.5. The normal extrahepatic biliary tract of the patient over 65 years tends to be 0.1–0.3 cm wider than that of the younger physiologic counterpart (448). In younger people, this same loss of elastic tissue may occur as a response to calculus disease and obstructive distention. The inner circumference of the duct increases 0.86 mm in women and 0.8 mm in men for each 10 years of age (448). A duct is considered dilated if it is larger than an ordinary lead pencil (385).

The narrowest portion of the common duct is at the point of its oblique penetration into the duodenal wall—the area indicated by the notch on the cholangiogram. The intraduodenal diameter of the 10-mm duct, for example, is abruptly reduced to about 5.4 mm and at the papilla it measures 0.5–1.5 mm. Hence, the most common site for the stone arrest or for stone impaction is in the area just proximal to this anatomic impedance—*i.e.*, in the suprasphincteric zone. Not only is the lumen narrowed, but the intraduodenal portion of the duct often takes a sharp turn in its most terminal segment, penetrating the lumen at a right angle. This anatomic narrowing has a dangerous potential. A probe may perforate out of this area into the duodenal wall, resulting in an intramural hematoma or choledochoduodenal fistula. This misadventure has been implicated as a cause of postcholedochotomy choledochoduodenal junctional stenosis (Fig. 1-3).

Pancreatic Segment of the Choledochus

A partial anatomic basis for some of the discrepancies in pancreatitis associated with biliary disorders relates to the frequency and intensity of the pancreatic complication and its morbidity and mortality. Experience with cholangiography has repeatedly demonstrated that acute inflammatory episodes in the biliary tract may be associated with distortion and angulation of the infraduodenal (transpancreatic) portion of the common duct. The pancreatic swelling can result in lateral displacement, reverse C-shaped distortion, or tubular stenosis of this segment of the duct.

Associated alcoholism aggravates the pancreatic affection. Long-standing, neglected choledochal disease is more commonly seen in municipal hospitals than in private practice. Obviously the source of the case material influences the patterns of the disease. The variability in the individual clinical response can also be related to the purely anatomic fact that the transpancreatic segment of the common duct can be significantly compressed only if it courses through the pancreatic substances; in 20–25% of individuals the partial or complete extrapancreatic course of the duct obviates the possibility of compression and allows only for lateral displacement. This is certainly a major factor influencing the incidence of pancreas-linked hyperbilirubinemia and of the duct configuration on the cholangiogram (Fig. 1-4) (620).

In about 5% of patients the duct of Santorini is the major pancreatic duct. This duct always lies within the pancreatic head parenchyma and exists at the minor duodenal papilla, cephalad to the major duodenal papilla. The minor papilla is patent in only 60% of instances. In over 1000 cholangiograms in the Montefiore Hospital and Medical Center (MHMC) series, only once has the duct of Santorini been demonstrated draining the pancreatic head. Understandably, there has been no experience with surgery for the Santorini ductal system. The effect that a lithic or infectious process in the gallbladder may have on the pancreas having no dominant Wirsung system can only be a matter for speculation. Compromise of the minor papilla in the duodenal stump closure has been suggested as a factor in the genesis of postgastrectomy pancreatitis (203).

The pancreatic duct normally joins the posterior medial wall of the common bile duct. Some cholangiograms demonstrate the point of duodenal penetration as a notch. A similar notch is often seen in the cholangiogram at the site where the common duct pierces the duodenal wall.

The Vaterian Segment

Boyden (82), with his restudy and translation of early historic sources based on gross anatomic autopsy data, has clarified the early concept about the Vaterian segment. Contemporary studies now rely on *in-vivo* cholangiography and manometry. The former, especially with cinefluorographic methods, allows detailed study at motion-picture

FIG. 1-3. Nomenclature of the choledochus and cystic duct. **A.** The areas of the choledochus are named in reference to the duodenum: **1)** The supraduodenal segment; **2)** the retroduodenal component; **3)** the infraduodenal or transpancreatic segment; **4)** the intraduodenal or Vaterian (Odditic) segment. The cystic duct is of the short angular type. **B.** The width of the choledochus is measured across area **1.** This cystic duct is of the short parallel type. **C.** The long parallel type of cystic duct courses through the pancreas. **D.** This variety of cystic duct passes behind the common bile duct, through the pancreas to enter on the left side of the suprapapillary segment. This left-sided cystic duct rarely crosses the anterior surface of the choledochus.

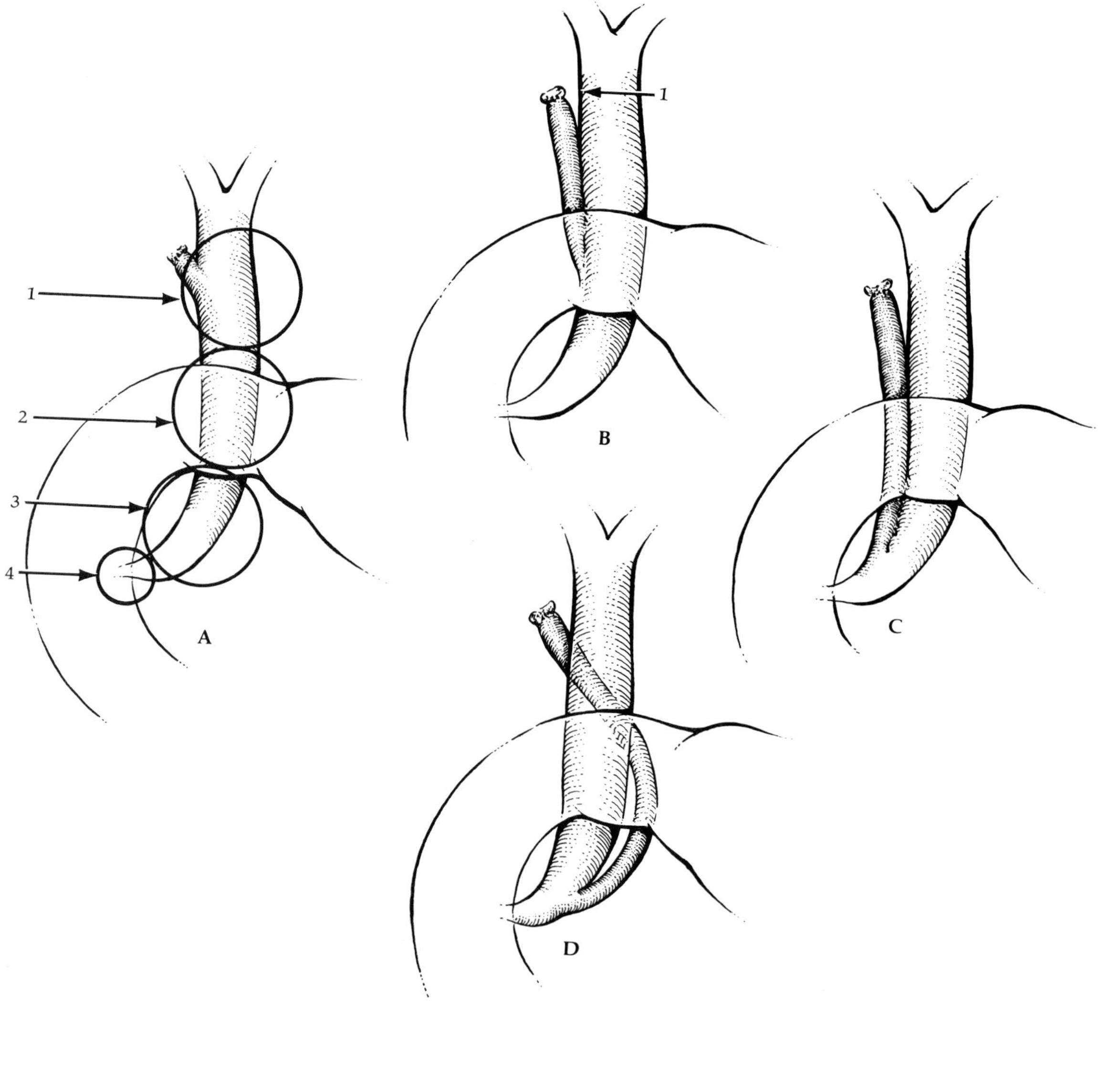

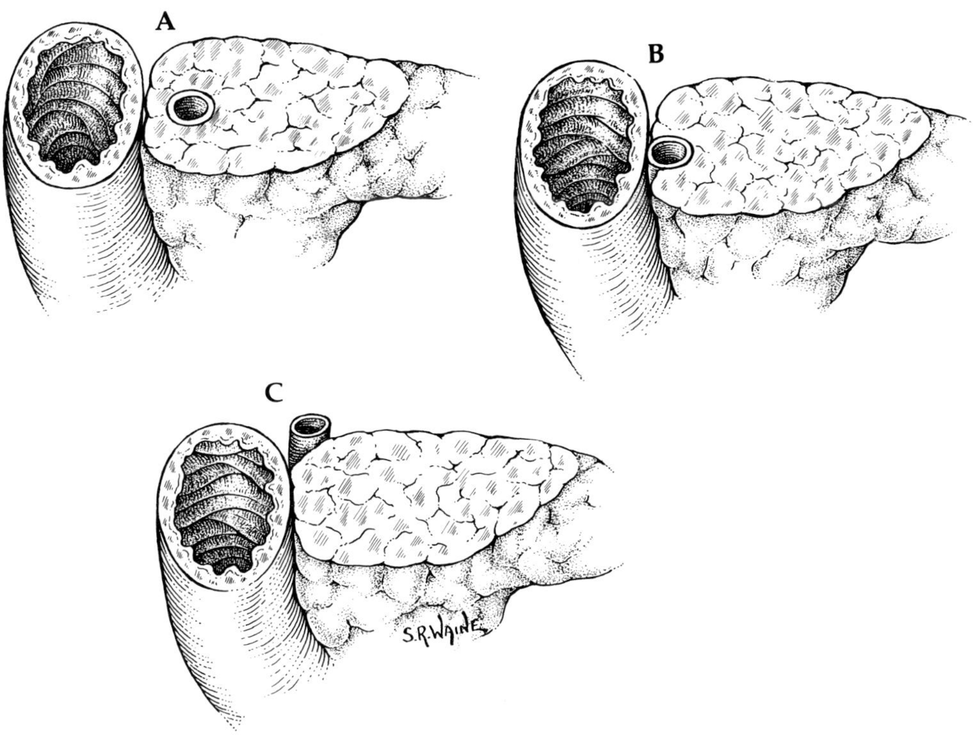

FIG. 1-4. Relation of the common bile duct to pancreatic parenchyma. The clinical parameters of gallstone-linked pancreatitis are determined, in part, by the anatomic relation of the infraduodenal segment of the choledochus to the pancreas. **A.** The common bile duct is completely intraparenchymal so that any edematous reaction in the duct can produce a contiguous inflammatory response in the bile duct. A fibrous reaction in the pancreas can produce a tubular stenosis in this portion of the duct. **B.** The duct is extraparenchymal but intracapsular. Swelling of the pancreas in this area results in a C-shaped distortion, with displacement of the choledochus to the left. **C.** The lay of the duct is completely extraparenchymal and extracapsular so that pancreatic swelling need not influence the function or the configuration of the common bile duct.

speeds. Techniques utilizing debimetry (flow rate per unit of time at a specific pressure) and manometry permit calibration of the papilla and study of intracholedochal dynamics.

The most distal part of the choledochus passes obliquely through the duodenal musculature and exists at the major papilla in some relation to the duct of Wirsung. For purposes of discussion and to avoid the semantic issues, the area referred to as the Vaterian segment includes the distal choledochus, the choledochal sphincter, the distal pancreatic duct, the pancreatic duct sphincter (when present) the ampulla (when present), and the major duodenal papilla (575, 582).

Several particulars about the anatomy of the area require consideration. From a strictly anatomic viewpoint, an ampulla ("jug") exists only when the two ducts enter into a confluent dilated zone proximal to their common egress at the duodenal papilla ("nipple"). The ducts otherwise enter the duodenum separately. It is probable that the common septum between the two ducts acts as freely movable sail, allowing intermittent flow from each organ during partial septal occlusion of the orifice of the other (Fig. 1-5).

Boyden (82) established the anatomic fact that there is always an independent sphincter for the choledochus. He has convincingly demonstrated that this choledochal sphincter segment arises from mesenchyma and that it is embryologically, anatomically, and functionally distinct from the duodenum. For this reason, the effect of certain drugs on the choledochal sphincter differs from their action on the duodenal wall. The studies of Ono *et al.* (455) establish that the peristaltic activity of duodenal muscle has no effect on the choledochus. The motor activity of each of these segments of the duodenum is subject to an

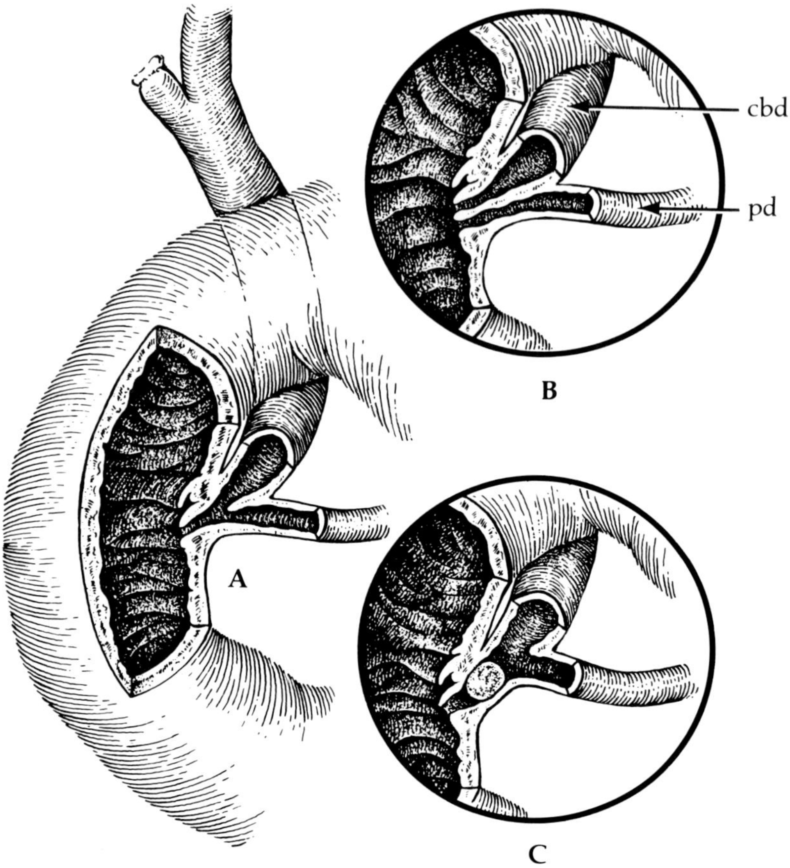

FIG. 1-5. The Vaterian segment. These are the commonest varieties of termination of the common bile duct **(cbd)** and pancreatic duct **(pd)**. **A.** There is a common septum at the confluence of the two ducts that shifts, partially occluding the orifice of the one that is not discharging. **B.** Each duct has a separate exit at the duodenal papilla. **C.** A stone induces the Opie phenomenon—the discharge of bile into the pancreas, a cause of hemmorhagic pancreatitis. This is the common channel.

independent neurohumoral control (334, 437, 521).

A distinct sphincter for the pancreatic duct has been described by Kreilkamp and Boyden (339) and Hess (263) as occurring in almost one-third of those in whom it has been sought. In the MHMC experience, it has not been recognized as a functional entity in over 1000 operative cholangiograms.

From a purely pragmatic point of view, much of the confusion about the interpretation of the operative and roentgen findings in the common duct relates to the native concept that the entire common duct acts solely as a passive conduit. This is not true. The choledochal sphincter portion of the Vaterian segment is always active. It measures 1–1.8 cm in length and is constituted by well-developed longitudinal and circular smooth muscle. The former opens the duct lumen and the latter closes it. These contractile (systolic) and relaxed (diastolic) phases of the choledochal function are pertinent to the interpretation of the cholangiogram (277, 434, 301).

All of the ducts exit at the major papilla; this orifice is 1–1.5 mm wide. It is the narrowest portion of the extrahepatic ductal system. All the bile and pancreatic exocrine secretion passes through it.

Intraduodenal Anatomy

The duodenal papilla is ordinarily on the posteromedial aspect of the descending duodenum, 7–10 cm from the pylorus. The degree of polypoidal projection into the bowel lumen varies. Occasionally the papilla appears merely as a small wrinkle between the mucosal folds. It usually has a papillary or hemispherical configuration. A bile stain in the area is a guide to its location.

The gush of bile in the duodenum, as evoked by forceful squeezing of the gallbladder during surgery, is a way of identifying the orifice. A dorsal frenulum or a characteristic mucosal fold is often present. It is easier to locate this orifice by endoscopic retrograde cholangiopancreatography (ERCP) than by direct inspection duodenostomy.

Intraoperative cannulation of the normal duodenal papilla more often effects an entrance into the pancreatic duct than into the common duct. During operation it is easier to cannulate the common bile duct via this route if a sphincterotomy is performed first. The pancreatic duct orifice is harder to identify by inspection than it is to cannulate. The septum separating the thicker common bile duct from the thinner pancreatic duct tends to obscure the posteromedial orifice of the pancreatic duct. The minor papilla may be mistaken for the Vaterian, but it is always cephalad. I know of one instance in which a sphincterotomy was mistakenly performed in the minor papilla (504).

In the ampulla, the columnar cells of the duct are arranged in fronds based on a loose fibrous-tissue stroma. These assume a polypoid character. They are especially obvious with the dissecting microscope. Such configurations can be misinterpreted as tumor or inflammatory polyps.

An occasional problem is differentiating between a normal duodenal papilla and the true perivaterian polyps described by Bagenstoss (30) and Dardinski (160) and the hypertrophied or inflammatory reaction that is papillitis caused by the ampullary response to an adjacent inflammatory reaction having its source in pancreatitis or active duodenal ulceration.

Ordinarily no reflux of intestinal contents occurs through the papilla, not only because it is closed in the interdigestive phase but also because of the obliquity of the intraduodenal choledochus. At autopsy it is not possible to overfill and distend the duodenum to the point where it will reflux into the biliary pancreatic ductal system. However, there are instances of sphincter incompetence as evidenced by the reflux of barium from the duodenum into the biliary tree. I have seen this in the normal as well as the diseased biliary tree. Of itself, this reflux can be an innocuous roentgen observation without clinical significance, but I have seen two instances of pneumocholedochus associated with this reflux (501, 505, 547, 551).

In this series there has been no case in which a duodenal diverticulum could be implicated as the cause of distal choledochal obstruction (227, 470) although there have been instances in which the duct entered the diverticulum as the path into the duodenum. Symptomatic cases are reported by Flament (201).

SEQUELAE OF PRIOR CHOLECYSTECTOMY AND COMMON BILE DUCT EXPLORATION

The sole function of the gallbladder is the storage and concentration of bile and its intermittent discharge into the duodenum. The abrogation of this function has no deleterious effect. The organ is expendable. However, the removal of the viscus is associated with changes that are both anatomic and physiological (604).

Anatomic Sequelae

These changes are usually innocuous. In certain instances pathologic sequelae can ensue from faulty healing. The abdominal wall incision is expected to heal firmly *per primum*. However, it can be the site of hernia, painful scars, or retained foreign bodies. The upper abdominal skin can be anesthetic from the division of two or more intercostal nerves. It is possible, but not usual, for the costal cartilages or lower costal rib flare to have been damaged or dislocated by the retractors or positioning on the operating table. Traumatic chondritis can be symptomatic. A divided costal cartilage which has slipped and is overriding can produce a painful snap.

The hepatic flexure of the colon and the pyloroduodenal segment become broadly adherent to the gallbladder fossa. This may be avoided if the omentum had been interposed. The omentum becomes adherent to the peritoneal surface of the scar or to the liver bed.

The duodenum adheres to the duodenal impression of the liver and actually overrides the right lateral edge of the hepatoduodenal ligament. Small-bowel adhesions are uncommon if the surgery has been confined to the supracolic compartment of the abdomen. Supraumbilical oblique incisions are especially salutary in this regard. This is in contrast to long vertical incisions or additional procedures that have been executed in the infracolic zone.

A dilated common duct is abnormal. This observation is the single most significant anatomic finding in PCS. It is now definitely established beyond speculation that the human common bile duct does not dilate in response to cholecystectomy alone (282, 284, 355, 372). Previous data derived from observations in dogs, goats, and rabbits are not pertinent to man.

A dilated common bile duct invariably has an obstructive cause that was either present at the time of the initial surgery and persisted or developed anew after the operation. It has its own cause, unrelated to cholecystectomy (315, 316). A chronically obstructed dilated duct does not revert to normal size after choledocholithotomy.

Burden (98) has demonstrated that the postcholecystectomy common duct can show an increase in its mucous glands and that these come to assume a deep intramural locus. This has been viewed as a compensatory way of forming accessory bile vesicles. These are changes akin to the Rokintansky-Aschoff sinus of chronic cholecystitis.

Schein *et al.* (529) have documented the changes in the common duct by intraoperative direct excisional biopsy. When the gallbladder is acutely and chronically inflamed, the reaction in the common bile duct is one of the edema and congestion. The parietal sacculi, the pitted areas in the epithelium, are maintained. This change is especially apparent by endoscopy, and can be known by no other method than direct observation.

The common bile duct reaction to calculi is a cellular infiltrate and focal subepithelial scarring with fragmentation and replacement of the elastic fibers. This is a specific response to intraluminal calculi and is not an effect of the cholecystectomy *per se.* The anatomic changes in the reexplored choledochus are those of the prior interventions and of persistent disease (48, 220).

It would be difficult to determine the duct reaction to cholecystectomy alone without having direct access to biopsy material taken at the time of the original operation and a second biopsy taken sometime later from the same patient. I am not aware of such a study.

The normal common bile duct can be distended to 2.5 times its normal width and will recoil when the perfusing pressure is reduced. Cinefluorographic studies in man have shown that the width of the duct can be evaluated only if the perfusion pressure is known. Evidence of a dilated cholecochus under high perfusion pressures does not reflect the *in situ* status. In anatomic terms the elastic recoil depends upon the integrity of its elastic fibers. If these are fragmented and replaced by scar, the duct has no more circumferential recoil than a broken rubber band (448).

A greatly dilated duct may overlap itself; in its most prominent form the duct appears curled. Firm caudal traction on the duodenum is required to demonstrate the full length of this type of duct.

The dilated duct does not return to normal caliber if obstruction has been present for more than 4 weeks. Dilation of a duct that empties normally on intravenous cholangiography and is free of calculi and contour distortion is due to innocent residual of previous disease. The dilated duct that has impaired emptying may be a source of symptoms. A technically good film is required for this discriminatory judgment; it must show the entire opacified column, free of bone overlap and of gas-filled bowel.

The duct wall is evaluated by indenting its anterior surface. Induration is an indication of reactive fibrosis. This diagnosis is associated with loss of peritoneal sheen and sparsity of capillary branches of the epicholedochal arterial plexus. In general, a dilated, relatively thin-walled duct suggests a passive response to distal obstruction. Courvoisier's law applies to the common duct as well as to the gallbladder. At thickened dilated duct indicates associated or antecedent inflammatory change—cholangitis.

The site of prior cystic duct amputation is usually identifiable. Adhesions of this remnant to the choledochus or to a long cystic artery stump or to the right hepatic artery are normal. In the absence of residual suture material, the prior choledochotomy incision is not always discernible.

The duodenum overlays the previously explored duct and becomes adherent to the liver at the duodenal impression, obscuring the common bile duct; it must be mobilized to expose the duct. The duodenal adhesion is to the liver, not to the duct, unless there is a fistula. Pericholedochal adhesions are usually sparse.

The clear posterior space between the distal supraduodenal choledochus, the hepatic artery, and the portal vein is usually maintained. It remains a safe zone for circumferential mobilization of the duct because the hepatic artery and the portal vein are well to the left.

The head of the pancreas harbors the infraduodenal segment of the choledochus. It is embraced by the C curve of the duodenum and often is described as firm or indurated. The tactile sense of a diseased pancreatic head is often one of exaggerated lobulation with perceptible interlobular septation and thickening of its capsule and rounding of its edges. This finding and its implications varies from one palpator to another and is often a way of "hedging" an observation and its therapeutic implication. Its significance as a solitary finding is highly dubious. In this area the common duct and the pancreas are often best palpated by introducing a catheter through the cystic duct remnant. That method of palpation, supplemented by a cystic duct cholangiogram, reliably establishes the indication for secondary duct exploration.

Pericholedochal lymphadenopathy in the retroduodenal area near the dorsal surface of the pancreas is a nonspecific finding. I have encountered it with and without choledocholithiasis. It is more prominent in inflammatory disorders than in purely functional or obstructive states. It is especially prominent in the presence of cholangitis or inflammation in a gallbladder remnant.

The lateral crescent of the hepatoduodenal ligament becomes thickened and loses its translucency. The common duct can no longer be visualized through a diaphanous edge. The epiploic foramen is often obliterated or is the site of synechiae.

Biliary surgery involving the gallbladder, the common duct, and the duodenum does not denervate any of the viscera, nor does it neurologically affect the pyloric or the choledochal sphincter mechanism. A complete hepatic plexectomy is required to affect sphincter dynamics. This is never accomplished in ordinary biliary surgery since the upper cord of the plexus are high in the lesser omentum, in the juxtadiaphragmatic area. Exposure of this area requires retraction of the left lobe of the liver. It is rarely the area of biliary surgery.

The sympathetic innervation is derived from T-4 to T-11; this is likewise out of the field. The operative stripping of the nerve fibers on the cystic duct and common duct, to expose and define these structures, is insufficient to effect complete denervation (252). Peri- and paracystic duct neuromas are a normal sequel of periarterial dissection. Flow rates and sphincter tone are not affected by this. No information is available regarding the possible symptomatic significance of partial denervation. Perhaps this partial corticovagal interruption is of consequence in certain susceptible individuals.

It is conjecture to suppose that because cholecystectomy makes the choledochal sphincteric segment unnecessary for gallbladder filling, the latter therefore becomes symptomatically atrophic, spastic, dyskinetic, hypersensitive, or less tolerant to normotensive or hypertensive intraductal changes.

The absence of the gallbladder, as such, does not affect the potential for choledochal reflux; this depends solely upon the anatomy of the Vaterian segment. The tonic effect of morphine, meperidine, and codeine on the choledochal sphincter is maintained without the gallbladder.

This sphincter normally functions to allow for preferential filling of the gallbladder during the interdigestive phase and for concentrated bile to pass into the duodenum in the early postcibal state. This sphincter mechanism now is no longer reciprocally related to the gallbladder. The choledochal sphincter in the cholecystectomized person is at best useless, and in diseased conditions it is a definite impediment to the free flow of bile. Its derangements have been implicated as a cause of PCS (31, 157).

From a phylogenetic point of view, Kreilkamp and Boyden (339) have indicated that the anatomic complexity of the distal common duct is a function of the concentrating capacity of the gallbladder. Animals without a gallbladder have no choledochal sphincter (*e.g.*, horse) and animals with a relatively ineffective gallbladder concentration capacity (*e.g.*, rabbit) have poorly developed choledochal sphincters (171). These phylogenetic facts deserve consideration since they indicate that a continuous free flow of bile, unrelated to eating, is consistent with normal digestion. This observation is paralleled in the well-being of those who have a well-functioning choledochoduodenostomy.

Is there an advantage to the storage of bile in the gallbladder? Does this intermittent ejection enhance the digestive process in a way that differs from the surgically established continuous free flow state? No clinically recognizable syndrome can be directly ascribed to either of these bile flow variants.

Functional Sequelae

After cholecystectomy, hepatic bile is no longer stored in the gallbladder, and a concentrated quantum of bile is no longer expelled into the duodenum in response to the hormones elaborated there.

Loss of gallbladder mucus appears to have no effect on the lubrication of the common duct since its own glands produce a comparable fluid. Absence of the four- to tenfold concentration of hepatic bile has no digestive significance. The continuous flow of hepatic bile into the duodenum cannot be differentiated from the intermittent evacuation. The loss of bile storage and the absence of intermittent emptying appear to have no clinical impact.

Specific and significant histologic changes due to common duct disease of a nonsuppurative type are not identified by hepatic biopsy. Diffuse nonspecific changes, such as a portal inflammatory reaction, fatty metamorphosis, nuclear vacuolation, or focal necrosis are thought by Falkmer and Sjostrom (196) to be of minor importance. The continental parlance of a "touch of liver" in association with gallbladder disease is not histologically identifiable. Some microscopic changes that have been described are due to anesthetic agents (198).

Certain of Puestow's (484) physiologic observations on the unrestrained unanesthetized dog with an isolated duodenal segment on the anterior abdominal wall do not appear to have consistent clinical relevance.

Thus, after cholecystectomy in the dog, the orifice of the common bile duct remains open and the flow of bile is continuous, except during fasting. This is not true in man, whose sphincter activity is not altered by cholecystectomy or cholecystostomy. Flow is determined by the intraductal pressure generated by the liver and by the resistance of flow through the duct and sphincter at the terminal end of the duct (246).

There appears to be a psychic or cephalic phase to bile flow in some dogs, in which the mere sight and smell of food causes a flow of bile. Ordinarily the ingestion of food initiates a bile flow that lasts for 1–3 minutes; a second flow starts 10–30 minutes later and lasts a few hours. In other dogs there is no interval biphasic bile flow.

Total bile volume and its bicarbonate concentration is not altered by cholecystectomy (600). Bile salt concentration and volume output does not increase after feeding, as it does when the gallbladder is present. The bile flow rate response to food intake is not altered by cholecystectomy (435, 546).

It is hoped that it will become possible to treat cholelithiasis by altering the lithogenicity of hepatic bile. There is some evidence that lithogenetic bile is secreted only intermittently by those with cholesterol gallstones and that this hepatic potentially lithogenic bile is not present after cholecystectomy (390, 410, 436, 552). In the cholecystectomized patient, the solubility of cholesterol in hepatic bile is more stable than it was before. A diminished bile salt pool is compensated for by more efficient enterohepatic circulation, and a sufficiently high bile salt level is maintained so that the ability to solubilize cholesterol is not in jeopardy. Therefore, the appearance of new cholesterol stones after cholecystectomy is very unlikely (151).

The demonstration that cholesterol solubility in bile is a function of the relative concentration of bile salt and phospholipid in relation to bile cholesterol has introduced a new potential for the treatment and prophylaxis of cholesterol gallstone disease.

During complete interruption of the enterohepatic circulation there is a transient supersaturation of cholesterol in bile. Cholecystectomy renders bile less lithogenic for cholesterol stone formation. In the nonobese patient, bile salt and phospholipid secretion increase, while cholesterol secretion is not affected. The cycling frequency of the bile salt pool doubles after surgery so that a third of the pool cycles each hour.

In the grossly obese patient these favorable

changes do not occur because increased cholesterol secretion invalidates the effect of the cholecystectomy-related increase in bile salt secretion.

Roentgenographic Sequelae

An intravenous cholangiogram of the normal state should show both hepatic ducts (161). Occasionally the normal left duct is not visualized because it is the more anterior of the two and the filming is done in the supine position. The common duct should have a curvilinear configuration and the opacified column normally measures no more than 10 mm in width. The contrast material should be evacuated into the duodenum within 60 minutes, as a maximum, after the injection. The contrast material should appear less dense or be completely evacuated on the 2-hour film. No portion of the gallbladder should be apparent. A thin tubular cystic duct remnant should be stone-free and should also be emptied by the time of the 2-hour film. The common duct and its tributaries should be uniformly opacified, free of calculi, curvilinear, and without segmental areas of narrowing or dilatation.

2 Clinical Physiology of the Normal and Diseased Common Bile Duct

The absence of direct access was at one time the greatest limitation to the study of the physiology of the normal common bile duct. The ability to catheterize the ampulla via an orally passed duodenoscope has now become an established procedure. When one considers how frustrating it can sometimes be to find the ampulla at laparotomy, it is astonishing to the surgeon that it can be successfully done endoscopically.

This singular advance as a route for cholangiography and pancreatography has been established and is successful in about 90% of instances. It is a great advance in the roentgenographic demonstration of the cause of biliary obstructions.

METHODS AND MATERIALS

The reports on this approach to sphincter section and choledocholithotomy portend an entirely new approach to the diagnosis and treatment of certain choledochal disorders. Even if it gets no further than it has now come, this diagnostic access to the jaundiced patient has already proved rewarding.

The value of endoscopic cannulation of the ampulla as a clinically diagnostic tool is well established, especially as a method for visualizing the pancreas and common duct in the jaundiced patient, in whom the only other recourse had formerly been percutaneous transhepatic cholangiography or the "mini-lap." The differential application of the two methods is considered in the section on endoscopic retrograde cholangiopancreatography in Chapter 3. A partial evaluation of the common duct transit time and *in-situ* dynamics have been achieved with the timed intravenous cholangiogram.

The study of motility and sphincter factors requires the insertion of a catheter somewhere in the extra- or intrahepatic biliary system. This step introduces an element of trauma, and in that sense the conditions are not "physiologically normal." For practical purposes the data derived from these observations are clinically pertinent and have been repeatedly confirmed. Studies, in patients, of the normal mechanisms of passage of contrast material, and presumably of bile, into the duodenum; the details of pancreatic duct opacification; the contractile and relaxed phases of choledochal sphincter function; and the mechanisms of biliary colic have added these functional parameters to the morphologic interpretation of the cholangiogram.

Surgical decisions must have their physiologic basis in the studies of the human biliary tree (477, 531, 613). Observations made in the dog are not always applicable, as there are important species differences. The dog has two independent pancreatic ducts entering the duodenum, the canine choledochal sphincter is not as well developed, the common duct–pancreatic head relationship is different, the hepatic ducts are multiple, and there is no comparable right and left hepatic duct. The dog's portal vein normally contains bacteria, and the canine common duct normally dilates after cholecystectomy. There are also important differences in postural, dietary, and feeding practices that influence biliary function. As a correlative aside, note that the normal, hormonally induced hydroureter of pregnancy does not occur in quadripeds. Hormonal influences on the gallbladder of women have been identified as a determinant in opacification during the progestational phases of the menstrual cycle (7, 111). Does this influence also affect the dog? One must question the relevance of biliary "dog-matics" to man.

The MHMC studies of the physiology of the common duct have been performed in patients whose gallbladders or common ducts had been intubated. The duct was considered "normal" if it had no stones and was less than 1 cm in transverse diameter and if the patients had no clinical or anatomic evidence of pancreatitis and cholangitis.

All radiographic physiologic studies were performed at least 10 days after operation and it was accepted that there had been associated pathology in the gallbladder and the trauma of intubation. Studies of thick-walled calculus containing common ducts with associated pancreatitis or cholangitis were considered to reflect the physiology of the diseased common duct.

Pressure and motility studies employed manometry with saline perfusion at body temperature. This was supplemented by 25% sodium diatrizoate perfusion cholangiomanometry monitored under cinefluorography with exposures at a rate of 15 frames per second. This technique added the physiological correlatives to the documentation of the roentgen aspects of choledochal activity under varying conditions.

PHYSIOLOGIC STANDARDS

1. Resting common duct pressure is most conveniently determined by inserting a widebore polyethylene tube into the common duct via the cystic duct and recording the height of the bile-filled column. This is the interdigestive intracholedochal tension that keeps the duct filled, its walls apart, and is insufficient to open the spincter.

2. Passage pressure is the force required to traverse the choledochoduodenal junction, and is expressed in centimeters of saline. The determination is made by gradually lowering the elevated reservoir of the manometer until the fluid level in the column stops falling. The Caroli manometer is a useful device for making this determination at the time of operation. It can also be done with a 50-cc syringe, as described by White, *et al.* (630). This is readily available and is the preferred method in the unprepared situation.

This pressure has been monitored in association with cinefluoroscopy, making it possible to visualize the actual transit of contrast material as the manometric level is recorded. Although this cineradiographic technique would be the ideal method of intraoperative end point determination, the equipment is not available in all operating rooms.

The determination of duct size by cholangiography has to be monitored because the duct width is related to the pressure at which the contrast material is injected. A duct can appear greatly dilated if the perfusion pressure is increased over the passage pressure. Hence the width of the duct as it is opacified at passage pressure is regarded as the baseline. One of the problems with hand injection cholangiography, as opposed to monitored methods, is that the force may so distend the duct that this iatrogenic dilation cannot be differentiated from disease. If the pancreatic duct is incidentally opacified, it signifies that the minimum passage pressure for the delivery of contrast medium into the duodenum was exceeded and that the duct width on the film may be the exaggerated response to excessive perfusion distention (Fig. 2-1).

The demonstration of duct elasticity and recoil potential can be obtained on sequential films taken at varying perfusion pressures. Diffuse duct dilation is a purely passive phenomenon in response to distal obstruction of any cause. The cine studies demonstrate, in ducts that have this potential, that dilation and recoil take place as an immediate response to alterations in perfusion pressure.

A dilated duct is never a normal finding. This is a fact even when its cause is not clear. It is in this ill-defined clinical area that certain ambiguous terms have been employed that suggest an inflammatory or combined inflammatory and neurogenic etiology as an entity, not only in the PCS but also in the genesis of primary biliary malfunction leading to stasis and stone formation. The experience with 160 examinations has revealed that the manometrically observed end point does not vary more than 1–1.5 cm from that observed fluorographically. This is within the area of clinical usefulness.

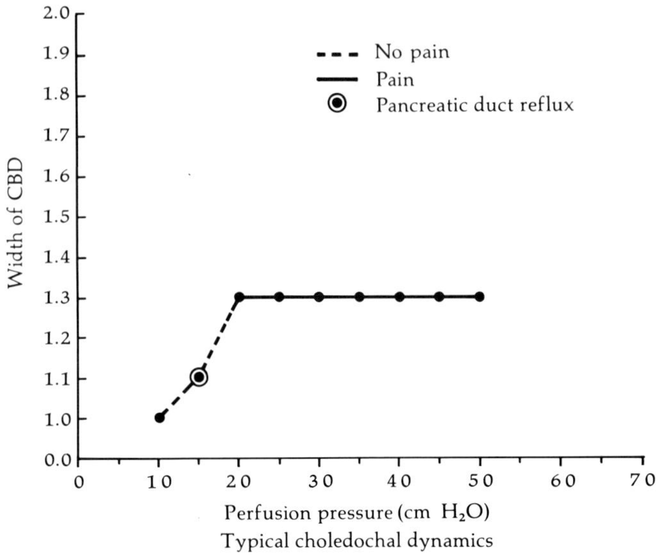

FIG. 2-1. Choledochal dynamics in man. Graphic indication of the relation of perfusion pressure in the common bile duct **(CBD)** to pancreatic duct opacification and the induction of pain. Pancreatic duct opacification is painless and occurs before the bile duct undergoes maximum dilatation. Pain is induced with maximum choledochal distention. It is also apparent that the width of the common duct, as measured on the cholangiogram, depends in part upon the perfusion pressure. (Schein CJ, Beneventano TC: Surg Gynecol Obstet 126:591, 1968. By Permission of SURGERY, GYNECOLOGY & OBSTETRICS)

The passage pressure in the normal duct is 13 ±7 cm of saline. The upper range has been observed very frequently. In the context of the published literature it is perhaps 5 cm higher than the level documented by other observers. This intraoperative experience has confirmed the cinefluorographic observations that the diagnosis of an elevated passage pressure is firmly established only when the level is above 20 cm. Obviously a specific gravity correction factor is required if the manometric determination employs a contrast material rather than saline. It is preferable in clinical practice to do all the determinations with saline. After that determination, the reservoir empties and is refilled with contrast material for the cholangiographic study. This standardized determination obviates the supposed spasm initiated by the iodine in the contrast medium.

COMMON BILE DUCT DILATATION

The determination of duct width is the single most critical factor in making intraoperative decisions and choosing between surgical alternatives. During the operation the unopened choledochus should be measured just above the angular cystic duct junction with a ruler or caliper, or by comparison with a Bakes dilator. This eliminates the possibility of including the width of the opacified parallel cystic duct. A duct wider than 1 cm is considered dilated. When the common duct is 1.4 cm or wider, the presence of a significant organic cause can be confidently postulated (185). The normal common bile duct in its pristine or postcholecystectomy state is never empty. It always contains a quantum of bile that awaits discharge into the duodenum. In this regard, it is unlike the normal ureter, for example, which is normally totally collapsed.

Duct dilation is the residuum of previous obstruction or evidence of persistent obstruction. In an interesting report, Glystorff and Faber (230),of Denmark, point out that when the common duct was evaluated before and after operation in 400 patients, those who returned with postoperative pain all had dilatation of the duct. No patients experienced pain if the diameter of the duct was decreased. In my opinion dilation suggests that there is a persistent obstructive disorder.

Bodvall and Overgaard (72) found that if the common bile duct was 7 mm, the duct contained stones in 55% of cases; if it was 10 mm, in 70%; and if it was 20 mm, all had calculi. The old idea that a normal-sized common duct does not contain stones is not borne out by that study, in which 10% of patients with ducts of 5 mm in size had stones (Table 2-1).

Reiss and Pikielny (494) evaluated the size of the common duct 1 year after operation and compared it to the preoperative condition. In 17% the duct had dilated; these patients were all symptomatic. The majority—

TABLE 2-1. SIGNIFICANCE OF CHOLEDOCHECTASIA IN CHOLEDOCHOLITHIASIS*

Common bile duct	
Width (cm)	**With stones (%)**
< 0.5	0.5
0.5–1.0	11.0
1.5–2.0	80.0
> 2.0	92.0

* Based upon MHMC experience correlating the width of the common duct with the incidence of stones.

78%—showed no changes; in 5% the duct became narrower, but no markedly dilated duct receded.

Intrahepatic ducts do not dilate as readily; this occurs only with prolonged obstruction. Experimentally it takes about 3 weeks. The duct that is both infected and partially obstructed becomes indurated, and dilatation is not as prominent as in the uninfected situation.

When calculi are arrested anywhere in the suprasphincteric area, the entire extrahepatic proximal duct passively dilates and permits unimpacted stones to fall back into the dilated zone. When the obstruction has persisted long enough to destroy the elastic fibers, the duct remains dilated and the stone can assume varying positions in the duct. Contrariwise, stones of appropriate size can remain impacted in the Vaterian segment or suprasphincter zone without moving into the proximal dilated area. Less commonly a stone becomes fixed in the choledochus in an area that develops a decubitus ulceration or a diverticulum. Although this is most commonly observed in the infraduodenal segment, it is also encountered in the left hepatic duct just proximal to the carina. In the latter position, the impacted stone may be the reason that the duct fails to opacify.

How long does it take for the choledochus to dilate? Under conditions of T-tube perfusion at pressures exceeding passage pressure, distensive dilation can be instantly initiated. In the clinical situation, the data can only be inferentially derived from the time interval between the preoperative intravenous study and the findings at operation. These data cannot be derived from observations of the sequence of events in the patient whose duct is intubated. The common bile duct has been observed to increase from 1 cm to 1.2–1.4 cm in 3–5 days. I have not been able to document an earlier change, but in the acutely obstructed state, permanent dilatation can probably be induced in hours.

These considerations concern diffuse and uniform dilation of the entire duct as a response to distal ductal obstruction or to a mobile stone in the common duct that, at some time in its transit, had come down into the duct's funnel end. These anatomic changes are not always paralleled by clinical jaundice. As a rough rule of thumb, only about 50% of patients with common duct stones are, or have been jaundiced.

Localized strictures in the common duct in the patient who has not been previously operated upon are an entirely different matter. These localized strictures are rarely the result of calculi, and when they are, there is an associated diffuse proximal choledochal ectasia. More commonly, they represent extracholedochal compression (as in the tubular strictures of pancreatitis), systemic disease (as in the sclerosing cholangitis associated with ulcerative colitis), compression at the porta hepatis (by metastatic carcinomatous lymphadenopathy), a primary bile duct cancer, or an iatrogenic stricture (222, 244).

Some strictures are in areas that preclude direct visualization or palpation; cholangiography then is the sole way of specifically defining the problem. Because the entire length of the structure must be defined, it may be necessary to perform a two-site puncture cholangiogram. The proximal injection is made directly into a dilated intrahepatic duct, and the distal injection into the gallbladder or common bile duct. This procedure demonstrates the site of the stricture, the extent of its intrahepatic component, its length, probable etiology, and the anatomic potential for correction. The MHMC experience has repeatedly demonstrated that the cholangiographic pattern is so specific that it is a much more accurate diagnostic aid than inspection, palpation, and even biopsy.

In the normal situation and in the majority of people there is no communication between the right and left bile duct systems. In certain diseased states and in the presence of marked choledochal ectasia the two systems can communicate. Possibly, certain collateral bile ducts function only in the presence of obstruction and breech normal lobar barriers. Thus, injecting contrast material into a dilated left ductal system may make it possible to visualize the right side and vice versa.

Hyperbilirubinemia, bile in the urine, and an elevated serum alkaline phosphatase may be associated with unilateral hepatic duct obstruction. This situation is most commonly encountered with biliary duct strictures and cancer of the duct; in the MHMC series it has also been seen with a solitary stone block of the left hepatic duct. In some circumstances the unobstructed lobe is diseased and cannot excrete conjugated bilirubin.

The common bile duct has no cilia or peristalsis. Its self-cleaning mechanism depends upon its own glandular mucus and the washout from hepatic secretory pressure. The duct never empties completely, as a bolus. It is never flat. I have never seen turbulence in the duct. There are no peristaltic waves propelling the bile into the duodenum. The passage into the duodenum depends upon a functioning liver, a free lumen, and a negotiable Vaterian segment. Reflux from the duodenum into the bile duct is uncommon because of the obliquity of the terminal bile duct, but it does occur.

PANCREATIC DUCT CONSIDERATIONS

The common channel concept has always intrigued surgeons. A shared biliary pancreatic outlet permitting the regurgitation of bile into the pancreas or of pancreatic juice into the gallbladder has been invoked as an etiologic factor in the genesis of acute cholecystitis on the one hand and of acute pancreatitis on the other. The suggested obstructing factors include calculi, "spasm," stagnant bile, dyskinesia, and inflammatory states at the ampulla, variously referred to as papillitis, or odditis. There is much in this concept that remains ambiguous and uncertain and clinically rare (55, 461).

Within these uncertainties, some facts have been established (55, 67, 131, 459). Congenital factors rather than acquired distortion most often determine the possibility of reflux into the pancreas. The exception is the true Opie (457) phenomenon, in which a small stone blocks the outlet at the distal ampulla, resulting in a common channel proximally. The normal excretory pressure in the common bile duct is less than that in the pancreatic duct (245).

It has become necessary to view critically the postmortem anatomic dissections of the past. These are less reliable than the data obtained by radiographic techniques. The MHMC series has demonstrated that 46% of patients with cholelithiasis have the anatomic potential for pancreatic reflux. If this anatomic situation does not exist, reflux cannot be induced by increasing the pressure of the choledochal perfusion. The pancreatic duct will either be perfused within the anatomic and physiological parameters that are normal for the area, or reflux cannot be negotiated (469).

The experience with cinemanometric cholangiographic perfusion of the pancreatic duct supports the following observations:

1. In no case is pain induced by pancreatic duct reflux, and in no instance is the patient aware of its occurrence.
2. There is no linear correlation between the length of pancreatic duct opacified and the perfusion pressure.
3. The pressure for pancreatic duct filling is always greater than choledochoduodenal passage pressure. The pressure for pancreatic duct reflux averaged 23 cm saline with individual variations between 15 to 40 cm.
4. In no instance can pancreatic reflux be induced at less than the passage pressure.
5. In all instances of perfusing the pancreatic duct, filling occurs before the common duct becomes maximally distended.
6. The contrast material empties from the pancreatic duct together with that from the choledochus; there is no differential in excretion from either channel.
7. In no patient in this monitored cholangiographic experience was reflux associated with or followed by clinical evidence of pancreatitis.

In no instances in which pancreatitis has been diagnosed in association with biliary disorder has the T-tube instillation of contrast material indicated disease of the pancreatic duct by demonstrating lakes, parenchymal strictures, an aveolar ductal pattern, or pancreatitis demonstrated at a biliary operation

7–14 days previously. These observations warrant the conclusion that the cholangiopancreatoductogram alone is of little value in assessing the pancreatic aspects of an associated biliary calculus disorder (Table 2-2).

THE CHOLEDOCHAL SPHINCTER

Cineradiographic examination under manometric control has resolved some queries regarding choledochal motility. The MHMC studies have failed to demonstrate a single instance of peristalsis in the common bile duct tube. Obversely, there is always rhythmic sphincteric activity at the distal end of the common duct. The muscle fibers of this sphincter, in the intraduodenal segment of the choledochus, regulate the flow of bile into the duodenum.

This sphincter has intrinsic myogenic tonicity and is subject to vagal influence. Schwegler and Boyden (545) have shown that the muscular component of the common bile duct arises from mesenchyme 5 weeks later than the intestinal musculature. Lutkens (377) has postulated that the neural regulation of the biliary tract resides in the cystic duct plexus and that operative interference with this area gives rise to motility disturbances. Vagal section and cholecystokinin have antagonistic effects on this sphincter.

Nash (440) describes clusters of mucous glands between the muscle bundles of the sphincter. This area can be infected as a component of acute papillitis or harbor a chronic infection whose fibrotic sequel results in choledochoduodenal junctional stenosis.

In man, bile flows intermittently into the duodenum in association with gallbladder contraction. When the contractile force of the latter is sufficient to overcome the normal resistance of the choledochal sphincter, bile from the vesica fellea is forced into the duodenum. If the gallbladder has been removed or is diseased so that it is no longer capable of effective contraction, the passage of bile depends upon the secretory pressure of the liver. This pressure is normally on the order of 30 cm H_2O.

Choledochal sphincter activity usually has been demonstrated from the choledochal side, but it has also been evaluated from the duodenal side. Nebel (442) has reported a manometric reading obtained by using a single lumen pull-out catheter inserted into the orifice of the papilla of Vater at duodenostomy. He located a high-pressure zone just within the papilla. Sphincteric pressures measured 15–43 mm Hg with the mean pressure of 31 $\pm$ 2 mm Hg. Similar studies have been done by operative endoscopic retrograde choledochotomy.

Species without gallbladders have no choledochal sphincter, and their bile flow into the intestine is continuous. A problem in PCS resides in those patients who, having been deprived of gallbladder propulsive function, retain a clearly diseased sphincter. In the postcholecystectomy state there is no need or advantage to the presence of a sphincter at the distal end of the duct. The horse has neither a gallbladder nor a choledochal sphincter and does not appear digestively faulted. Sheep have a gallbladder, but the bile flows continuously into the bowel (150). Patients who have had a sphincter-exclusion operation, such as in continuity choledocho-

TABLE 2-2. STANDARDS FOR EVALUATING THE CHOLANGIOMANOMETROGRAM

Common bile duct (normal values)	
Width	Not greater than 1 cm
Passage pressure	13 ($\pm$7) cm H_2O
Flow rate	More than 15cc/min
Pancreatic duct opacification	Normal in 40% of individuals
Volume of extrahepatic system	3–8 ml
Contractile segment	0.7–1.4 cm in length
Left-sided entrance of systic duct	8–10%
Emptying into third part of duodenum	10%
Duodenal papilla (radius)	$<$ 0.5 cm (average 0.3–0.4 cm)

duodenostomy, do not have symptoms that can be specifically ascribed to the continuous rather than intermittent flow of bile (Fig. 2-2) (208).

Many studies have been performed to evaluate the effect of various drugs on the sphincter mechanism with the hope of discovering therapeutic applications. A favorite procedure has been the use of morphine to produce sphincter contraction and evaluating the effect of so-called sphincter relaxants on the preparation. This in no way simulates the patient's problem, and it may be that the presumed relaxant effects are often due to opium antagonism rather than to a direct action on the sphincter.

The problem is more than a matter of mere semantics. Is there truly an entity of duct spasm (353, 352)? If so, it can only be in the distal segment, for that is the only part that has muscle. Can one differentiate between spasm and a prolonged systolic contractile phase of distal choledochal function? Tetanic spasm in association with pain is not a feature of biliary muscular contractility. Thus, gallbladder contraction in response to a fatty meal is never spasm; there is no pain or convulsive muscular movement. Therefore, the

FIG. 2-2. Morphology of the choledochal sphincter. **A and B.** Maceration specimens of the transmural portion of the distal bile duct and duodenum. These muscle fibers are the anatomic basis for the biphasic (diastolic and systolic) function of the choledochal sphincter. (Schreiber H: Arch Klin Chir 206:220, 1944)

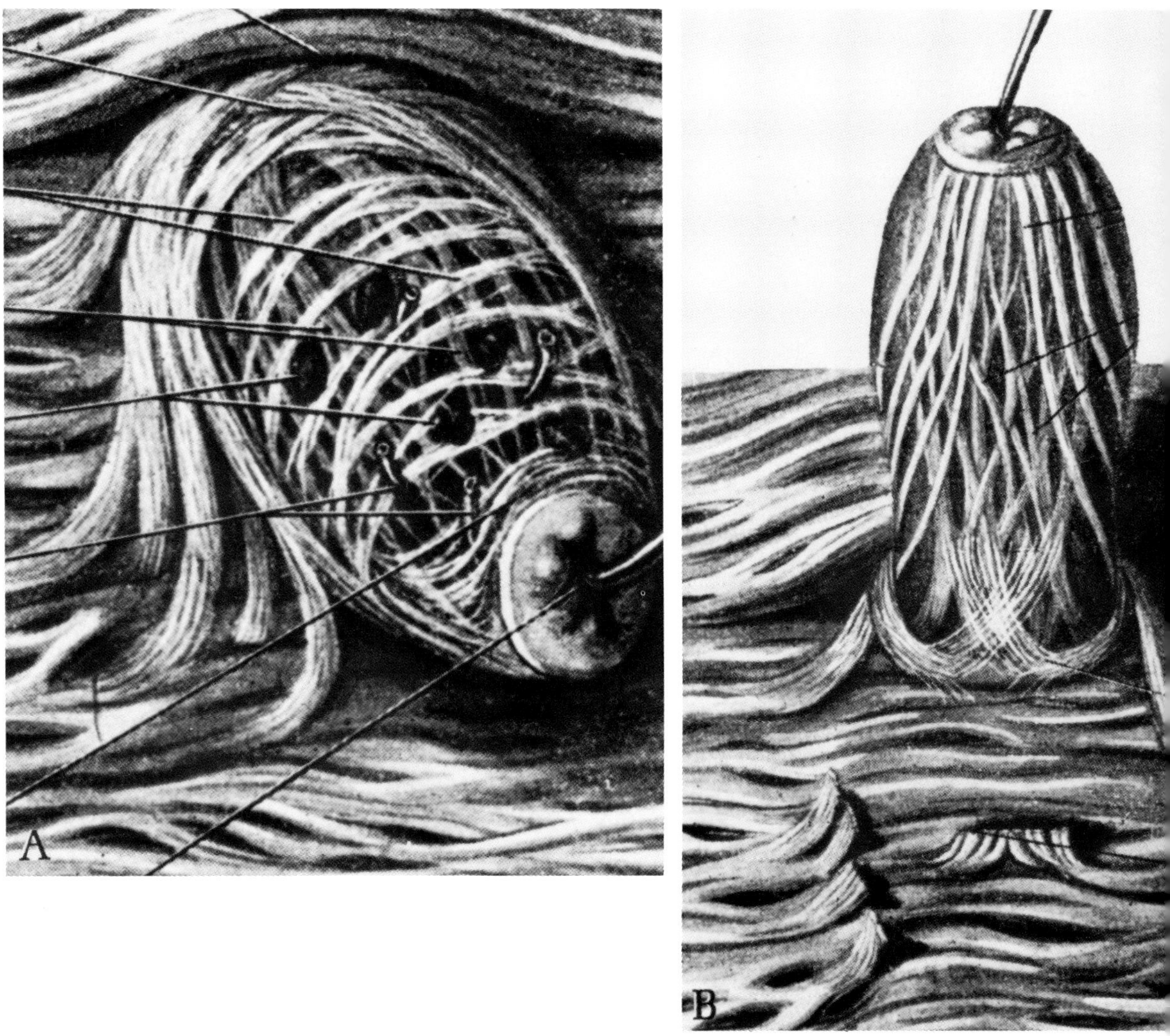

conventional dose of some drugs that are supposedly antispasmodic have little relaxing effect on the biliary tree.

In a study of this problem, Shore *et al.* (561) inserted a Thomas cannula into the duodenum of a trained dog. It was possible directly to observe sphincter activity through the cannula. This was a more physiological preparation than the exteriorized loop used by Puestow (484) and introduced fewer variables. These observations in the otherwise normal animal demonstrated that the biliary sphincter is closed during fasting, that fat relaxes it and hydrochloric acid causes it to contract, and that alcohol contracts the sphincter that had been relaxed by a fatty meal. The normal bile flow response to a fatty meal is interrupted by the introduction of acid into the duodenum.

These findings might be significant in the problem of biliary dyspepsia occurring in the patient with a pyloroplasty or incompetent pyloric sphincter who still has significant gastric acidity (46, 296). The intermittent phasic contraction and relaxation of the choledochal sphincter produces changes on the cholangiogram that are clearly demonstrated by cineradiographic techniques. In the ordinary single-exposure cholangiogram at operation, only one aspect of this morphologic variation is demonstrable. Cognizance of the range of changes is essential to the correct interpretation of the cholangiogram.

Duodenal peristalsis does not play a role in the configuration of the common bile duct as it is visualized by radiographic examination or as it is evaluated manometrically. Ono *et al.* (454) have convincingly demonstrated that the choledochal sphincter in man functions independently of the duodenum. Bipolar electrodes inserted into each area indicate that the electric activity at each site differs, and that the bile flow is not influenced by duodenal contractions (294, 596). Bile flow occurs when there is no electrical activity in the sphincter of Oddi and ceases when there is electric activity in this area.

Franksson (204) has demonstrated that the choledochal nerves go to the papilla but not to the duodenum. McGowan *et al.* (412) maintain that exaggerated duodenal contractions accompany prolonged "spasms of the sphincter" and that the morphine can evoke this abnormality in patients with biliary dyskinesia. These investigators postulate that certain varieties of postcholecystectomy pain are due to duodenal distention in association with a contraction ring in the third part of the duodenum. This nonspecific contractility can be manifested as bloating, abdominal fullness, or nausea.

The retraction of the longitudinal fibers of the sphincter interrupts the flow of contrast material to the extent that a roentgenographic void appears. The simultaneous contraction of the circular muscle sequentially closes that duct lumen and often produces a limbus. This contractile phase is referred to as the systolic aspect of sphincter activity during which there is no bile flow. In the diastolic phase of sphincter function, the lumen is open and bile is discharged into the duodenum. The pattern of this change is constant and repetitive for any one person, but the same general morphologic changes occur in all persons. The intraoperative significance of these roentgen manifestations is discussed in Chapter 5.

This circular muscle is one important factor limiting the spontaneous extrusion of stones. The roentgen contours in the sphincter zone (Fig. 2–3) are not altered by truncal vagotomy, contraselective vagotomy, or epidural sympathetic block.

The duration of each phase of the sphincter cycle is calculated by the formula: Number of exposures/rate of filming = duration of cycle. The rate of filming is 15 exposures per second.

The analysis of the cine strip on a variable-speed projector permits detailed study of the roentgen configuration at single frame and, at slow motion, as well as physiologic speed. The duration of the systolic phase ranges from 0.5 to 4.3 sec at passage pressure perfusion. The duration of the diastolic interval at the same pressure is between 1.7 and 5.3 sec. At passage pressure levels, the duration of a full "normal" cycle ranges between 4.7 and 7.3 sec.

When the perfusion pressure is elevated, the duration of each phase of the cycle is lengthened. This occurs in no predictable or uniform fashion and results are so variable that they escape mathematically significant formulation.

These findings contradict those of Caroli (109) who found that with increaed choledochal pressures the prolongation is most pronounced in the diastolic phase. Caroli describes a repetitive basal rhythm of 3 sec to each phase of sphincteric activity. The

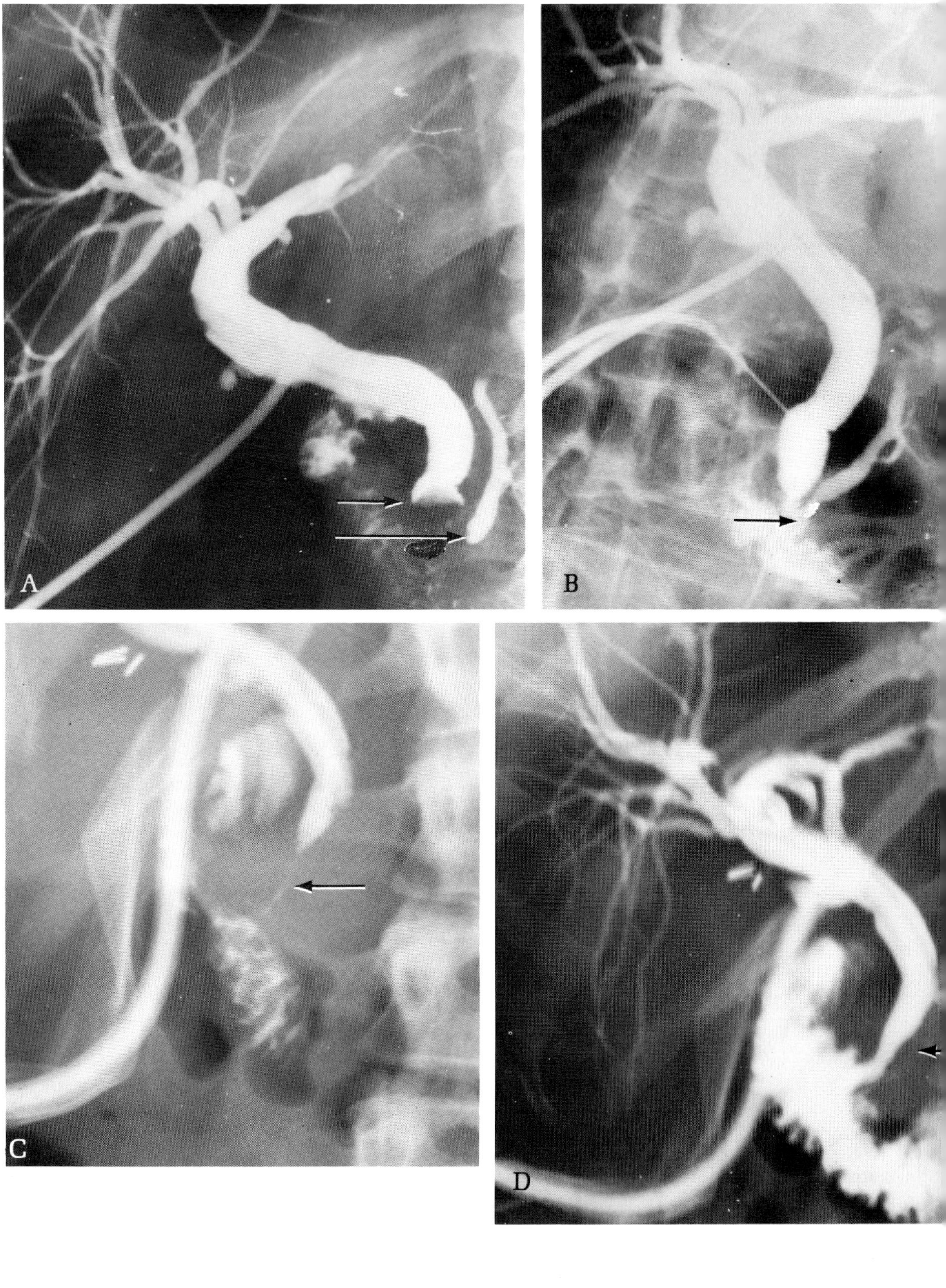

◀ FIG. 2-3. Cholangiographic features of the choledochal sphincter. **A.** T-tube cholangiogram demonstrates that the choledochal sphincter has contracted (systolic phase), producing a concave impression at the distal end of the bile duct **(short arrow).** This simulates a stone and has been referred to as a pseudocalculus sign. Note, however, that there is contrast material in the duodenum. The pancreatic duct is seemingly blocked **(long arrow)** as a result of the contractile function of the pancreatic duct sphincter. **B.** A second film taken a few seconds later shows that the pseudocalculus sign has disappeared **(arrow),** and the contrast material traverses the sphincteric segment. The pancreatic duct is also normally opacified. **C.** T-tube cholangiogram demonstrates long-segment narrowing of the distal end of the common bile duct **(arrow).** On a single film this would suggest a stricture at the distal end. The duodenum is opacified, and the proximal common bile duct is not dilated in proportion to this suggested stricture. **D.** A film taken a few seconds later demonstrates that the distal common bile duct is completely normal **(arrow).** On single-exposure films, the phases of sphincteric function can be misinterpreted.

MHMC examinations, however, revealed a marked variation in the duration of each phase of the cycle in different patients at the same intracholedochal pressure, as well as in any single patient at varying pressures.

NEUROLOGY OF THE CHOLEDOCHAL SPHINCTER

The potential clinical application of neurophysiology data to the surgery of the abdominal viscera has been delayed or ignored. Witness the time lag between Pavlov's 1897 demonstration of the role of the vagus in gastric physiology and its definitive surgical application to the treatment of peptic ulcer.

The nerves in the biliary area are numerous, large and obvious to the surgeon. They have to be stripped off adequately to liberate the cystic duct. Interlacing nerve cords wander on the choledochus. Burnett *et al.* (102) demonstrated that in the diseased gallbladder 50–75% of the ganglia are in various stages of degeneration even though the intramural plexus is intact. I am not aware of similar studies in the ductal system. Boyden (80) and Villemin (602) demonstrated experimentally that there is a hormonally sensitive intrinsic neural mechanism in the sphincter even after all the extrinsic nerves have been cut. The significance of these observations has not been integrated into clinical practice. The present discussion considers the MHMC clinical experiences regarding the influence of the anatomic nervous system on biliary dynamics and pain mechanisms.

The hepatic vagal plexus consists predominantly of motor fibers to the extrahepatic biliary tree. Its trunks originate mainly from the intraabdominal left vagus nerve and pass through the cranial end of the gastrohepatic mesentery (367). Experience with 40 patients subjected to complete hepatic plexus vagectomy in the course of cholecystectomy and common duct intubation demonstrated a fall of passage pressure gradient by 32–56% in comparison to presection levels. There were no exceptions. This decreased resistance occurs immediately and is directly related to the denervation of the choledochal sphincter (Fig. 2-4). The denervation is not accompanied by alterations in the roentgen morphology of the choledochal sphincter, nor has the duct become dilated on subsequent examination. There are no muscle fibers in other portions of the common duct to undergo atrophy. The therapeutic aspects of this permanent neurogenically induced sphincter relaxation procedure are discussed in Chapter 18.

The influence of the sympathetic autonomic nervous system on human choledochal function was studied in patients who had had a cholecystectomy and common duct intubation. Complete bilateral sympathetic interruption was achieved by epidural block extending to T-4.

Total sympathetic block does not influence choledochal dynamics. The passage pressure is unchanged, and pancreatic duct opacification is not altered. In this regard the vagal and sympathetic systems have neither equal nor contrary effects on the choledochal musculature. Sympathetic block does markedly increase the tolerance to pain provoked by excessive choledochal perfusion pressures. The range of pain threshold tolerance is increased by 25–133% (average 52.8%) and is a result of anesthesia of the afferent pain pathway, which is mediated via the sympathetic system. The increase in tolerance of pain is unrelated to a basic change in choledochal dynamics, and it is assumed to be the physiologic basis of the therapeutic efficacy of sympathectomy on certain painful affections of the biliary-pancreatic systems (Fig. 2-5) (156). Ray (490), upon observing the effect of biliary distention in patients who

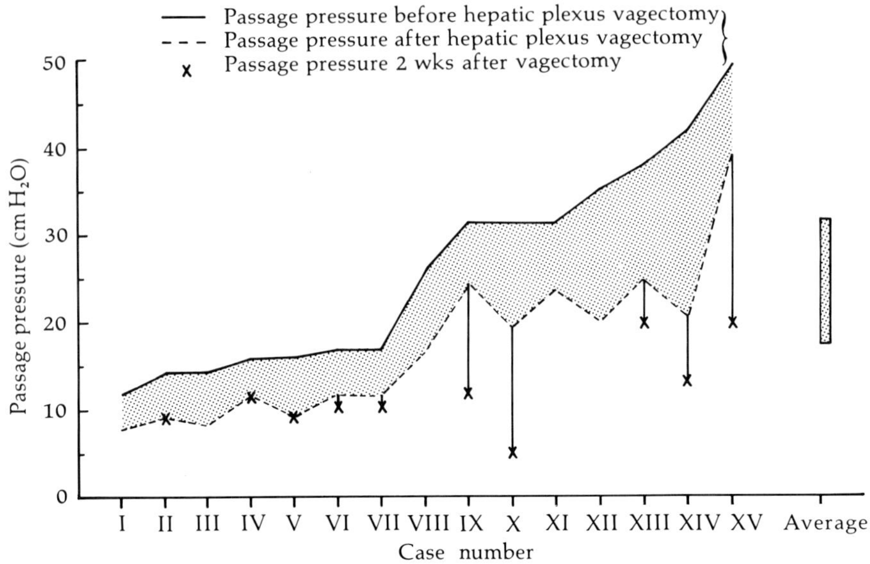

FIG. 2-4. Effect of elective complete hepatic plexus on the choledochal sphincter in man. Resistance to the passage of fluid through the sphincteric segment is invariably decreased. The **shaded area** indicates the magnitude of this change. There have been no exceptions to this decreased resistance if all the hepatic plexus fibers have been severed. (Schein CJ, Beneventano TC, Rosen, RG, et al.: Surg Gynecol Obstet 128:241, 1969. By Permission of SURGERY, GYNECOLOGY & OBSTETRICS)

FIG. 2-5. Effect of sympathetic block on choledochal dynamics. The bile duct of each of nine patients was perfused to the pressure-induced pain threshold before **(x)** and after **(|)** sympathetic block. The pain tolerance was increased in each individual, the average pain-producing perfusion passage pressure gradient going from a base line of 46 cm H_2O to 60.9 cm. Sympathectomy has an analgesic effect on the pain provoked by choledochal distention because it interrupts the afferent pain pathway. (Based on Schein CJ, El Tawil V, Dardik H, Beneventano TC: Am J Surg 119:261, 1970)

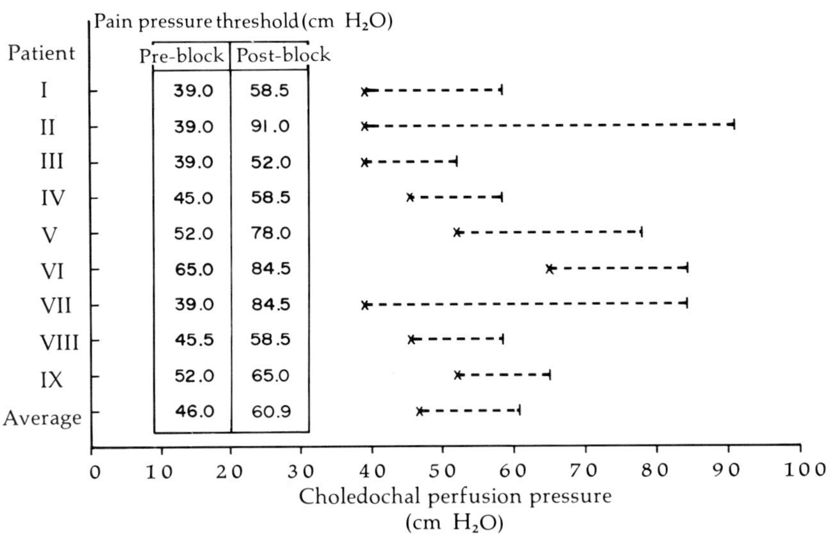

had had sympathectomies, regarded the greater splanchnic nerves as the major sensory pathways.

The study of the canine biliary dynamics by vagotomy and thoracolumbar sympathectomy has elicited a similar response to that observed in patients (14, 15, 224, 279, 556). Therefore, the study of the biliary tract adrenergic receptors in the dog might have reference to the human situation. Dardik *et al.* (159) at MHMC have demonstrated that beta stimulation by isoproterenol infusion produces a decrease in passage pressure that can be reversed by a specific beta blocker such as propranolol. In general, alpha blockage following vagotomy has no consistent effect on the passage pressure. In the dog and probably in man, the beta adrenergic system dominates this aspect of the choledochal sphincter resistance. It may be that the sphincter behavior in certain cholecystectomized patients exhibits a malfunction that is comparable in its symptomatic effect and as difficult to document as the associated problems of esophagitis, functional constipation, or pylorospasm. This group of symptoms can dominate the clinical picture, yet the early objective documentation is difficult to verify.

PAIN MECHANISM IN THE COMMON BILE DUCT

Many patients will tolerate the dyspepsia and dietary limitations imposed by biliary disease, but few want to endure repeated bouts of biliary colic. Pain is a cardinal indication for secondary biliary surgery. The intraoperative evaluation of the biliary system is directed at determining its etiology and the best operative procedure for eliminating it.

Biliary pain can always be produced by rapid distention of the common bile duct such as might occur behind a stone. This has been studied manometrically (531, 534). It became clear that there are two phases in this pain production, the pain-equivalent phase and the precise painful phase. The pain-equivalent state is related to lesser degrees of distention and is of the pure visceral type, described as fullness and discomfort in the mid-upper abdomen. It is tolerable but associated with a sensation of feeling "sick," of gut awareness, and of digestive discomfort. This phase is experienced at a perfusion pressure 5–10 cm below that of the precise painful phase. The latter is intense, localized to the upper abdomen, and lasts as long as the elevated perfusion pressure is maintained. It is rapidly ameliorated when the perfusion level is reduced (174).

Lumsden and Holden (376) recognize three phases in the act of vomiting. The first is nausea, then retching, and finally emesis—the forcible expulsion of the stomach contents. This same sequence of events is observed in mechanically produced biliary distention. Retching in man is frequently accompanied by contraction of the descending duodenum. Retching consists of spasmodic abortive respiratory attempts with the glottis closed; there is a simultaneous inspiratory effort of the chest muscles and diaphragm with contraction of the abdominal muscles. The act culminates in a powerful, sustained contraction of the abdominal muscles and descent of the diaphragm that raises the intragastric pressure so that when the cardia opens, gastric contents are propelled up and out.

There are several significant clinical corollaries to these observations:

1. In no instance can pain be produced at the passage pressure level. In 20 patients this pertained even when the passage pressure was markedly elevated.

2. The minimum pain pressure threshold correlates with the observation that the duct has dilated from 1.2 to 2.4 times its baseline width at that perfusion pressure. Though the duct width cannot be increased beyond this maximum diameter, continuing perfusion at still higher levels intensifies the pain. Detumescence of the duct immediately relieves the agony. In 20 patients the pain was evident when the intraductal pressure ranged between 26 and 56 cm (average 36 cm). This corresponded to a passage pressure of 13–26 cm (average 22.8 cm) greater than the individual patient's passage pressure.

3. The pain perfusion pressure level is always equal to or greater than that required to produce maximal choledochal distention.

Despite the variations in pain tolerance, the perfusion pain pressure threshold can be directly correlated with the severity of an associated cholangitis. When the latter is marked, the pain threshold level is lower. Choledochal perfusion under manometric control in this regard can be used as a way of charting the course of cholangitis. When the inflamed common duct is distended pain can be evoked by pressures within the physiologic range. Distention of that same infected duct at lower perfusion levels produces pain-equivalent nausea, retching, and a vague epigastric sense of being ill. As the perfusion pain level becomes reduced, it may be inferred that the biliary inflammatory process is less intense. The perfusion is done via the T tube as a postoperative procedure and can be viewed as intraductal palpation for tenderness.

CHOLANGITIS

The surgeon is concerned with that variety of cholangitis that has its etiology and major expression in the extrahepatic bile ducts. The changes in the liver and periductal structures are secondary. The inflammatory process invariably has its etiology in obstruction or stasis, separating the problems of surgical cholangitis from the realm of the physician concerned with primary liver disease as it affects the intrahepatic bile radicles.

It is difficult to determine the incidence of cholangitis because the obvious diagnosis is most easily made in cases of suppuration—in which, literally, there is an intraductal abscess. In these instances the clinical picture is striking, characterized by chills, fever, jaundice, mental changes, and septic shock. The suppurative phase constitutes a surgical emergency; it can be fatal (497).

However, there is also a catarrhal or phlegmonous type of major duct cholangitis that is pathologically evident as the congestion that accompanies common duct stones or Vaterian segment obstructions. This variety can only be definitely diagnosed by direct or choledochoscopic investigation of the bile ducts. In the presence of common duct stones, an accompanying edematous reaction strongly suggests this process.

In the MHMC experience this type of cholangitis has been observed in virtually all instances of choledocholithiasis associated with fever and leukocytosis. The entity is most common in older patients with long standing disease. In the series reported by Bismuth *et al.* (62), the average age was 72.

Renal failure in association with suppurative cholangitis is so common that it has been designated as "uremigenic cholangitis," caused by the decreased renal perfusion associated with sepsis. It is also probable that the excess conjugated bilirubin renders the kidney more suspectible to the ischemic insult.

Charcot (124) described cholangitis in 1877 as a disorder with jaundice, chills, fever, and right upper quadrant pain. In 1959 Reynolds and Dargan (497) stressed the clinical recognition of the septic implications of the process as a closed abscess also associated with shock and mental stupor. I would emphasize that there is an antecedent stage, characterized by fever and bacteremia, in which the intraductal reaction is primarily phlegmonous and associated with marked regional pericholedochal lymphadenopathy. The process involves the entire ductal system but is especially prominent in the Vaterian segment where it is variously identified as odditis, papillitis, or sphincteritis. In the MHMC experience, no diffuse gangrenous, granulomatous, or perforative ulcerative process has been recognized although each of these has been encountered locally, at—or just proximal to—an obstructing stone (Fig. 2-6).

At choledochoscopy, the increased vascularity of the duct wall is evidenced as subepithelial congestion. Often the effort to clean out the duct by irrigation is so diligent that the significance of the washed-out exudate is little appreciated in the evolution of a situation that might be very dramatic. Shreds of mucus are evidence of inflammatory glandular hypersecretion.

The undisturbed fibrin strands in the duct are visualized as irregularly arranged interlacing synechiae that stretch across the lumen. These resemble multilevel clotheslines in a tenement yard. Such intraductal webs constitute a strainer or net in which small calcui are caught and become embedded. These are a factor in the genesis of stasis bile conglomerates and in the recurrences of clinically recognized cholangitis. The insidious nature of the process, as well as its tendency to recur, is again related, in part, to the harboring of organisms and calculus material in these webs.

The pericholedochal lymph node is the sentinel lymphatic filter of the area. In the presence of cholangitis the node becomes greatly enlarged, soft, and friable.

Surgical cholangitis is never a primary

FIG. 2-6. Spectrum of pathologic findings in cholangitis. The clinical presentation of calculus-related cholangitis can range from an unsuspected pathologic finding to a moribund septic state.

CHOLANGITIS

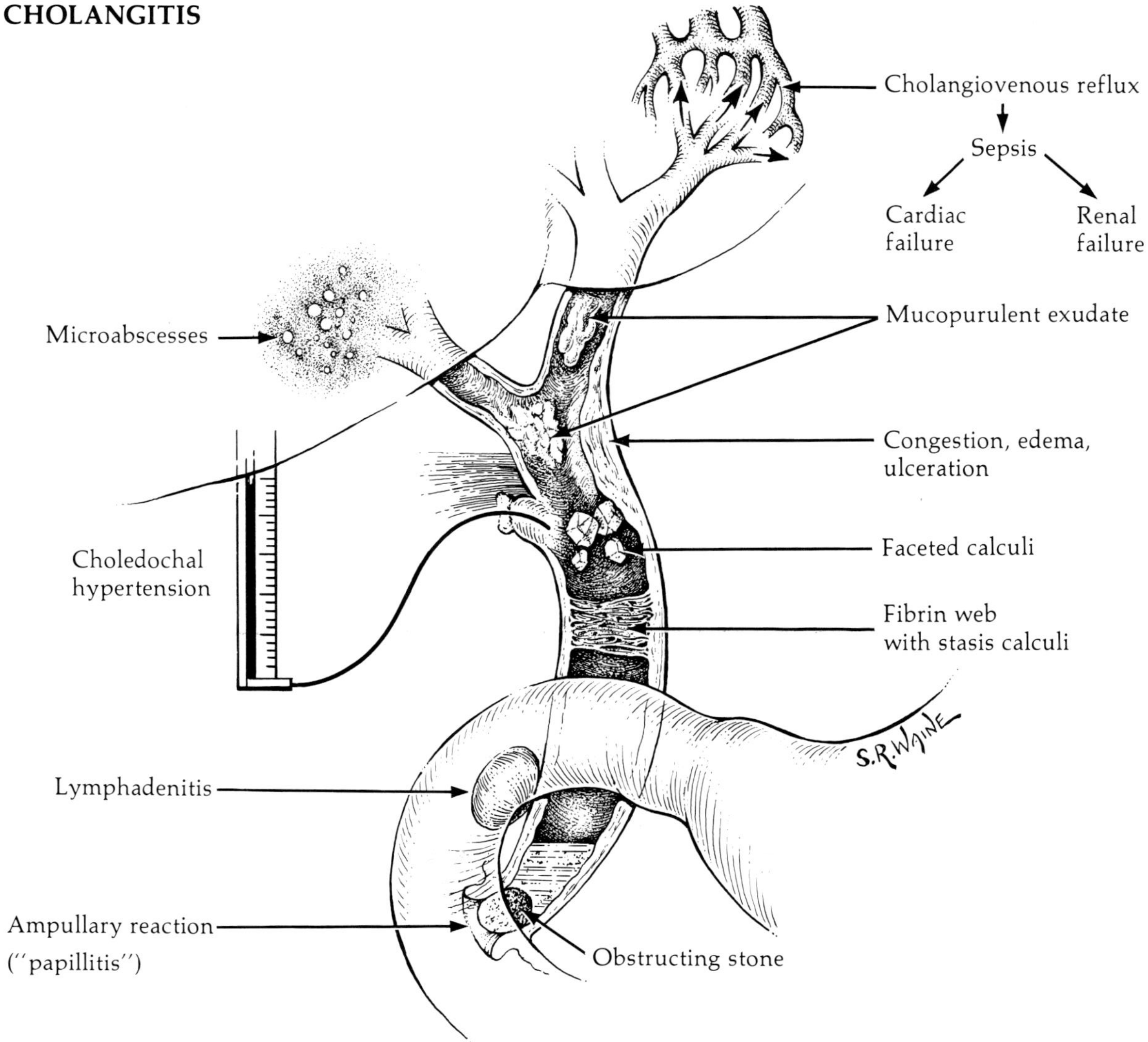

disease. It is always secondary to obstruction or stasis, more commonly incomplete than total. In the MHMC series the most frequent causes are choledocholithiasis, cystic duct remnant cholecystitis, choledochoduodenal junctional stenosis, and biliary enteric anastomatic strictures. The dominant features are pain, fever, leukocytosis, and an increase in alkaline phosphatase, SGOT, and serum bilirubin. The last is not always clinically evident. Abdominal pain and tenderness are not prominent features in phlegmonous cholangitis. Bacteremia is demonstrated in more than half the patients when repeated cultures are taken at the time of the chill or the febrile reaction. The usual organisms are *E. coli, Klebsiella, Proteus,* and *Pseudomonas* (228, 271, 299, 414).

The bacteriologic data of the past has little relevance in view of the present reported incidence of nearly 90% positive bile cultures in association with common duct stones alone. Recovery of anaerobic organisms is increasing with newer technologic advances. There is a distinct difference between bacteria in the bile and an infected biliary tree. The bacteriology of the biliary infection is directly correlated with the flora of the upper gastrointestinal tract (323, 383). The route of infection is via the portal vein; the organisms are then excreted into the bile.

The antibiotic treatment of cholangitis must be predicated on the bacteria sensitivity. Ampicillin is useful since it is active against *E. coli,* clostridia, and streptococci, and there is the additional advantage in that it is excreted in the bile. *Klebsiella* organisms are resistant to ampicillin, but an aminoglycoside such as kanamycin can be effectively used with ampicillin. Tetracycline can produce liver damage, and chloramphenicol is toxic for bone marrow.

Chetlin and Elliott (127) report that 9 of 22 deaths in 1421 biliary operations were due to sepsis. Septic complications were 40 times more frequent in patients with positive bile cultures. Positive bile cultures are to be anticipated in patients over 70 years of age with obstructive jaundice and/or common duct stones. These patients should receive antibiotics suitable for coliform bacteria. This "duct prep" for surgery should precede all secondary biliary tract operations (195).

Patients often present after having had several episodes of cholangitis, each apparently successfully treated with antibiotics. In other instances, because of the absence of clinical jaundice, the patient was diagnosed as having "flu," urinary tract infection, or fever of unknown origin. The relation between the antecedent biliary disease and the presenting episode was not appreciated.

The pathogenesis in most cases is fairly clear. There is incomplete bile duct obstruction, with a seeding of organisms into the bile from the bowel via the portal vein. Many patients with choledochal bacteria do not have cholangitis, as we define it clinically. In the presence of obstruction, the duct has no cilia and no peristalsis—*i.e.* no predictably effective self-cleaning mechanism.

One attitude toward the treatment of acute cholangitis of the nonsuppurative variety is analogous to an approach to acute cholecystitis. The patient's electrolytes should be restored and his cardiac and pulmonary status evaluated. He should be put into best possible condition, started immediately on antibiotics, and have surgery performed within 24–48 hours after this base-line improvement has been attained. Since this is invariably an obstructive phenomenon, the patient is best operated upon during the same hospital admission in which his condition is stabilized, rather than allowed to have another bout of cholangitis, the results of which can be unpredictable. The treatment of acute cholangitis should be definitive on the initial admission that confirms the diagnosis.

In PCS the most common cause of cholangitis is a retained common duct stone or ampullary stenosis. However, a suppurative gallbladder remnant can simulate cholangitis. In the Johns Hopkins series reported by Saharia and Cameron (518), the average interval to cholangitis in the 19 patients with primary common duct stones was 9 years. This suggests that an inadequately drained common bile duct, although its cholecystogenic stones had been adequately removed, becomes the seat of stasis, primary calculi, and partial obstruction, eventuating in cholangitis.

The suppurative variety of cholangitis is less frequent than the phlegmonous type but presents more dramatically with the clinical syndrome of Gram-negative sepsis and stupor. That aspect of the entity is rarely seen before age 55, and one can usually elicit a long history of biliary problems. The cholangitis is most often a complication of advanced disease (309), and it is in this situation that urgent surgical drainage is required. The mortality following medical treatment for this variety of infection is high, but not 100%. The suspicion that suppuration is unlikely to respond to antibiotics alone is suggested by leukocytosis in the range of 20,000 ($\pm$9500) and mean bilirubin of 9.1 ($\pm$3) mgm%. Shaking chills occur in 80% of patients, and in 60% the fever is in the 103–104° range. The indication for drainage or revision is especially pertinent if the antecedent procedure was a choledocholithotomy or biliary enteric anastomosis.

When infection is present, the degree of obstruction and intraductal pressure are the variables that determine outcome. With persistent, complete obstruction alone, the segmental liver area becomes atrophic and fibrotic. In partial obstruction, infection intervenes as miliary intrahepatic abscesses or a solitary liver abscess. Elevated ductal pressure allows bacteria to violate the bile–blood barrier. Generalized sepsis ensues. Experimentally, Huang *et al.* (281) have demonstrated that bacteria-containing bile may become bacteremia when the intraductal pressure is 25 cm H_2O. In the MHMC experience, many patients had resting pressures at that level who had no clinical symptoms to suggest acute cholangitis. At operation such patients did not always have an edematous and congested duct. In some, the duct wall was not even thickened. This disparity between the pressure measurement and their clinical implication is further discussed in the section on the practical applications of cholangiomanometry in Chapter 6. In the former circumstance organisms can be recovered from the hepatic veins and the thoracic duct (172). Both are sterile if the ductal pressure is less than 20 cm H_2O.

Several patients in the MHMC series have been in the care of courageous internists who have treated cholangitis with combinations of penicillin and chloromycetin with improvement in their general condition. They have then advised surgical correction in this "better general condition." The lethal factors are combinations of sepsis, liver failure due to microabscesses superimposed on an already diseased organ, and renal failure due to acute tubular necrosis. The intrahepatic liver abscesses are better tolerated and more easily treated than is the septicemia.

The prognosis for urgent surgery is poor if the cholangitis is associated with renal failure, with a blood urea nitrogen at 100 mgm% or acidosis with serum bicarbonate less than 15 mEq/liter. The question is when the patient should be dialyzed. One should delay the operation for as long as necessary to allow the renal status to return to normal either spontaneously or by hemodialysis. The order of priorities are as follows: 1) antibiotic treatment of the infection; 2) correction of the renal failure; and then 3) the definitive operation.

The differential diagnosis is sometimes difficult. One must consider the septic problem as having an alternate source in the lungs, genitourinary tract, or colon. The chest film and the urine examination serve for rapid screening. Sometimes the syndrome is mimicked by pancreatitis. If the serum bilirubin is below 3 mg/100 ml, I have found it prudent to do an intravenous cholangiogram or echogram while the patient is being hydrated and bolstered with intravenous antibiotics. The sonogram is a noninvasive method of demonstrating dilated intrahepatic ducts, a dilated common duct and the associated pancreatic reaction. On rare occasions, a patient has the complete clinical picture with apparently dilated but otherwise normal extrahepatic ducts. I have chosen to explore such patients and have found the effort well advised. I have found infected stasis bile with Vaterian segment stenosis, or a suppurative retained gallbladder remnant, or both.

Ascariasis in the common bile duct that has previously been explored for stones has been reported in areas where this infection is ordinarily not encountered (454). In a report from Jerusalem (467), following the 6-day war, three such cases of ascariasis were encountered with the worms found in the bile ducts. Prior to this time no case of *Ascaris lumbricoides* of the biliary system had ever been reported in Israel. The preoperative diagnosis was not made although the defect was visualized in the cholangiogram. The dead or live worm or fragments of worms were found to account for the cholangitis although there were also stones. It has been suggested that the prior damage to the integrity of the choledochal sphincter mechanism made it possible for the parasite to ascend into the extrahepatic bile duct.

If the patient is jaundiced, I have operated as soon as the general condition has improved, but not necessarily stabilized, with intravenous fluids, antibiotics, and hydrocortisone. There is often no opportunity for the determination of antibiotic sensitivity. I have used intravenous clindamycin or chloramphenicol or a combination of ampicillin and chloramphenicol when there is reason to suspect anaerobes. One experience with liver-related damage following the use of tetracycline has restrained my use of this antibiotic.

Obstructive cholangitis is a surgical disorder. The medical treatment is adjunctive. When the diagnosis is made, Naunyn's (441) early admonition still pertains: Remove the etiologic factor and prevent further biliary stasis. The surgery should be definitive, for each bout is associated with further liver damage. The neglected chronic patient ends up with biliary cirrhosis and portal hypertension.

A specific consideration applies only to the cholangitis that occurs with the biliary enteric anastomosis performed for iatrogenic bile duct stricture. For technical reasons, there can be difficulty in getting an absolutely accurate mucosal approximation. One has to accept the fact that bouts of cholangitis will occur. The anastomosis is to be regarded as adequate if there are less than two attacks of cholangitis per year, provided that these respond to antibiotics.

The surgical procedure requires opening the duct, removing the calculi, and correction of the stasis factor. In the presence of a greatly dilated duct, choledochoduodenostomy should be performed. My general policy has been also to do this wide anatomatic decompression on all dilated ducts with stasis stones and on all dilated ducts with cholangitis. There have been no technical complications associated with this operation carried out in the presence of severe and suppurative cholangitis. It is unlike the situation of having to deal with inflammatory free margins, which are a problem in intestinal disorders.

The inflammatory reaction in the Vaterian segment has been documented by both clinical biopsy and roentgenographic observations. Because this confluence of the pancreatic and common bile ducts with the duodenum is the narrowest portion of the extrahepatic biliary tract, inflammatory swelling here can be both prominent and influential. The reaction seen in x-ray films is characterized by an inflamed papilla that, on the contrast film, projects into the duodenum. It is especially obvious on the cholangiogram but is also seen on barium opacification. The change in this area is not specific for cholangitis; this "papillitis" or "ampullary reaction" is also seen in acute cholecystitis, acute pancreatitis, and in active duodenal ulcer.

This Vaterian process is reversible in the vast majority of instances, as evidenced by a return to normal of both the intrusion and the choledochal hypertension. Two biopsies

FIG. 2-7. Cholangiographic cholangitis. Cystic duct cholangiogram shows multiple small sawtooth ulcers **(arrows)** that are characteristic of advanced acute ulcerative cholangitis. This is an uncommon but characteristic cholangiographic finding.

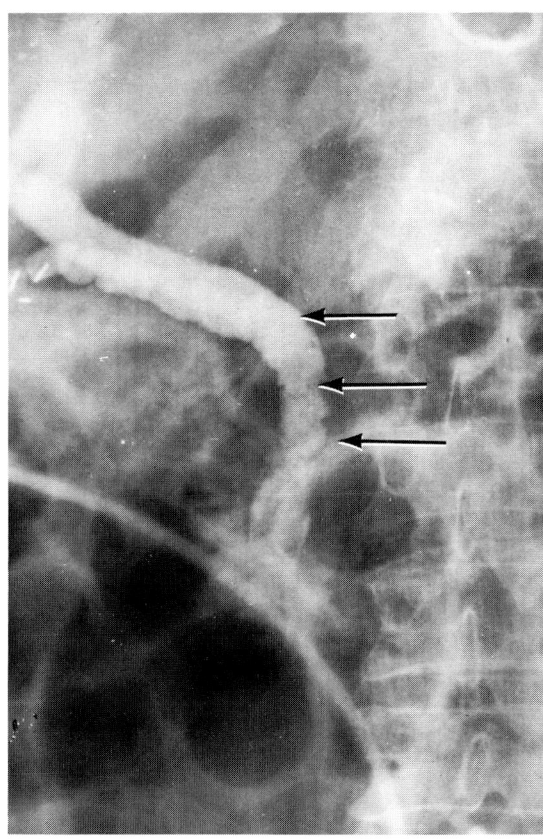

of this area in the acute stage when a "tumor could not be ruled out" revealed edema and congestion.

Another source of biopsy material has been the effort to define histologically the clinical entity of chronic ampullary fibrosis or choledochoduodenal junctional stenosis. Biopsies from this area have been reported from several sources but the findings are inconsistent (4, 65, 160, 167, 236, 237). The clinical entity has been histologically correlated with granulomatous reactions, muscular hypertrophy, inflammatory cell infiltration, and fibrosis, as well as with a completely normal histologic picture. This area of the ductal system is much better defined clinically, manometrically, and radiologically than it is in terms of its histologic response (Fig. 2-7).

3 Assessment of the Postcholecystectomy Patient

A knowledge of the details surrounding the first operative procedure is part of the diagnostic scaffold for evaluating the present illness. It is also best to review all the prior objective data: the initial cholecystogram, the operative cholangiogram (if there was one), the pathology report, and the operative record.

DIAGNOSTIC INTERVIEW

1. Were the initial symptoms those of colic, infection, or obstruction? These represent the best indication for the prior surgery and give the best results. It is reasonable to expect that if the cause was truly in the biliary tract, the patient should have been relieved. Otherwise there should be a demonstrable anatomic abnormality.

2. Was the operation an emergency or an elective procedure? Although the urgent galbladder operations can relieve the acute complications of gallbladder disease, intraoperative problems may have prevented the complete biliary toilet.

3. When did the symptoms recur, and how do they compare in type, localization, character, intensity, and frequency with those that were present before the first operation? If the symptoms were never significantly relieved, the surgery was not definitive or the diagnosis was in error.

4. Were there subjective complaints? There is a large category of such complaints that are nonspecific and toward which an operative approach is not required. Some patients have been treated for the dyspeptic syndrome, often with borderline abnormalities on the cholecystogram. The demonstration of cholelithiasis does not necessarily indicate a cause-and-effect relation to symptoms. I have elicited these non-specific symptoms as having been the indication for elective surgery: headache, belching, flatulence, fatty food intolerance, migraine, asthenia, inability to sleep on one side, insomnia, chronic constipation, irritability, weight problems, epigastric discomfort, "liverish" feeling.

5. Was the postoperative course unusual? A postoperative complication can suggest a persistent abdominal wall or intraabdominal problems. Hence, it is important to know about wound infections, postoperative jaundice, excessive biliary drainage, prolonged ileus, or reintervention for bleeding or jaundice. Major complications can be the first indication of an intraoperative accident. This is suggested by excessive biliary drainage or early jaundice. A deep wound infection or evisceration often precedes a postoperative hernia. An initial unexplained febrile reaction can later present as an established subphrenic abscess; this can appear months afterwards.

6. Were there any associated disorders or incongruous symptoms at the time of the initial procedure? It is particularly pertinent to consider an associated duodenal ulcer, alcoholism, diverticulitis, hiatus hernia, hemolytic disease, severe psychiatric problems, or personal instability. An occult cancer is especially likely to be in the colon or pancreas.

OPERATIVE SPECIMEN

The pathologist's report should be reviewed to establish the objective evidence of gallbladder disease and the extent of gallbladder removal. Special attention is directed to these questions:

1. Was the entire gallbladder removed? This can be documented distally only if a portion of the cystic duct has been included in the operative specimen. A determination that is as important in this regard as is the demonstration that the distal extent of a gastrectomy for peptic ulcer includes duodenal cuff in the specimen (192).

2. Were stones present and what type were they? The diagnosis of acalculus cholecystitis is an equivocal indication for cholecystectomy. A PCS is not unanticipated. Operations for this entity are indicated only under very special circumstances.

If the stones were present in the original operative specimen, the following inferences are pertinent: a large round solitary gallstone is rarely accompanied by common duct stones; faceted stones rarely occur singly; stasis calculi in the common bile duct occur in response to local choledochal obstruction and are unrelated to the gallbladder.

3. Did the gallbladder show an inflammatory reaction? This observation is important as a way of distinguishing between the normal gallbladder, the uninflamed gallbladder that is the seat of cholelithiasis (*i.e.*, so-called primary cholelithiasis), and the stone-containing gallbladder that has been or is the site of infection. The latter is evidenced by marked serosal edema, congestion, Rokitansky-Aschoff sinuses, mural fibrosis with clusters of inflammatory cells, focal endarteritis, marked percholecystitic adhesions or focal suppuration. Lymphocytic infiltrates in the submucosa alone are not abnormal (357, 576).

OPERATIVE NOTES

The surgeon's formal report of his findings and detailed description of the operation ideally should be as complete and precise as a musical score of a performed work so that the reader has a sense of being at the procedure.

One is alert to the description of anomalies, whether a transfusion was required (this often indicates the blood loss more vividly than does the operative note), and the duration of the operation—unusually long (3 hours) or too short (15 min) procedures are extremes that may have significance. One notes the nature of the suture material (silk can be the nidus of a foreign body), the use of hemostatic gauze in the liver bed (this can be the source of inflammatory reaction), and the method of abdominal wall closure. The description should include findings relative to the liver, pancreas, stomach, and esophageal hiatus. The descriptions of the pericholecystic reaction and of the common bile duct are critical. If the latter was not explored, the thickness of the wall and possibly the nature of the choledochal aspirate should be noted.

The anesthesia sheet can be informative. It objectively documents the blood pressure–pulse reaction and problems in relaxation or with fluid replacement.

The nurses' notes can be a source of information with reference to the tissues removed, biopsies taken, the instrument and laparotomy pad count and the monitoring procedures.

If the operative note is well done, the reviewer gets a sense of the procedure and of the difficulties encountered. Unfortunately, the descriptions can be routine, terse, evasive, or incomplete and ambiguous, and sometimes incongruous with other data in the record. Even so, it provides the ambience of the circumstances.

This assessment of the initial procedure and its circumstances can establish whether 1) the initial symptoms and signs had their likely origin in the biliary tract; 2) the biliary operation was complete or inadequate; 3) there is an iatrogenic factor in the postoperative complaints; and 4) the present complaints are related to persistent disease in the biliary tract or have their origin elsewhere.

PHYSICAL EXAMINATION

The physical examination must be particularly detailed and complete because it is directed at uncovering new findings that may lead to a totally different diagnosis as well as evaluating the status of the hepatobiliary system. One evaluates liver size, an abdominal mass, the stigmata of cirrhosis, hernia sites, painful subcutaneous granulomas, areas of hypesthesia, or costal tenderness. One searches especially for localized tenderness in areas in which discomfort is aggravated by cough or bearing down.

X-RAY STUDIES

Only those changes that cause or are the result of disease linked to biliary disorders are considered here. Obviously other distinct abnormalities can be the sole responsible factor. In this regard choledocholithiasis, hiatus hernia, and diverticulosis coli are associated, not interlinked, diseases, albeit certain of their symptom complexes may overlap.

Upper Gastrointestinal Series

1. Hiatus hernia with reflux can produce dyspeptic symptoms. In Baker and Williams' (39) study of patients with associated hiatus hernia and gallbladder disease in whom reflux was demonstrated, the incidence of esophageal symptoms was 60%; fewer than 20% of these patients were improved by cholecystectomy alone. In the series reported by Rhind and Watson (498) 70% of patients were relieved. The cure rate in women is 45%, better than the 29% reported in men. In general the patients who are improved are those who have heartburn without roentgen evidence of a gastroesophageal reflux, whereas those with reflux are not cured.

This validates the hypothesis that there is an association between esophageal symptoms and gallbladder disease, and in some patients cholecystectomy improves these symptoms. However, in patients with radiologic evidence of reflux, the chances of improvement are fewer (566).

2. Antral gastritis can be secondary to cholangitis, pancreatitis, or a subhepatic infection.

3. Pseudodiverticula of the first part of the duodenum are the result of extraduodenal traction.

4. A common duct groove in the first portion of the duodenum suggests choledochalectasia.

5. An excessively prominent ampulla is also referred to as a "papillary sign." This is a reversible edematous response to an anatomic contiguous inflammatory process. It is observed in association with biliary or pancreatic inflammation or peptic ulcer. Its roentgen appearance is distinct, but its cause is nonspecific.

6. Widening of the curve of the duodenum indicates enlargement of the head of the pancreas. It is a late sign of pancreatic cancer but an early sign of pancreatitis or of pancreatic pseudocyst. Edematous duodenal mucosa with a hair-on-end appearance, can be encountered in a variety of disorders (183).

7. Widening of the retrogastric space with anterior displacement of the stomach indicates pancreatic enlargement. Fluid levels in the area suggest pancreatic suppuration or a lesser sac abscess.

8. Duodenal ulcers occur or have occurred in 10–15% of patients with cholelithiasis. The clinician has to evaluate the differential role of each in patient management. Simultaneous combined treatment is often required to achieve symptomatic cure (132).

9. Perivaterian diverticula, on the medial wall of the descending duodenum, occur in about 2% of routine studies. I have not encountered an instance in which this finding could be symptomatically implicated in the postcholecystectomy state. However, there are reports to the contrary, most of them related to the fact that the common duct enters the duodenum through the diverticulum. In the vast majority of instances this is of no clinical significance (201).

Barium Enema Examination

Studies using barium enema are performed to exclude other diseases. They rarely offer any indication of biliary disease. The hepatic flexure bears a constant relation to the gallbladder area: It always overlies it. In the patient with PCS this flexure is adherent to the gallbladder fossa. Focal irritability or stasis in the area can be reflected in this segment of the colon as part of gallbladder remnant inflammatory disease.

Intravenous Cholangiography

Cholangiography is the single most pertinent examination in PCS. Its applicability has moved the character of diagnosis from speculation to objective demonstrability. There is no objection to a policy of preceding this intravenous study by an attempt to visualize the extrahepatic biliary tree solely by the oral route as applied to routine cholecystography or by echography.

The intravenous study and its technique, variants, and findings have been particularly well described in Wise's still pertinent monograph of the Lahey Clinic experience (638). There are several factors to be considered if one is to get a satisfactory examination: 1) It should not be undertaken if the patient has a specific history of allergy or previous iodism. Others have a more aggressive approach to the patient with "minor" allergies. I prefer not to take the risk. 2) There will be no visualization if the serum bilirubin exceeds 3.5 mg/100 ml. 3) The patient should be well hydrated. 4) A preexamination purgative should be adequate to eliminate all gas shadows in the area. 5) The study should be continued until the contrast material is observed to enter the duodenum; if this does not occur in 4 hours, 12- and 24-hour films should be obtained.

One reviews these films with particular reference to the size of the duct, the presence of calculi, visualization of the gallbladder remnant, the adequacy of emptying after 60 and 90 min and for evidence of contour deformities. It is important to know that delayed visualization of the bile ducts can occur in hepatic dysfunction. Therefore, films should be taken up to 8 hours after the start of the examination if there is no prior diagnostic film. On the other hand, prolonged infusion time and increased dosage do not improve the radiographic results in this regard. The 24-hour film can be diagnostic even when those taken up to 4 hours show no opacification of the biliary system (Fig. 3-1).

The intravenous study has the advantage of obviating the air-bubble artifact, the pseudocalculus sign, the problem of associated gastrointestinal motility, or absorption disturbances with failure to deliver the contrast substance to the liver. It has the disadvantage of being of little value in the presence of a pneumocholangiogram. Tomographic cuts are often necessary, especially in the obese.

Gunnarson (241) has used the morphine intravenous cholangiogram as a provocative test. He noted an average 24% increase in the width of the common bile duct in the cholecystectomized patient with severe symptoms. The asymptomatic patient had no response or a far lesser one. A provocative dose of morphine may selectively elevate the SGOT in the symptomatic patient, with the highest level attained in 5–8 hours and the effect lasting for 24 hours. This associated chemical determination has no exclusionary diagnostic value.

Puncture Cholangiography

The postcholecystectomy patient who is jaundiced is no longer managed by observation of the liver enzymes. The present approach is a rapid, diagnostic, direct invasive roentgenologic definition of the abnormality in the bile ducts.

The percutaneous transhepatic cholangiogram is the procedure of choice in regard to ease of performance and minimum equipment. The technique allows for an anatomic diagnosis whenever the dilated bile duct can be punctured. It carries certain disadvantages: 1) Sometimes a dilated bile duct cannot be entered. 2) There might be a significant bile leak. 3) Laceration of the liver is possible. In the MHMC series we encountered bile leaks of 300–400 ml, but they bore no significance in the total management of the patients, because the diagnostic procedure is carried out while on the way to the operating room. If an obstructed duct is visualized, the patient is operated upon promptly (Fig. 3-2).

The idea of combining direct visualization of the liver with biopsy and transhepatic cholangiography is advocated in Del Guercio's concept of the "minilaparotomy" (166). This procedure is performed with local infiltration anesthesia. An incision is made in the midline of the subxiphoid area. The liver is thus exposed for biopsy and direct puncture cholangiography. By this technique one can see and control hepatic leaks or bleeding.

Another closed procedure combining the advantages of biopsy and cholangiography is that reported by Berci *et al.* (51) as laparoscopy with transhepatic cholangiography. A laparoscopic observation of the liver is made. Then a direct, guided liver biopsy is performed. Under direct observation a puncture transhepatic cholangiogram is performed with cinefluoroscopic control (574).

ENDOSCOPIC RETROGRADE CHOLANGIOPANCREATOGRAPHY

A modification of the fiberoptic gastroduodenoscope now permits an experienced endoscopist to cannulate the Vaterian segment in the conscious patient (145, 318). With functioning equipment and experienced personnel, endoscopic retrograde cholangiopancreatography (ERCP) can be the initial differential diagnostic approach to the jaundiced patient. It requires no incision.

The modification of the forward-looking endoscope by a lateral viewer and a bridge for passing a teflon-coated cannula has made it possible for the truly experienced endoscopist to cannulate the Vaterian segment in about 85% of patients in 30–90 min (68). The procedure has received worldwide recognition as adjunctive to the diagnosis of biliary and pancreatic disease. The value in the former is perhaps even greater than in the latter aspects. The usual premedication consists of atropine, intravenous diazepam (Valium), and the use of atropine or propantheline bromide (Pro-banthine) or glucagon to promote duodenal ileus. The endoscope is passed with the patient in the left lateral decubitus position so that the entire esophagus and stomach and duodenum can be visualized and endoscopic

FIG. 3-1. Intravenous cholangiography. **A.** Intravenous cholangiogram, taken 2 hours after injection, before contrast material has been voided, shows selective dilatation of the supraduodenal choledochus **(a)** and of the left hepatic duct **(b)**. The infraduodenal segment is displaced to the left **(c)**. These findings are consistent with a choledochal reaction due to pancreatitis. **B.** Intravenous cholangiogram reveals dilation of the common bile duct and contrast material in the duodenum **(a)**. The left hepatic duct **(b)** cannot be visualized, and there is an irregularity at the carina. A normal variant failure of opacification of the left hepatic duct may occur when the examination is performed in the supine position, in which instance the anterior position of the left hepatic duct ostium explains the failure of opacification. The irregularity here suggests that this failure of opacification has a different basis. In fact it was due to an incarcerated stone impacted in the left hepatic duct just proximal to the carina. The deformity resulted from encroachment and perforation of the carinal septum.

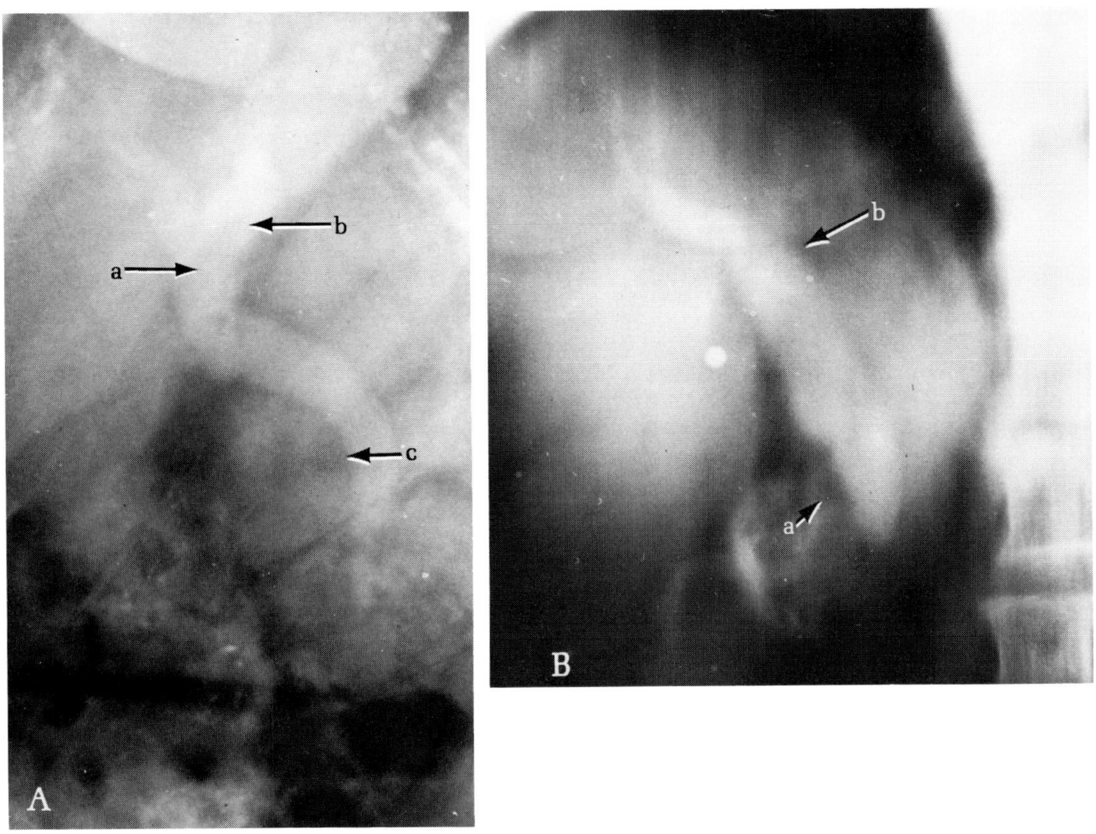

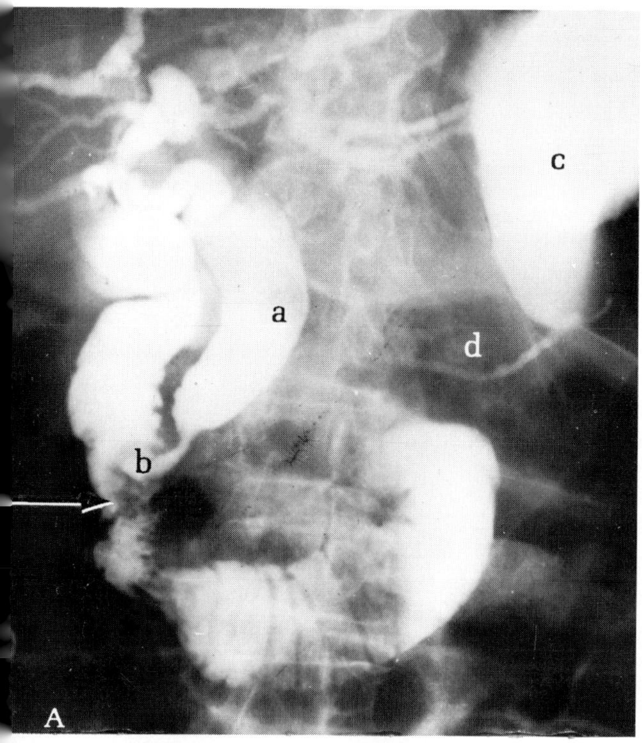

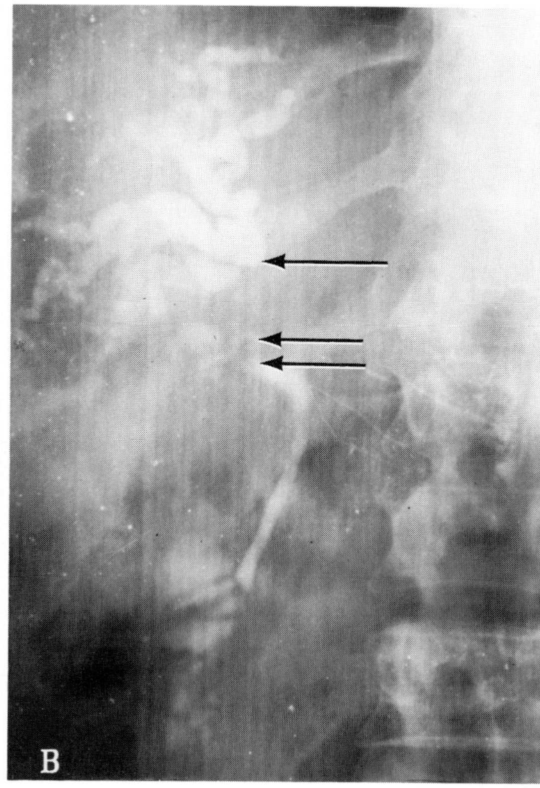

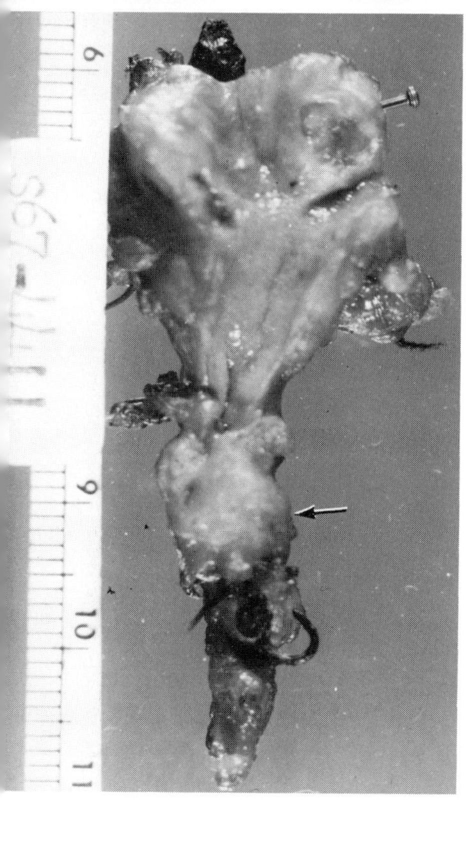

FIG. 3-2. Transhepatic cholangiography. **A.** This transhepatic cholangiogram illustrates the compound nature of the problems that may be encountered: There is a solitary round stone **(a)** in a dilated common bile duct and true stenosis of the distal portion of the common bile duct **(b),** which is to be differentiated from long-segment sphincterization. The ampulla **(arrow)** is edematous, a "papillary" sign that frequently accompanies choledocholithiasis. The incompetent pyloric sphincter allows reflux of contrast material into the stomach **(c).** The entire pancreatic duct **(d)** is visualized and shows no abnormalities. The patient was managed by choledocholithotomy and choledochoduodenostomy. **B.** This patient, who had a cholecystectomy 5 years before, is now jaundiced. The transhepatic percutaneous cholangiogram shows dilated intrahepatic ducts coming down to a nipple stricture **(arrow).** There is a long defect between that area and the **double arrow.** The stricture is only partial because the distal normal common bile duct empties into the duodenum. This film is diagnostic of hepatic duct cancer. No biopsy confirmation is required. **C.** Resected choledochus of the same patient whose cholangiogram is shown in Figure 3-2B. The carcinoma is polypoid. The specimen consists of the entire supraduodenal choledochus and hepatic duct carina.

abnormalities uncovered *en passant*. The patient is then rotated into the prone position for the cannulation of the ampulla.

The only contraindications to the procedure are recent acute pancreatitis and the suspicion or the demonstration of hepatitis antigen. In regard to the latter, there is a danger of transmitting the disease from one patient to the other via the endoscope.

The major papilla is identified by its proximal semicircular, hooded fold. The cannula usually enters the pancreatic duct preferentially, and visualization of this area is accomplished by the injection of 2–3 cc of the contrast medium. The cannula may have to be repositioned to enter the biliary tract. The intact biliary tract has a capacity of approximately 30–40 cc contrast material. The biliary tract retains the contrast material for a sufficient time to allow for leisurely x-rays, but the contrast material runs out of the pancreatic duct rather rapidly (Fig. 3-3).

Septic complications, including pancreatitis, have been reported. Certain cautions in the procedure are suggested by Davidson *et al.* (162): 1) The operation should not be delayed more than 12–24 hours after an obstruction is demonstrated. 2) Any patient who develops significant abdominal pain and fever following this procedure and who does not respond promptly to nasogastric suction and antibiotics should undergo laparotomy. The question of routine prophylactic antibiotic therapy prior to endoscopy has not been answered.

This retrograde cholangiogram gives an especially good view of the distal common bile duct. There is some hazard to injecting contrast material beyond a stricture, as it has been associated with postendoscopic bacteremia. Stones are readily visualized. Even more importantly, a completely normal study can make for the secure diagnosis of a normal biliary tract.

In the obstructed duct this examination has less value, for in that situation it is important to know what lies proximal to the stone—stenosis or tumor. Such information is required not only to make an accurate diagnosis, but also to plan the surgical corrective procedure. This is ordinarily best achieved with the percutaneous transhepatic cholangiogram.

The main pancreatic duct is 16–20 cm long and the width at the head averages about 3.5 mm; at the body, 3 mm; and at the tail, about 2 mm. The excellent roentgen demonstration of this ductal system however, does not always correlate with the disease. The pancreatic duct can be roentgenographically normal despite chronic pancreatitis or pancreatic cancer (564, 565). Therefore, ERCP alone cannot be used as the sole screening test for pancreatic pathology. The recent endoscopic retrieval of pancreatic fluid for cytology may improve the yield (446).

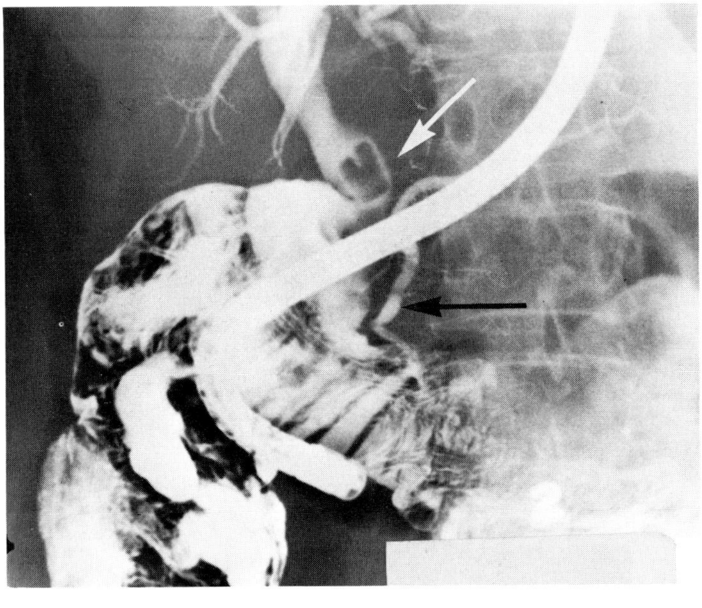

FIG. 3-3. Film of an endoscopic retrograde cannulation in a jaundiced patient. A solitary calculus is in the common bile duct **(white arrow).** The pancreatic duct is normal **(black arrow).**

The ERCP procedure involves expensive equipment. Considerable experience is required to achieve 85% diagnostic accuracy. It has less general utility than puncture cholangiography done with the skinny (Chiba) needle.

ULTRASOUND STUDY

Ultrasound is a totally noninvasive diagnostic technique, requiring no preparation and no contrast material. The source of the contrasting black and white images is the reflected ultrasonic pulses stimulated by a piezoelectric transducer. The echoes arise between tissues of different densities. Scans are done in both transverse and longitudinal sections, with cuts taken at 1- to 2-cm intervals. A total biliary or pancreatic scan takes about 20 or 30 min to perform. The procedure is totally pain-free. The definitive role of ultrasound in the diagnosis of biliary or pancreatic disease is still in evolution, but its value has already been definitely established. Because of the relatively innocuous nature of the procedure, it is frequently suggested as the first "screening" approach to the jaundiced patient (Table 3-1).

In the patient with PCS, one can definitely discern pancreatic enlargement and large gallbladder remnants and the stones therein, provided they are over 0.5 cm in diameter. It is an excellent and reliable method of demonstrating dilated intrahepatic ducts that indicate obstructive choledochopathy. The normal gallbladder is visualized as an echo-free structure about 3–cm above the umbilicus. Its true size and the thickness of its walls are best seen in the longitudinal section. Stones are indicated by echoes within this normally echo-free area. The method is especially valuable in discerning the associated intrahepatic disorders, such as a hepatic abscess, and pancreatic cysts (Figs. 3-4, 3-5, 3-6).

TABLE 3-1. RAPID DIAGNOSTIC APPROACH IN THE CHOLECYSTECTOMIZED PATIENT PRESENTING WITH POSSIBLE OBSTRUCTIVE JAUNDICE

Indication	Diagnostic procedure
Bilirubin	
< 3	Intravenous cholangiography
	Duodenal drainage
> 3	Transhepatic cholangiogram
	Ultrasound
	ERCP*
Associated problems	
Pancreas	Angiography
	Percutaneous biopsy
Liver	Ultrasonic scanning
	Peritoneoscopic guided biopsy
	Angiography

* Endoscopic retrograde cholangiopancreatography.

The intraoperative use of A-mode ultrasound to demonstrate intraductal calculi has not proved practical because of the artifacts that complicate the interpretation (270).

Computerized axial tomography (CAT) is an additional modality for the noninvasive evaluation of the viscera. The role of CAT scanning has already been well established for the brain. Its unique role *vis a vis* echography for the evaluation of the liver, gallbladder, bile ducts and pancreas has not yet been established. There are overlapping potentials. CAT scanning can define these changes: enlarged liver, dilated intrahepatic bile ducts, hepatic tumors, dilated common bile duct, biliary calculi, pancreatic enlargements and peripancreatic swellings. These can be visualized in both longitudinal and transverse section.

At this time such non invasive modalities appear to have an advantage over intravenous cholangiography as the initial diagnostic tool.

Despite this, transhepatic cholangiography is the single most accurate method of defining the problem anatomically and etiologically.

PSYCHIATRIC EVALUATION

The relation of the psyche to biliary disease is not so well defined as it is to peptic ulcer and to ulcerative colitis. This role of the liver is part of the oldest medical tradition. The bilious personality is part of fiction and folk lore. The absence of precise documentation that is clinically pertinent is a therapeutic deficit. Certainly the demonstration of a cephalic phase in biliary-pancreatic secretion and its analog in the application of this information to the treatment of duodenal ulcer suggests that an important aspect of the etiologic factor in biliary dysfunction is open for study.

McMaster and Elman (418) observed that with the perception of food, the gallbladder of the dog contracted and the choledochal sphincter relaxed. However, Crain and Walsh (148) failed to observe this gallbladder activity in sham-fed dogs who had an esophagotomy or gastric fistula. Puestow's (484) biliary fistula preparation demonstrated that excitement sometimes delayed or inhibited the discharge of bile. Johnson (357) observed that the duo-

FIG. 3-4. Ultrasonography. This is a transverse ultrasonic scan 7 cm below the xiphoid process. **A.** A large pseudocyst (**arrow** indicates posterior surface) involves the body and tail of the pancreas in a patient who had had a previous cholecystectomy. **B.** A longitudinal scan 7 cm to the right of the midline shows a calculus in a gallbladder remnant **(arrow).** (Courtesy, Dr. Ruth Rosenblatt, Department of Diagnostic Radiology, Montefiore Hospital Medical Center)

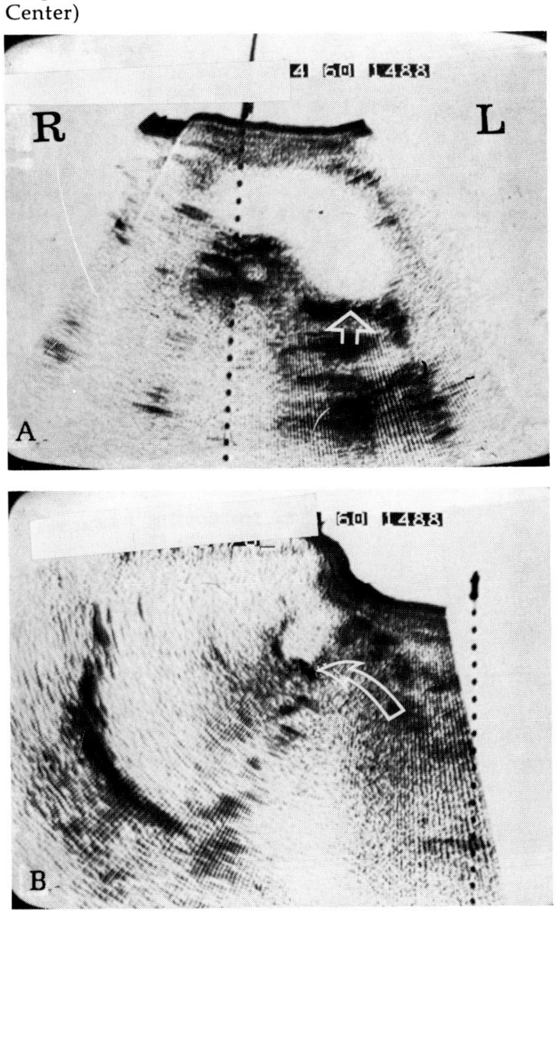

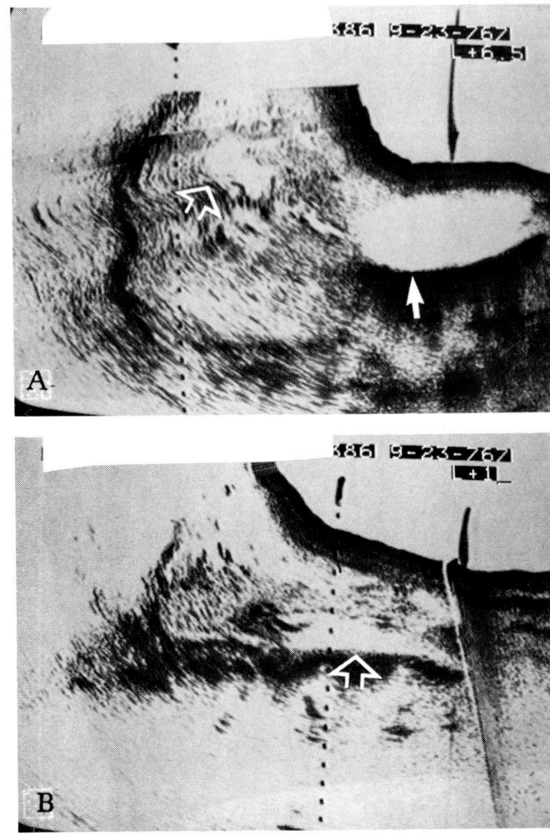

FIG. 3-5. Ultrasonography. The value of ultrasonography in evaluating jaundiced patients who have previously been operated upon is indicated in these longitudinal section studies. **A.** The gallbladder is greatly enlarged **(arrow at right)**; it is the Courvoisier type. The intrahepatic bile ducts are dilated **(arrow at left).** This suggests the diagnosis of tumor of the head of the pancreas. The diagnosis may then be confirmed and the area mapped out by transhepatic cholangiography. **B.** An ultrasonic longitudinal scan 15 cm to the right of the midline demonstrates a small gallbladder. The intrahepatic ducts are dilated **(arrow).** (Courtesy, Dr. Ruth Rosenblatt, Department of Diagnostic Radiology, Montefiore Hospital Medical Center)

denal drainage of dog bile was inhibited by fright.

The problem in the PCS is whether and in what manner the "normal" Vaterian segment is influenced by neural endocrine factors of psychic initiation. Pavlovian type influences on the biliary tract remain to be evaluated.

In clinical practice, it is an empirical fact that emotional problems can trigger symptoms in the right upper quadrant. It is not uncommon to see symptoms presumed to be

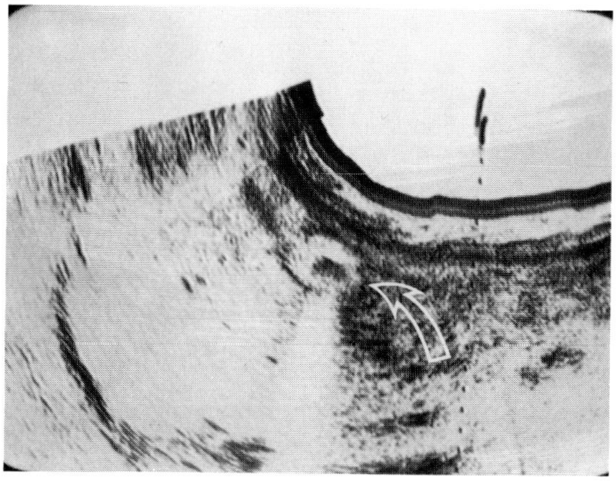

Fig. 3-6. Ultrasonography. A longitudinal scan 15 cm to the right of the midline shows a small gallbladder remnant containing a large solitary calculus **(arrow).** (Courtesy, Dr. Ruth Rosenblatt, Department of Diagnostic Radiology Montefiore Hospital Medical Center)

linked to biliary disorders appear in relation to stress situations, migraine headaches, and menstrual irregularities. It is my observation that this association occurs more frequently in depressive states than in hypomanic or hyperkinetic situations.

There is often a disparity in the affect that these people present: They have a whole catalog of symptoms, but smile or remain bland throughout the interview. These patients often describe detailed biliary symptoms acquired, unwittingly or not, in their shuffle from one medical facility to another.

A neurotic focus may find its locus in the biliary tract as well as in the duodenum, heart, or colon. Dreiling (178), in a study of 96 PCS patients, could find no organic disease in 82%, and two-thirds of these had never had a symptom-free interval. Sixteen percent of this group had a major psychosis (schizophrenia, depression) or a psychoneurotic anxiety state, conversion hysteria, or cancer phobia. This observation is important because many postcholecystectomy patients continue to present again and again despite unrewarding prior surgical procedures.

One situation to which the physician must be especially alert is depression, which can be the presenting symptom of cancer of the pancreas. Some patients who have recently undergone a cholecystectomy present again with obstructive jaundice. The clinical examination or second laparotomy reveals the ominous association of depression, biliary symptoms, and pancreatic cancer.

A significant problem arises when residual anatomic disease is demonstrated in a psychopathic personality: The organic may aggravate the psychic. If there is definite symptomatic anatomic residual disease that is amenable to surgery, the patient should be advised to have this corrected, with the understanding that only the specifically related complaints are likely to be alleviated. The basic personality remains.

I have encountered neurotic patients whose threshold for personal problems improved when they were surgically relieved of bouts of biliary colic or the knowledge that stones were retained. Whether to make these patients "calculus free" has to be determined in consultation with an organically oriented psychiatrist. A neurotic patient may also have a surgically curable disorder. Others who have had biliary surgery are just mentally sick; reoperative surgery can be a futile assault.

The symptomatic patient in whom the physical findings and radiographic study are normal should have an analysis of duodenal bile. If no cholesterol crystals are demonstrated, a provocative test should be done. If these too are normal, surgery should be withheld. A repeated study is warranted if the symptoms are still typical, as objective findings lag behind the disease. I have done no secondary operations unless there was a definitive objective abnormality. I have not regretted this approach, for in the face of normal results on x-ray studies and studies of bile cytology it is unlikely that the patient has an anatomic disease of the extrahepatic biliary tract that is amenable to surgery.

When abnormalities are encountered, they rarely occur singly, choledochalectasia is the commonest denominator. These are the commonest combinations:

Gallbladder remnant and choledocholithiasis

Choledocholithiasis with primary and secondary stones and choledochoduodenal junction stenosis (CDJS)

Choledochal fistula with choledocholithiasis

Cholangitis with choledocholithiasis or CDJS

Pancreatitis and choledocholithiasis and gallbladder remnants

A single disorder may dominate the clinical finding, but one has to suspect the associations.

DYSPEPSIA

Johnson's study (307) revealed dyspeptic complaints in 30% of patients who had undergone operation: heartburn, flatulence, eructation, bloating, bad breath, and altered taste sense. These complaints deserve consideration in this evaluation. Usually these symptoms do not develop after operation; they simply persist. Patients voice considerable discontent that the prior operation did not deliver the dividend of relief from these symptoms. They regard the operation as incomplete and felt cheated.

Numerous studies (70, 173, 307) have shown that there is an equal distribution of dyspeptic symptoms among those with normal and abnormal cholecystograms, further emphasizing the observation that chronic dyspepsia cannot be attributed to the biliary tract, and that the association is fortuitous or inexplicable.

Argon wash-out studies have been performed to study flatulent dyspepsia (358). Argon introduced into the proximal small bowel washes out all the native gases in the intestine. These are collected at the rectum. Normal subjects pass 400–2000 ml gas per day per rectum and have only about 100 ml of gas in the intestinal tract at any given moment. In the patient with severe bloating, abnormalities have been encountered. Often much of the infused argon moves retrograde and can be aspirated from the stomach. Only in some persons is this increased sensitivity appreciated as bloating. Flatulence is fundamentally a motility disorder.

An important question is which of the two sources of intestinal gas—that swallowed or that produced intraluminally—is the principal offender. If it is the latter, then dietary manipulation might be of some value. Certain foods are notorious for gaseous provocation: cabbage, broccoli, brussels sprouts, cauliflower, kale, sauerkraut, turnips, carrots, beets, peas, beans, lentils, and other legumes.

The components of intestinal gas are principally nitrogen, hydrogen, methane, and carbon dioxide. Oxygen and nitrogen constitute the contribution of swallowed air to the intestinal gas pool. In intestinal obstruction, the major source of distention is the nitrogen. In normal subjects, only 50% of the bowel gas is atmospheric; the rest is produced within the lumen. Thus the century-old observation of the relationship, for example, of beans to flatus, resides in the fact that these cannot be digested by the normal intestinal tract and they react with colonic bacteria to produce gas. The inflammable properties of flatus in certain individuals, although not in all, is related to the methane production. The specific regulatory factors here have not been elucidated.

Patients suffering from flatulence have normal volumes of gas in the fasting state. Lasser *et al.* (350) have evaluated the problem at a more crucial time in the patient's symptomatology—that is, postprandially. In that state, the volume of intestinal gas did not differ from that in normal controls. The difference was in the increased hydrogen content.

These flatulent patients did not produce abnormal volumes of gas. Those with bloating pass the gas more slowly: The controls pass at 44 ± 6 ml/min; the flatulent, at 28 ± 4 ml/min. The slow transit can be associated with discomfort. Thus flatulent disturbances appear to be related to impaired intestinal motility for gas.

Kantor (317) has indicated that there is a considerable delay in the transit of certain proteins. Stinking gases such as skatole and indole may be produced. These can be absorbed and then excreted in expired air, constituting a basis for bad breath. It is probable that fetid gases are normally deodorized during their passage through the liver. This fits with the explanation for the "heavy" breath of hepatic insufficiency; it is a manifestation of the failure of deodorization of odorous intestinal gases.

Experimentally, it has been shown that if the small intestine has been filled with carbon dioxide, about 90% is rapidly absorbed if the portal vein is free. If the portal vein is ligated, only 40% of the gas is taken up in the same period of time.

It is not strange that one of the signs of a failing or congested circulation may be the inability to remove intestinal gases. Thus, flatulence in the elderly can be one of the manifestations of mesenteric arteriosclerosis or of an intermittent claudication phenomenon in the bowel, thus comprising two components—one, the inability to move the gas out, which is the dysfunction of impaired vascularity; and the other, an inability to move it on, which is a related or independent deficiency in peristaltic activity. In the younger flatulent patient, the defect may be only one of impaired motility.

The mechanisms of eructation, aside from air swallowing, has not been thoroughly clarified. Jaonnides (305) has evaluated the problem insofar as diaphragmatic function is concerned. The left hemidiaphragm ordinarily functions together with the right hemidiaphragm. In those who eructate it contracts at the same moment that the right diaphragm relaxes and rises proportionately. This intermittent contraction of the left with coincident relaxation of the right leaf straightens out the acute angle of the gastric cardia sufficiently to prevent the valve function that resides in this angle. With a slight pressure on the abdominal muscles the air very promptly finds its way up the esophagus and into the mouth.

Eructation is a disordered function of the diaphragm at the esophagocardiac angle and of air-swallowing and has no specific relation to gallbladder disease.

Johnson's studies (306, 307) show a direct correlation between flatulent dyspepsia and roentgen evidence of pyloric reflux. Eructation is regarded as associated with duodenal gastric reflux that is often precipitated by intraduodenal fat. The primary defect is that the malfunctioning pylorus does not close in response to duodenal contractions. The normal pylorus acts to prevent reflux produced by an isolated duodenal contraction. This reflux was not observed in any of the asymptomatic patients. Capper *et al.* (108) have a different viewpoint. They found normal pyloric function in only 2 of 18 patients with gallstones and suggest that the pylorus becomes incompetent years after cholecystectomy.

Benevantano and Schein's study (46) indicates that competence of the postcholecystectomy pylorus varies. In some patients it is always competent, in some it is intermittently competent, and in some it is incompetent all the time. Each of these states is viewed as a normal physiologic variant in the cholecystectomized patient.

The effectiveness of avoiding fatty food is presumed to be based on this alteration of gastroduodenal reflux. It is still not clear why or if patients, including those with biliary disorders, have this alteration in pyloric function and intestinal motility.

Eructation is seen both in health and disease. Among certain peoples, belching is considered a sign of good digestion and is an indication to the host that his food has been enjoyed and properly digested. The Goteborg follow-up study of the dyspeptic patient revealed that the symptoms are ameliorated in about two-thirds of those reviewed 5 years after operation. In a general way the prognosis in this regard is better for men than for women (623).

The diagnosis of the PCS patients by invasive techniques (cholangiography, biliary drainage, peritoneoscopy) has, on the whole, replaced indirect radiologic studies or evaluation of blood chemistries (624, 631). The aim is the demonstration of a culpable anatomic, physiological abnormality.

11 Intraoperative Diagnosis

4 Technique of Operative Cholangiography

THE PORTAL

The portal for cannulation is chosen in relation to the information sought and the accessible channel.

1. Instillation of contrast into the lumen of the gallbladder remnant is often of limited value in the intraoperative situation. Contrast material delivered by this route may fail to negotiate the cystic duct because of inflammatory edema, obstructive calculi, or inability to effect a satisfactory pressure within the punctured viscus. Direct palpation and inspection of the opened vesical is a far superior way to evaluate its contents.

This technique of cholecystocholangiography can be of special value, however, in assessing the ducts in problems related to the gallbladder remnant that contains no calculi or to the collapsed gallbladder. It can be usefully employed to detect hepatic duct tumors, to seek an "escaped" stone or to make the differential diagnosis between extrahepatic obstruction and intrinsic liver disease. This modality is most profitably employed in the postoperative cholecystostomy patient.

2. Cystic duct stump cannulation makes it possible to evaluate the entire biliary conduit prior to formal exploration. It is technically the most simple approach in the uncommon situation of the diseased common duct of normal width (Fig. 4-1).

3. Transhepatic cholangiography is undertaken to establish the presence of obstructive jaundice and to define its cause and anatomic characteristics. It also serves to demonstrate whether the right and left hepatic ductal systems communicate—an important consideration in patients in whom decompression by a single or double hepaticoenterostomy is being considered.

PREOPERATIVE TRANSHEPATIC CHOLANGIOGRAPHY

Transhepatic cholangiography prior to surgery is carried out in the x-ray department under fluoroscopic control with an image intensifier (114, 200, 633). The patient is fully prepared for surgery. There is complete understanding by the patient, the x-ray division staff, the attending staff, and the operating room personnel that immediately following this study the patient may be operated upon.

The procedure has had about 90% success in getting into the dilated intrahepatic ducts. With image intensification control, Arner *et al.* (28) were also able to opacify the ducts in 51% of 35 patients in whom the ducts were not dilated. This report parallels the MHMC experience that the accuracy and success of the method is vastly improved with television monitoring and use of the Chiba needle.

The patient must be cooperative, and there can be no bleeding diathesis. I have found it wise to administer intravenous ampicillin just prior to the examination. The patient is in the supine position, and the site of the costophrenic sinus is defined. One may use either the Teflon-covered needle, which permits aspiration of bile, or the "skinny" Chiba needle, which is assumed to be less traumatic but can only deliver the contrast media. The former has the advantage of making it pos-

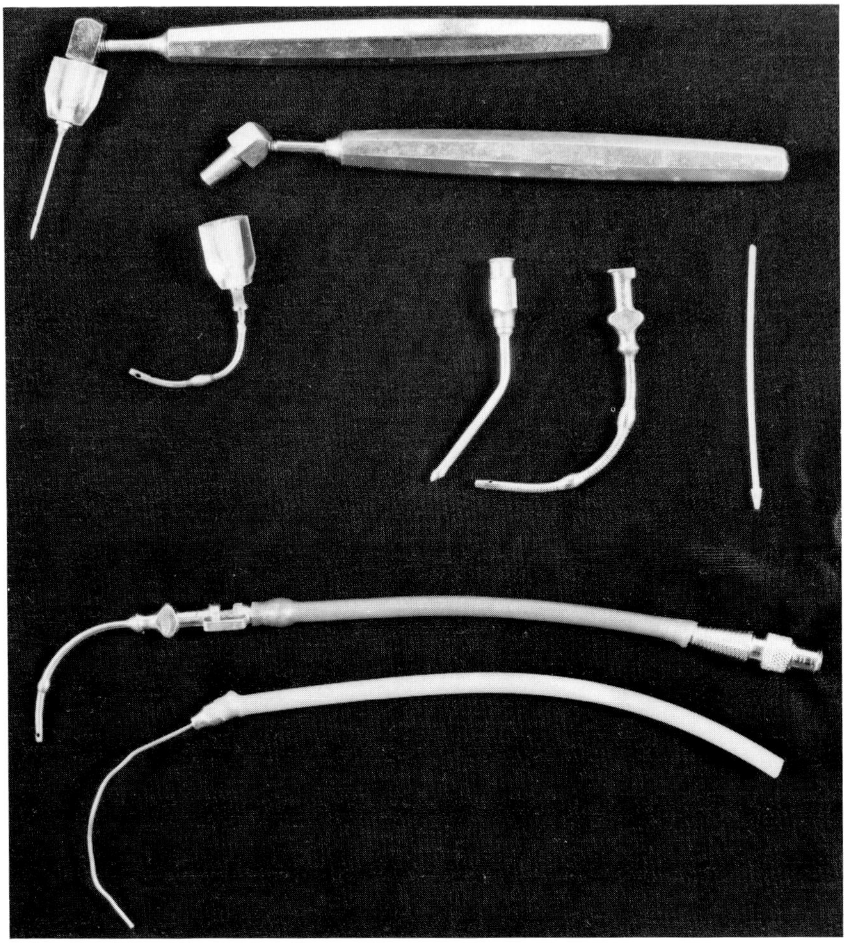

FIG. 4-1. Cannulas for intraoperative cholangiography. These cannulas have certain advantages over ureteral catheters, polyethylene tubing, mucosal sinus cannulas, and cardiothoracic tubing.

sible to aspirate bile for culture and sensitivity determination and to manipulate across and into biliary enteric anastomosis.

The Teflon-covered 8-in. needle is introduced just above the tenth rib in the mid-axillary line. It is advanced to within 1 in of its hilt. The needle is removed and the Teflon sleeve is attached to a 50 ml syringe. The soft plastic tube is slowly withdrawn until bile appears, indicating that the catheter is well positioned. If blood is aspirated, it is flushed out of the two-way stopcock, and the catheter is farther withdrawn. An initial test injection of contrast material confirms the fact that the catheter is satisfactorily seated. If the material gets into a vascular channel, it is rapidly flushed out. The bile duct pattern is highly characteristic. The catheter is left in place for drainage and the patient is transferred to the operating room.

In a review (633) incorporating 423 such procedures, there was a 1.8% incidence of bile leakage without peritonitis and a 3% incidence of bile peritonitis. These problems can be minimized if the catheter is left in for drainage in the normal instances and if prompt surgery is performed in those patients with diseased ducts. One should not do this examination without being prepared to act on the findings that are disclosed.

The aspirated fluid may be a green obstructed bile, a flocculent, green, stasis calculous bile, or the mucoid secretion of long-standing obstruction. If no operation is to be performed, culture, Gram stain, and cytology may help toward further management. The cannula can be withdrawn or left in, or it can be pulled out of the bile duct cavity and left in the subhepatic space as a drain or suction tube (330).

Molnar and Stockum (428) indicate an additional advantage to transhepatic cholangiography. If the patient is septic with obstruction, it is possible to leave the Teflon catheter in the bile duct or to guide it through a stricture for the purpose, not only of dilatation, but of maintaining ductal enteric continuity in a nonoperative way. It is an intriguing procedure to intubate strictured hepaticojejunostomies and postoperative biliary strictures under fluoroscopic control. In this way a diagnostic technique can be a therapeutic approach to relieve jaundice and pruritus while permitting the liver to recuperate from the effects of obstruction (595).

Recent modification in this technique has been prompted by the use of the Chiba "skinny" needle, which has completely replaced the sheathed needle. All MHMC studies are now done with this technique. The needle is slender, very flexible, unsheathed, and 15 cm long, with an outer diameter of 0.7 mm and an inner diameter of 0.5 mm. The advantage of this needle is obvious in entering the large dilated duct. The procedure is different from that employed with a large-bore needle that depends upon aspiration to identify the large duct.

The Chiba needle is introduced through an intercostal space in the right mid to anterior axillary line. A tape marker is placed over the eleventh thoracic intervertebral space, and the needle is passed parallel to the table and perpendicular to the right chest wall to a point in the liver just short of the fluoroscopic monitor. The stylet is removed, and the contrast solution is connected to the needle with a polyethylene tube. While the solution is injected at very slight pressure, the full inserted needle is slowly withdrawn from the liver. Injection into the bile duct outlines the biliary tree while injection into the hepatic venous system is immediately recognized by the rapid disappearance of the contrast material. The great advantage of this needle is that 1) the danger of significant bile leak is reduced, and 2) it is possible to enter nondilated ducts in more than half the cases after one to four passes of the needle. The former premise that only large ducts could be entered is not valid with the use of the skinny needle.

In 60 diagnostic examinations using this technique at MHMC, no mortality occurred. In four instances there was more than 100 cc of bile in the peritoneal cavity. One dilated duct was not entered after the customary four passes had been made.

The method has the advantage of clearly defining the biliary problem prior to dissection for identification and immobilization. At the operative procedure one often finds 50 ml of bile in the area lateral to the site of the puncture. This might be a problem in the patient who has a normal biliary system and does not undergo surgery. However, we have never encountered it. If the patient is operated upon, the biliary system is decompressed. It has not been necessary to do anything about the puncture site once the biliary hypertension has been relieved. There has been no morbidity associated with this technique in terms of continuing leak or an increased incidence of related intraabdominal abscess.

In the postcholecystectomy circumstance, the hazard of bile leak is reduced because the gallbladder is not present to be lacerated. Major leaks occur when that organ is punctured. The needle, which is in the bile duct, is an effective decompressing tube en route to the operating room. However, bile peritonitis may ensue even when the exploring catheter is left *in situ*. Therefore, operation should be scheduled soon after the transhepatic study if an obstructing lesion has been verified or if the diagnosis is still obscure (133). Lindenauer and Lattenschlager's concept of laparoscopic transhepatic cholangiography with electrocoagulation (364) goes far toward avoiding the leak factor, which is the only major complication of this percutaneous procedure.

Endoscopic retrograde pancreatic cholangiography is done via the oral route and is the preferred initial diagnostic procedure in the jaundiced patient who may not require surgery. These two procedures supplement one another (Table 4-1). The endoscopic method is more difficult to learn and the equipment more expensive, but the rewards are so great in terms of the information gained that it is now impossible to do biliary surgery without this adjunct. In all secondary biliary opera-

TABLE 4-1. COMPARISON OF METHODS FOR EVALUATING THE BILE DUCT

ERCP*	PTC†
Equipment more expensive	Routinely available
Training more specialized	Good mapping of proximal ducts
Not indicated if hepatitis is a consideration	Bile leak risk
Common duct cannot always be entered	Bile culture is possible
Inspection of ampulla possible	Temporary decompression possible
Complications uncommon	

* ERCP, endoscopic retrograde cholangiopancreatography
† Percutaneous transhepatic cholangiography

tions the surgeon does best to know the etiology and anatomy of the problem before he goes in.

An alternate diagnostic approach has been to puncture the liver for the cholangiogram as soon as the abdomen is opened. One then proceeds with the information that this provides. The case for intraoperative puncture is valid provided that the filming in the operating room can be of good quality. I have been satisfied with both techniques.

CHOLEDOCHOGRAPHY

Direct common duct puncture cholangiography can be facilitated by the use of the sleeved needle designed by Fourres. However, a leak about the puncture site will occur unless a purse-string suture is employed. This technique has proved to be the least useful approach to cholangiography preceding operative exploration of the common duct.

The T tube inserted after common bile duct exploration has been the most frequently used portal for studies undertaken to evaluate the effectiveness of the choledochal toilet or the decompression of an obstructed segment. Every explored common duct in the MHMC series has been evaluated by postmanipulative, intraoperative T-tube cholangiography. The only exceptions are in patients treated by a biliary enteric anastomosis.

Open transduodenal ampullary cannulation can be a portal for contrast introduction. However, the other methods are so much easier, this approach has not been employed in this series.

PERITONEOSCOPIC APPROACHES

Diagnostic studies can reach an impasse in which it is virtually impossible to differentiate between intra- and extrahepatic disease. Blind biopsy of the liver sometimes fails to solve the problem because one cannot be certain that a representative diseased area has been submitted for examination. It is in this limited sphere that peritoneoscopy has a role. The procedure may be used alone, in conjunction with liver biopsy, and/or in association with precise puncture of the viscus for the delivery of contrast material (420).

Our experience with the Hopkins lens system peritoneoscope has proved satisfactory in those instances in which it was employed. The Witmoser needle allows for the safe induction of pneumoperitoneum because the spring guards against entry into the bowel. The cautery allows for coagulation of the puncture site (487). In PCS the main indication for this approach has been in the differential diagnosis of liver disease.

Laparotomy is sometimes unnecessary. One patient was seen to have congenital cystic disease of the liver; another, metastatic carcinoma; and the third, hepatitis in association with common duct stones where the symptoms were due to the former (211).

The great advantage is in the facility for getting a guided liver biopsy when a prior biopsy has not validated what seemed a reasonable clinical diagnosis (Fig. 4-2). This procedure has the advantage of permitting simultaneous liver biopsy, observation of the liver, and transhepatic injection of contrast to visualize the entire biliary system. It is particularly impressive in revealing intrinsic liver disease in association with biliary lithiasis when both are present, but symptoms are related to the one, as Berci (49) and others (115, 515) have reported. An additional advantage over blind puncture is that any bleeding or bile leak is fulgurated under direct vision.

The excellent color photographs as arranged by Schaeffer in the text by Beck *et al.* (43) indicates the diagnostic potential of this modality. The liver is the easiest abdominal viscus to examine and to biopsy by this method.

MINI-LAPAROTOMY

Mini-laparotomy is performed in the x-ray department via an upper abdominal midline incision. Under local anesthesia one can cannulate the umbilical vein, as the route for a portal venogram, and perform direct biopsy of the exposed liver and direct puncture cholangiography (577). It is a rapid open diagnostic approach to the jaundiced patient. From a practical point of view it eliminates the delay of waiting for test results on the fecal urobilinogen, the occasional hazard of transfermoral arteriography, and the problems associated with the interpretation of frequent blood studies. Large satisfactory experience with this technique has been described by Del Guercio (166). It requires either an operating room in the department of radiology or a sophisticated radiographic unit with image intensifiers that provide for rapid film sequence in the operating room.

TECHNICAL CONSIDERATIONS

With a large gallbladder remnant, cannulation is best accomplished with a winged mushroom catheter inserted through the center of a double purse-string suture. If the organ is not to be removed, that catheter is left in place as a cholecystostomy tube.

There is a large variety of special cannulas designed for intubation of the cystic duct. It

FIG. 4-2. Guided liver biopsy. The peritoneoscopic technique for laparoscopic examination of the liver and gallbladder area and for guided liver biopsy is carried out under local anesthesia and mild sedation.

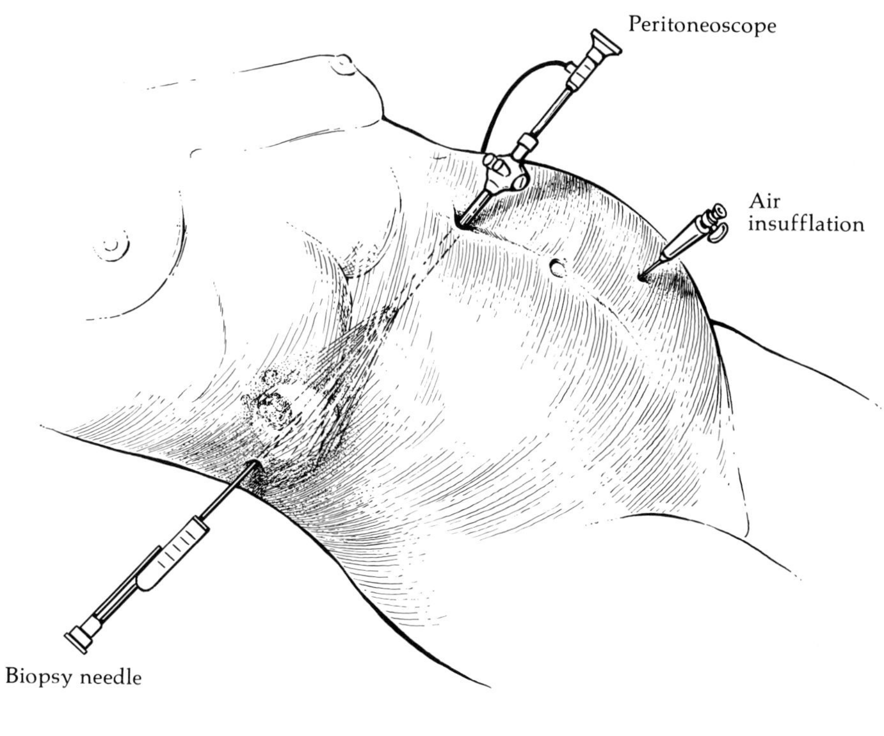

is often possible to achieve the same purpose with polyethylene tubing, a ureteral catheter, or a blunt needle. A stenotic cystic duct can often be sufficiently dilated with a probe to permit insertion of the cannula. It is important that the cannula be tautly secured to prevent leaks, that it not be advanced into the duodenum, that it not perforate the duct posteriorly, and that it be completely removed at the conclusion of the procedure. A long segment of cystic duct should be suitably dissected out to within 0.5 cm of the common bile duct. It is important that a small stone present in the cystic duct not be pushed into the common duct or retained in the stump.

For T-tube cholangiography the choledochostomy site should be tested to be certain that there are no leaks. The test is done with saline. The T-tube is always left in after the contrast examination. We do not recommend primary choledochal suture after formal common duct exploration and T-tube cholangiography even when the duct is radiographically normal.

In the section on pancreatic duct considerations in Chapter 2, it has been shown that the perfusion pressure and volume of the contrast medium influence the capability for visualizing the pancreatic duct. When this delivery is under manometric control, it is possible to calibrate these factors. If hand delivery is employed, one takes the precaution of avoiding bubbles and raises the loaded syringe until the barrel falls by gravity alone. Ordinarily the medium passes into the duct at less than 15–20 cm of saline above the level of the common duct. The contrast material should not be cold, excessively concentrated, too viscous, or delivered too rapidly.

Excessively forceful delivery of the saline perfusate or of the contrast material carries the risk of introducing bacteria from the duct into the vascular system, causing a syndrome characterized by chills and fever that is called the "cholangiographic reaction." This correlation of cause and effect is assumed because bacteria can be cultured from the bile in about 90% of individuals with choledocholithiasis or common duct obstruction. About 30% of patients with an unobstructed common duct have bacteria in the bile in association with choledocholithiasis. For clinical consideration, these occasional reactions are a transient phenomenon without sequelae, in our experience, if the T-tube drainage is maintained for 12–24 hours after the examination.

It is wise to preflush the ducts with saline. The volume of contrast to be instilled is determined by the estimated capacity of the ductal system: A 1-cm duct requires 6–8 ml; a 1.4-cm duct requires 10–15 ml; and a 2-cm duct, 20–35 ml of contrast. The rubber tube is clamped while the films are being exposed. Immediately thereafter the bile-stained contrast material is allowed to drain out of the cannula to minimize the volume of this hygroscopic contrast material that will get into the small bowel.

In the very early years the contrast material for the opacification of the biliary tract was compounded of bismuth and barium pastes. These materials were very poorly tolerated and frequently induced fever and cholangitis. They were especially hazardous because they were not sterile. If peritoneal spillage occurred, infection often resulted. With the development of the iodinated compounds, iodized oil (Lipiodal) came into use. This had the disadvantage of being exceptionally radiopaque and of being very slowly absorbed if the ductal system was obstructed or contrast entered the free peritoneal cavity. The density of this oily contrast material was so great that it frequently obscured small calculi.

With the introduction of such water-soluble contrast materials as sodium diatrizoate and methylglucamine diatrizoate, these problems were virtually eliminated. These agents may be used during operations employing sterile techniques. When spillage does occur, the material is rapidly absorbed from the peritoneal cavity and is excreted in the urine. The concentration of this water-soluble opaque material can be altered to suit the habitus of the patient. At MHMC a 1:1 saline dilution of commercially available 50% sodium diatrizoate is used. This 25% concentration provides an optimal density for the visualization of small calculi. Because the opaque material is hygroscopic, its dilution also lessens bowel distention secondary to osmotic fluid passage into the lumen of the small intestine.

As with other iodinated compounds, sensitivity reactions may occur. However, during operative cholangiography the severe sensitivity or allergic reaction is rarely encountered. Unless the patient is known to be hypersensitive to iodine compounds, we have not restored to routine preoperative intravenous, conjunctival, or skin testing. In patients who are known to have iodine allergies manifested by urticaria or bronchospasm, premedication with antihistamines can successfully suppress and control such allergic response. Atropine and steroids may be necessary in the premedication of some known hypersensitive patients. When there is renal damage or a previous history of anaphylactic reaction, cholangiography with iodinated compounds is not employed. In the MHMC experience no anaphylactic or allergic reaction has been recognized during operative cholangiography (554, 639).

It is quite correct to believe there is no relation between the allergies to seafood, eggs, and strawberries in relation to these iodine compounds. The vast majority of patients with such allergies would not react adversely to the contrast medium any more often than others without such allergies. The knowledge that is obtained by such an examination is important, and there should be little hesitation, with safeguards, to do this examination in the patient whose only allergy is to food. However, it is in this group that one may consider doing the sensitivity test. The hesitancy about performing such an examination is more often based on its medicolegal implications than on the published experiences.

If a real allergic background is present, it is best completely to avoid the use of iodinated compounds. Air, diluted barium, or tantulum have been used as the contrast material. In cases of serious allergy, intraoperative biliary endoscopy can be of special value as a complete substitute for opacification studies.

A 200-mamp portable x-ray unit with a manipulatable head is positioned over the protected sterile field. Beam columnation at the x-ray tube is used to reduce scattered radiation to the operating room personnel. A grid cassette is initially placed beneath the patient and positioned so that the entire right upper quadrant and abdominal area of interest will be projected upon the 14- × 17-in. film The patient is rotated 15 in. to the right during the filming, to rotate the spine away from the area being opacified. A flat film of the abdomen can be taken while the patient is being prepared, to be certain of proper positioning and to document artifacts. A technically adequate setup can facilitate the changing of cassettes without compromise of time or sterility.

The contrast material is either hand-delivered from a 50-ml syringe or from the reservoir of a manometer. The anesthesiologist must remain with the patient to monitor vital functions during the induced apneic phase of the radiographic exposure. He wears a lead apron. The remaining surgical personnel either leave the room or stand behind the portable lead screens away from the area of exposure. The radiation received by the anesthesiologist varies between 5 and 50 mr per examination. This exposure is principally to the face, hands, and head.

The first radiographic exposure is made just after the contrast material has been delivered. A second exposure is obtained with the patient in a 10° Trendelenburg position, and the third exposure is obtained in a 20° reverse Trendelenburg position. The time interval between films is about 2–3 min. The films are best developed in a rapid automatic processor so that they come out dry. The interpretation of wet films can be difficult because of the drip, inadequate fixation, and surface artifacts. On the other hand, a film that is completely adequate for immediate interpretation may not be suitable for a permanent record or for reproduction.

The most accurate, facile, and complete procedure entails the use of image intensification in the operating room, especially as it is used in relation to the operating table. The Kiefer table has the advantage of conveniently being able to move the patient up and down and to the right or left. There is an overhead x-ray tube that slides on a track. Here one can directly observe the course of the contrast material in the duct with true selective details and monitor the procedure as it is being done. The filming can be permanently recorded on 70-mm film strip. This is the most complete roentgen setup for intraoperative cholangiography (51, 235).

The close cooperation of the radiologist and surgeon contributes to the accurate interpretation of the film. Nothing is more disappointing than the missed lesion or calculus. Still more disconcerting is the negative exploration for a presumed calculus or tumor. The unnecessary prolongation of the procedure, the extension of the operation by unrewarding duodenostomy, common bile duct exploration, or the necessity for a second laparotomy to correct a finding missed during the first procedure tend to increase morbidity. A proper interpretation can be based only upon technically satisfactory film.

Royal Free Hospital's 1969 review of bile duct cancer indicates that 18 of 23 patients had had a prior laparotomy that missed the lesion (627). This is unfortunate, for it is a diagnosis that is accurately made on the cholangiogram. Longmire's monograph (368) further emphasizes the value of cholangiography in defining a lesion that is otherwise elusive.

5 Criteria for Operative Cholangiographic Interpretation

The 20-year experience at MHMC with intraoperative cholangiography supports the attitude that this diagnostic adjunct should be part of virtually every biliary operation (260, 522). There has been no unfavorable immediate or late complication observed in this study. No surgical finesse can equal the capacity of the radiographic examination to evaluate the intraduodenal and proximal hepatic ducts. The basic procedure is neither difficult nor expensive and requires no unusual equipment. Since all who insert a T tube obtain a cholangiogram after an operation, why not have it immediately available at a time when a missed stone or tumor may be demonstrated during the initial operation, which is the optimum time for its management?

The value of the intraoperative cholangiogram lies in reducing the problem of residual stones, in revealing anomalies at the choledochoduodenal junction, and in checking the adequacy of the biliary toilet. I have seen residual problems in patients in whom this objective adjunctive procedure has not been employed, but have never encountered a complication from its proper use.

Alternate viewpoints, insofar as these can be clearly elicited, feebly harp on an incidence of false positive and false negative interpretations, the delay and the difficulty in obtaining technically adequate films, the possibility of contamination of the operative field, and the hazards of repeated radiation exposure. All these problems are easily overcome with experience and trained personnel. None of these objections comfort the individual patient who, without this aid, is left with an incomplete operation.

ARTIFACTS

Errors in interpretation may be related to artifacts induced at the time of the study or to the misunderstanding of the normal function and pathophysiology of the extrahepatic conduit. Schulenberg (M-43) reported false negatives in 4.2% of 1000 cases. The MHMC experience is less than half of this, in the range of 1–1.5%. The film itself is never wrong; only the interpretation can be in error, except when the film is so poor technically that no accurate interpretation is possible (Fig. 5-1).

With good techniques, false positives most often involved an air bubble, blood clot, the fenestrated end of the T tube, barium flecks, the transverse process of the second lumbar vertebra, or calcified costal cartilages. An artifact simulating stone can be produced by the right hepatic artery's crossing the common hepatic duct just distal to the trifurcation (378).

The most common artifact is the air bubble, mimicking a stone. This can be avoided by allowing bile to flow out of the cannula's connecting tubes before attaching the tube that is already filled with contrast material. When the transfer is made from the saline flush to the contrast cholangiogram, the tubing should be clamped while full, and then the empty segment should be filled with contrast before the reservoir tubing is reattached.

Air bubbles are usually multiple and spherical, and they assume varying positions in the ductal system. They are not faceted. Changing the position of the patient dislocates the bubble. One may also discern an air column in the segment of the connecting

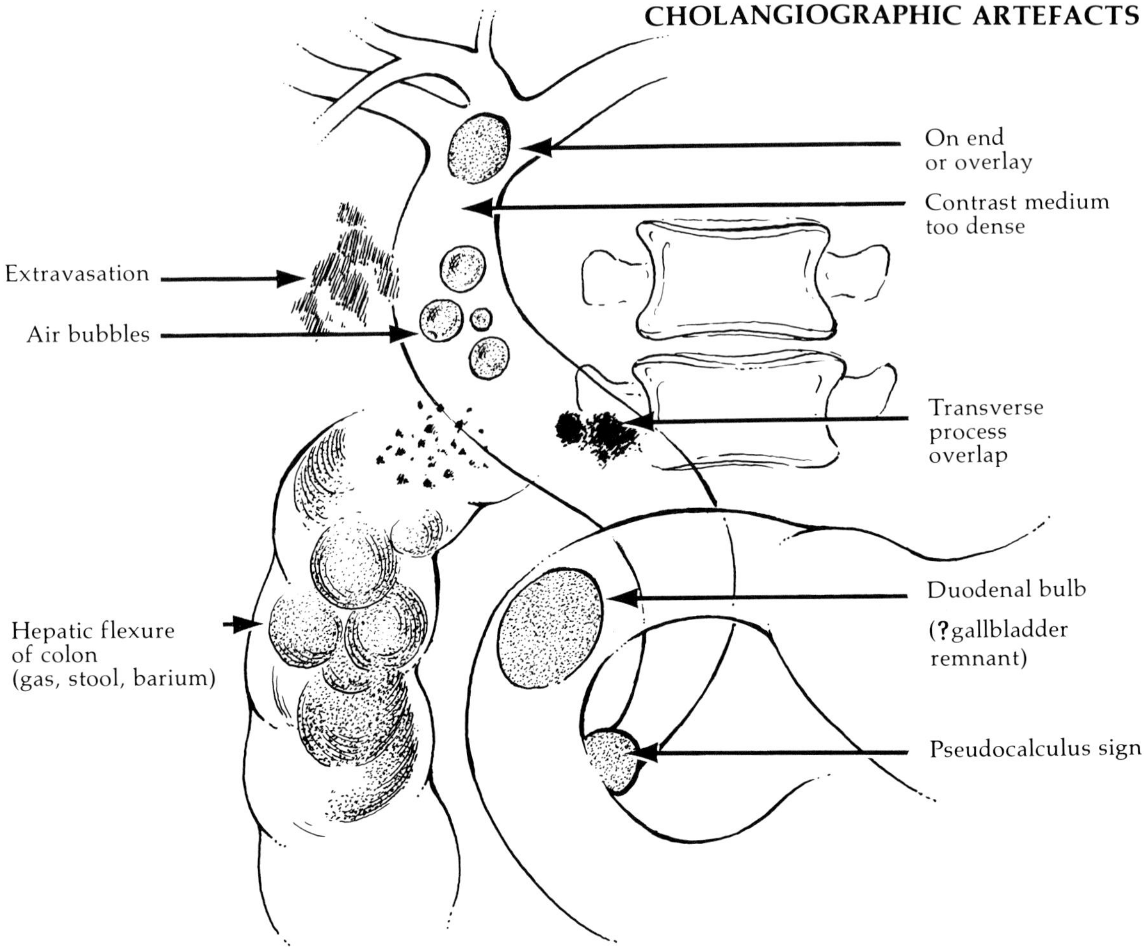

FIG. 5-1. Artifacts that may lead to improper cholangiographic interpretation. Such artifacts as those illustrated can be minimized by proper positioning of the patient, careful instillation of the contrast material, and sequential films.

tubing. When an air bubble is suspected, the ducts should be carefully flushed with saline and a more cautiously performed cholangiogram repeated with the patient positioned somewhat differently. It is not advisable to attempt to aspirate the bubble, as this only introduces air from the duodenum into the biliary tract (88). It also produces a foaming action of the bile that further obfuscates the study (Fig. 5-2).

Air is normally present in the hepatic flexure of the colon, and the common duct is opacified in its silhouette. Focal air sacculations in the colon can mimic calculi. A specific problem may be presented by a fortuitous fleck of barium retained from a gastrointestinal series or barium enema. The tip of the transverse process can project into the contrast-filled column of the obliquely positioned patient. Two or three sequential films in oblique, and slightly altered head-down and head-up positions will allow a differential diagnosis of stone from air bubble, gas in the colon, barium fleck, normal skeleton, and the pseudocalculus phenomenon.

CALCULI

Stones are either visualized as defects in the contrast-filled column or identified inferentially by the failure of a segment of the conduit to opacify. In either situation it is assumed that the column is obstructed by the stone and the edema caused by the associated mucosal reaction. The diagnostic radiographic criteria require the demonstration of a lucent defect surrounded by contrast material on all sides. If the defect is faceted or rimmed with calcium, the diagnosis is easier (360, 365).

Special precautions have been learned from a review of the experience with retained calculi when the diagnosis was missed on the previous cholangiogram (Fig. 5-3). Errors were usually due to a failure to appreciate that a stone may be obscured by the increased density of the normal overlap at the hepatic confluence, or that the stone can overlay a vertebra or transverse process, or that a gas-filled colon places the stone in a penumbra. A stone in the left hepatic duct may escape attention because there are so many other calculi in the choledochus. A lesion may be missed if one does not systematically examine the right hepatic duct and its two major divisions, the left hepatic duct to its bifurcation, and the entire choledochus (free of overlying densities) to and including the demonstration of contrast in the duodenum (153, 176).

A solitary faceted stone is less common than two or more stones. Nonfaceted primary choledochal stones are associated with intra-choledochal stasis that usually has its obstructive focus in the Vaterian segment. Stones are relatively uncommon in ducts of normal size.

DIFFERENTIAL DIAGNOSIS

Failure to appreciate the roentgen aspects of normal choledochal sphincter function have resulted in futile exploration of the common duct, frustrating duodenostomies, and unnecessary plastic surgical procedures on the Vaterian segment. Certain cholangiographic configurations can be misinterpreted as a stone, stricture, or tumor, depending upon which phase of the cycle is demonstrated. Misinterpretation of the pseudocalculus phenomenon, which is due to the normal contraction of the sphincter of Oddi, can be avoided. In contrast to the stone defect, this functionally determined configuration occurs only at the distal end of the duct, and contrast material does not surround all sides of that radiographic phenomenon. A crescentic semilunar defect at the distal end of the duct should alert one to the possibility of this alternative diagnosis.

Sequential films obtained during the diastolic phase of choledochal sphincter function will demonstrate the alternate phase with normal open walls and flow of contrast into the duodenum. Sequential views will indicate that a presumed defect is a physiologic variant. Defects proximal to the sphincteric zone cannot be produced by this physiologic phenomenon. This will avoid futile surgical manipulations whose sole indication is this roentgen configuration (45, 223) (Fig. 5-4).

It is possible to recognize differential patterns that are caused by specific etiologic factors. Thus, if the duct is uniformly dilated, the cause is either a calculus that had once obstructed the outlet or an obstruction in the Vaterian segment, *i.e.*, stone, tumor, or ampullary stenosis. A long uniform tubular stricture that may occur in the infraduodenal section of the common bile duct is due to pancreatitis (Fig. 5-5). This diagnosis is further supported if the duct is also angulated. Stenosis in the supraduodenal (gastrohepatic) segment with an irregular tapering in the previously unoperated patient is due to tumor.

The differential diagnosis of the cause of a localized area of stenosis must always be made in relation to the history. If this is a second biliary operation in a patient with symptoms of cholangitis or jaundice, primary consideration must be given to the possibility of an iatrogenic stricture (610). In a previously unoperated biliary tract, the differential diagnosis is between carcinoma of the bile ducts and inflammatory cholangitis or sclerosing cholangitis. The latter is such a rare entity that in the MHMC experience with more than 6000 biliary tract operations no primary case has been recognized. Those encountered were associated with ulcerative colitis. The difficulty is epitomized in the patient whose roentgenograms are shown in Figure 5-6. The roentgen criteria for carcinoma of the bile duct at the junction of the intra- and extrahepatic segments were definite (329, 485, 627). The patient's cancer was nonresectable because of direct wide extension into the liver parenchyma. A positive biopsy was not obtained even though tissue was taken from the involved area. The patient lived 4.5 years after intubation across the stricture. His longevity was a challenge to the roentgen criteria, and during his lifetime it was suggested that the condition could be

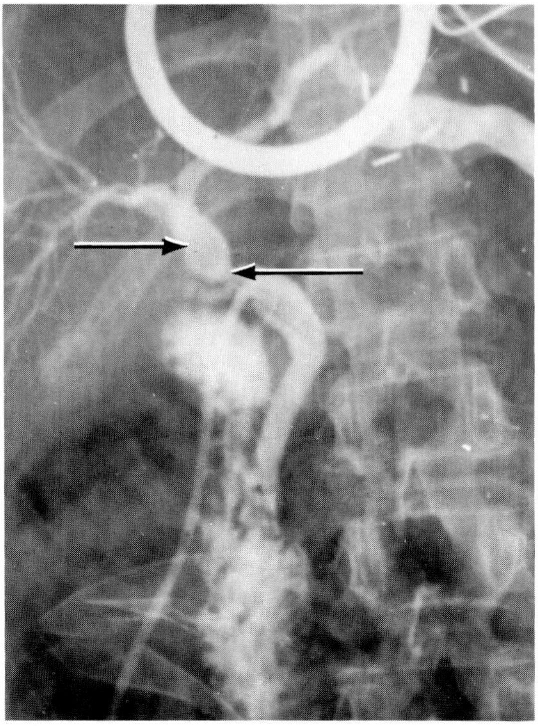

FIG. 5-2. Misinterpreted cholangiogram. A female patient was to have a secondary biliary tract operation on the basis of the interpretation of this film. The presumed stricture **(right arrow)** is an artifact due to the crossing of an aberrant hepatic artery. The presumed stone **(left arrow)** is an air bubble. Note that there are other air bubbles in both limbs of the T tube.

FIG. 5-3. Technically poor cholangiographic study. **A.** This intraoperative cholangiogram was interpreted as normal. Although the film is of poor quality, the bile duct is not significantly dilated, and the contrast material is seen to enter the third portion of the duodenum. Even on this film **(arrow)** it is apparent that there is some abnormality at the distal end of the duct, which was interpreted as duodenal mucosal change. **B.** A subsequent T-tube cholangiogram demonstrates several stones retained in the ampulla **(arrow)** with surrounding area of edema of the duodenal wall. The proximal pancreatic duct is minimally dilated. The contrast material readily passes into the duodenum. Note that the common bile duct loses its normal curvilinear contour when the ampulla is in the third portion of the duodenum.

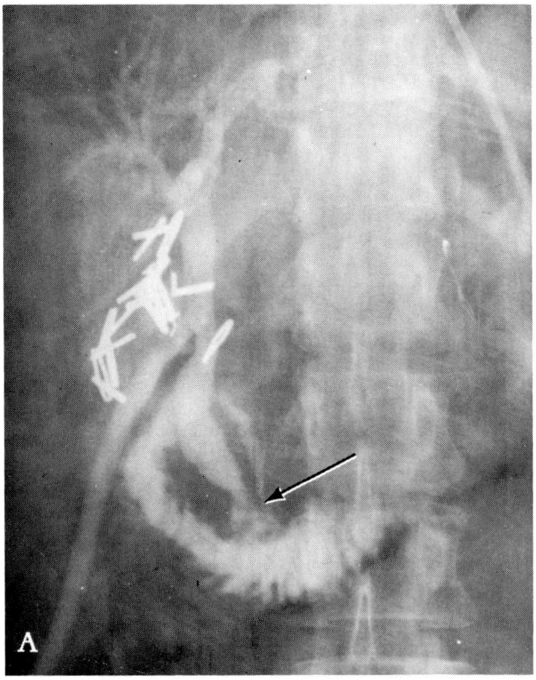

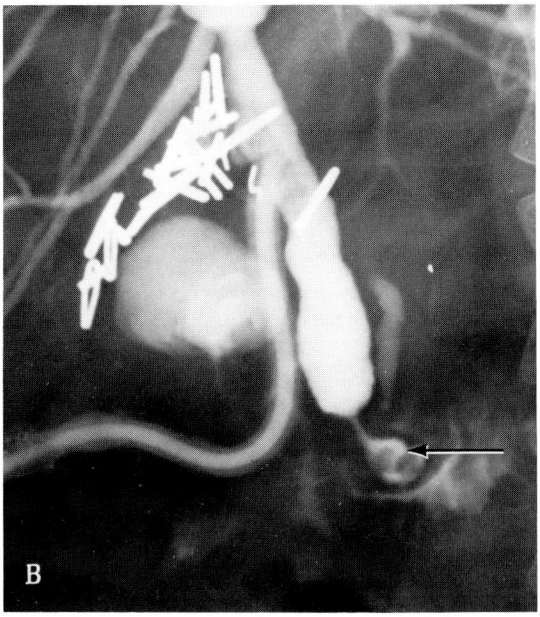

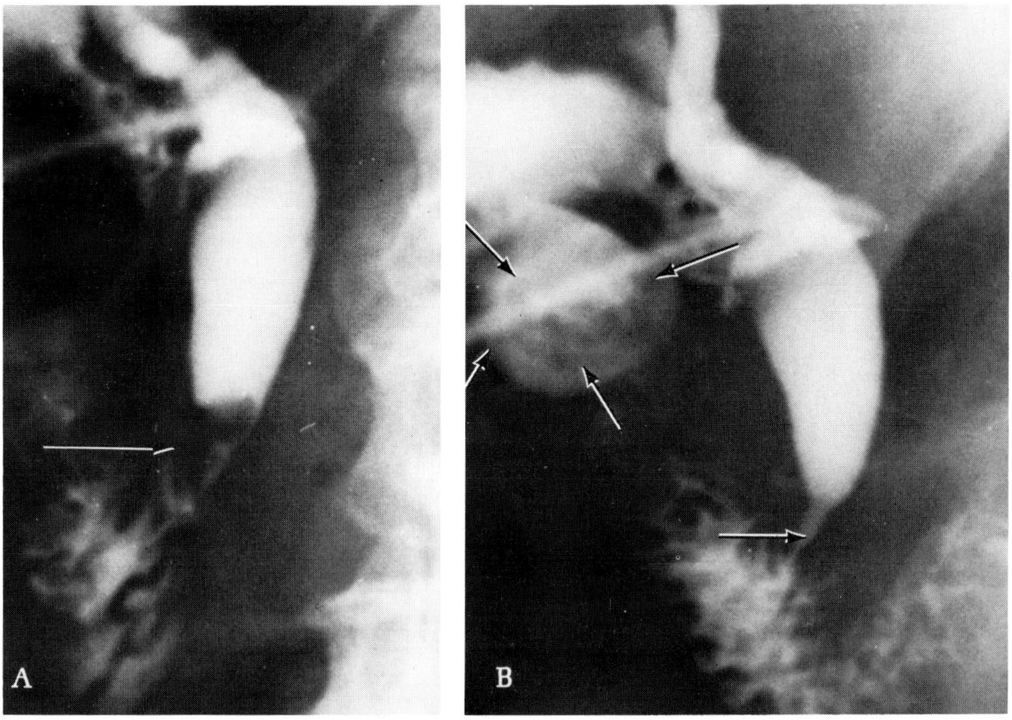

FIG. 5-4. Pseudocalculus phenomenon. **A.** The defect at the distal end of the T-tube cholangiogram suggests the presence of a stone **(arrow).** Note, however, that a complete circumferential outline is not present, a finding suggesting a functional change. **B.** In this film, taken a few seconds later, there is no stone. This is the resolution of the systolic phase (Fig. 5-4A) of choledochal sphincter function **(bottom arrow).** The failure to have sequential films available presents an erroneous indication for common duct exploration. The air- and contrast-filled duodenal bulb **(arrows, upper left)** can be misinterpreted as a calculus gallbladder remnant.

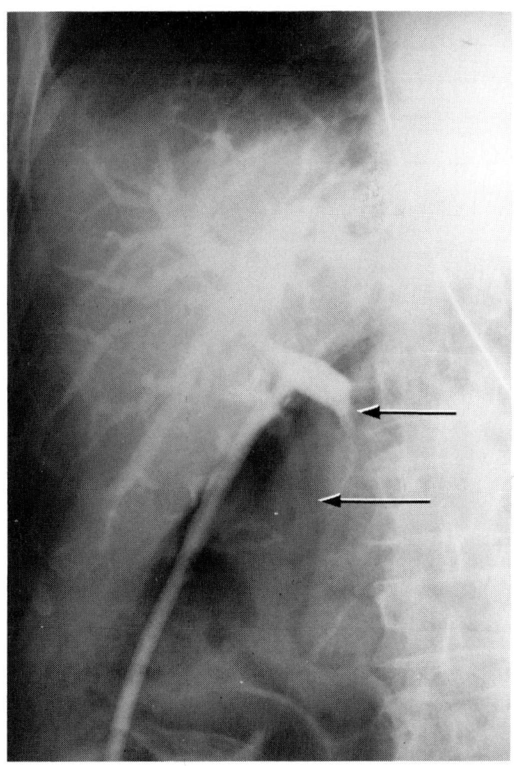

FIG. 5-5. Innocent tubular stenosis. A cystic duct cholangiogram obtained at the time of cholecystectomy, reveals tubular stenosis of the entire transpancreatic portion of the common bile duct without dilation of the choledochus and intrahepatic radicles **(arrows).** The decision not to explore the common duct was reinforced by determining that the passage pressure and the residual pressure in the common bile duct were completely normal. This patient has remained asymptomatic for 8 years.

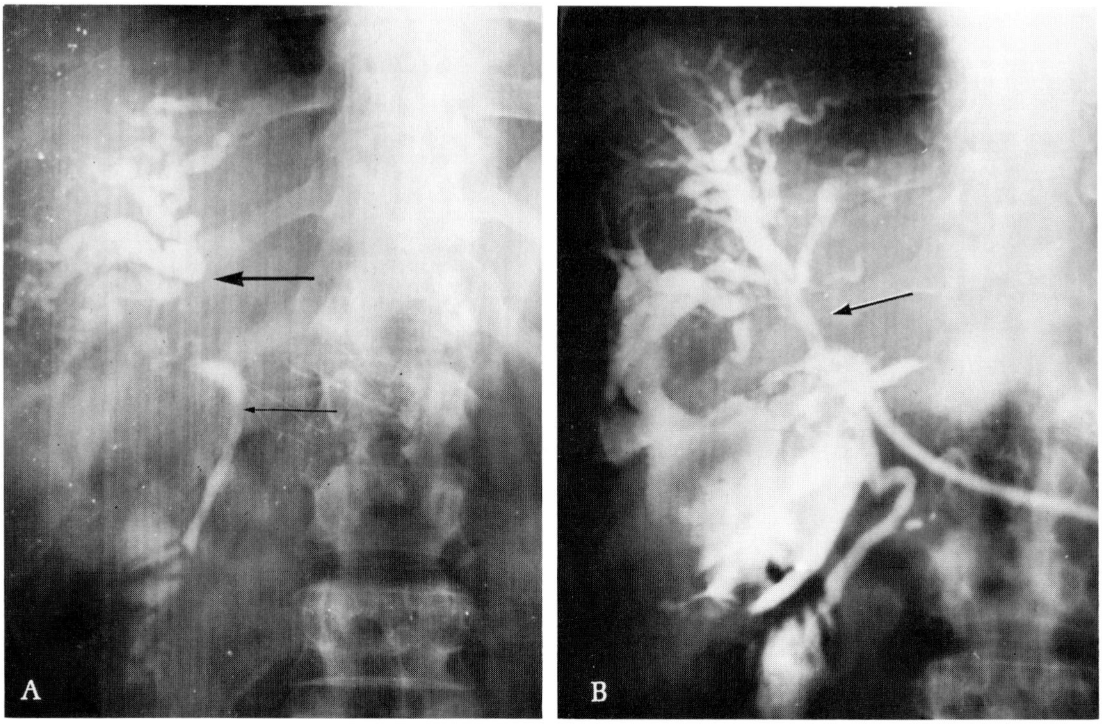

FIG. 5-6. Carinal obstruction. **A.** A transhepatic cholangiogram of a jaundiced patient shows an obstruction at the hepatic duct carina **(large arrow)** with a nipple deformity. The distal common bile duct is normal **(small arrow).** These cholangiographic findings are specific for bile duct cancer and no biopsy is necessary. **B.** A postoperative film reveals the rubber tube **(arrow)** with which the tumor has been cored to relieve the patient's jaundice. This particular tumor was both intra- and extrahepatic. Because the patient died 4½ years after intubation, the diagnosis was challenged. Autopsy demonstrated carcinoma of the hepatic duct. The cholangiographic findings are specific.

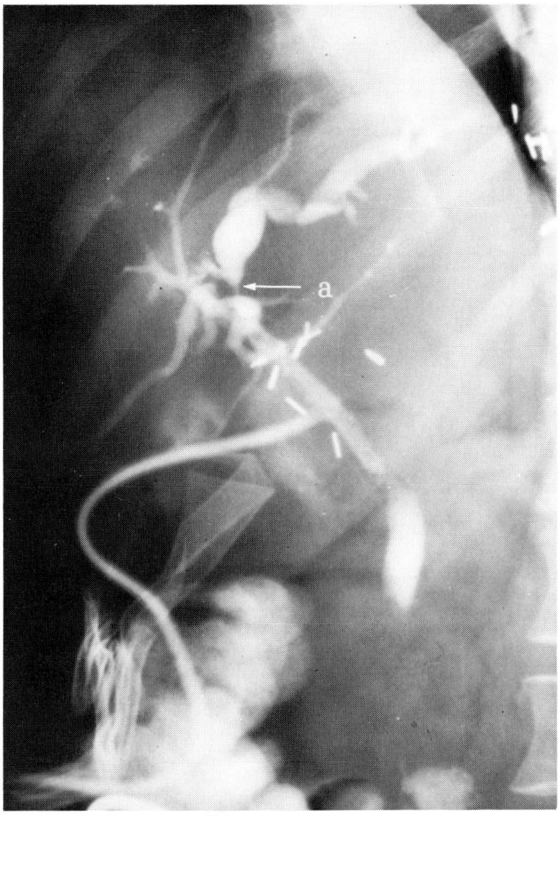

FIG. 5-7. Cholangiogram with calcified gallbladder. This patient had had a cholecystectomy for a porcelainized gallbladder. The T-tube cholangiogram shows a stricture of the left hepatic duct **(a)** with proximal dilatation in that segment **(arrow).** This finding is characteristic of bile duct cancer.

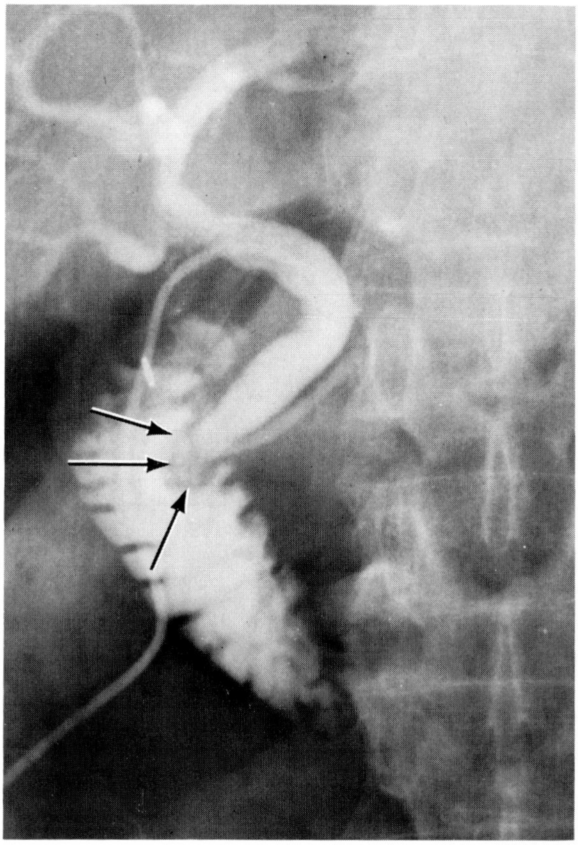

FIG. 5-8. Ampullary reaction ("papillitis"). Cholangiogram after completion of choledocholithotomy shows a crescentic defect **(arrows)** on the medial border of the descending duodenum. The defect is an edematous ampullary reaction. It is also referred to as Odditis or papillitis. This roentgen sign is not specific for biliary pancreatic disease and may also be seen in association with duodenal ulcer.

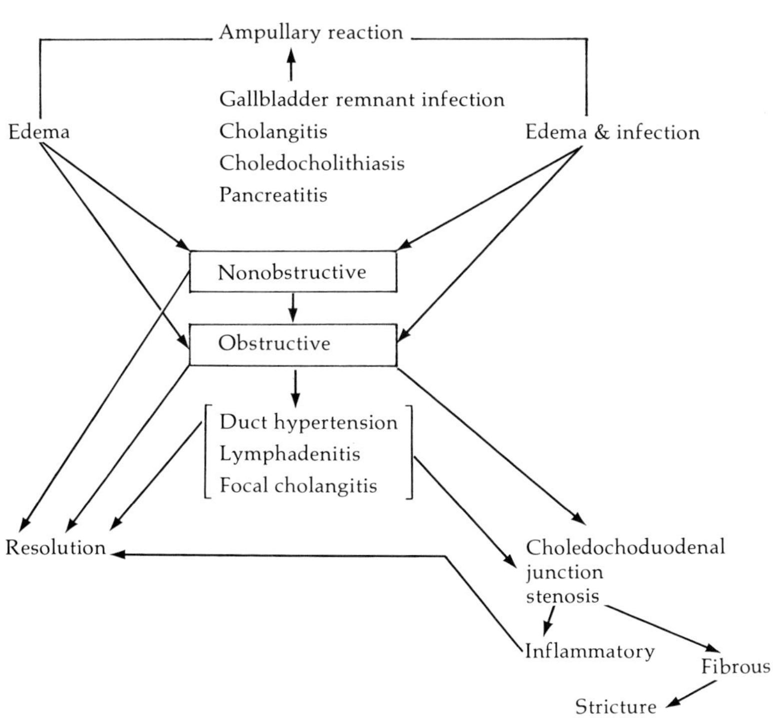

FIG. 5-9. Schematic indication of causes and subsequent effect of stone-linked ampullary reaction.

sclerosing cholangitis. The postmortem examination revealed a sclerosing adenocarcinoma of the bile ducts.

A short segment stricture with distal collapse and proximal dilatation, especially when there are no calculi, can be interpreted as cancer, and the surgical management may be undertaken on the basis of the cholangiographic pattern without a biopsy (Fig. 5-7). Cholangiography by the dual puncture technique serves to demonstrate details regarding the length of stricture and its relation to the hilum. The difficulty in obtaining a positive biopsy in this problem is related to the fact that most of these tumors do not present as an intraluminal polypoid mass that allows for intraductal biopsy with a laryngeal forceps (473). Quite the contrary; most cancers of the hepatic ducts have a dominant subepithelial scirrhus component. The palpatory finding of a localized sclerosed area in conjunction with the type of cholangiogram shown in Figure 5-6 is characteristic. Presumed idiopathic sclerosing cholangitis has proved in most instances to be a sclerosing duct cancer (13, 251, 256, 609).

There are certain commonly encountered cholangiographic patterns that have been correlated with a specific etiology:

1. The contrast material fails to enter the duodenum on sequential films, but no stone is visualized. The uncertainty here relates to the possibility of not recognizing an impacted stone. An ampullary sign in association with acute cholecystitis or cholangitis is evidence of a distal edematous reaction (Fig. 5-8). If the catheter probe or saline irrigant negotiates the choledochoduodenal junction, then it is usually correct to assume that the obstruction is not fixed.

The failure of contrast medium to enter the duodenum should not be the sole indication for duodenostomy. On the other hand, a nipple-contoured defect or irregular narrowing with rat-tailing will suggest the diagnosis of a tumor of the ampulla or distal common duct.

The absolute differential diagnosis between papillary edema, small incarcerated stone, ampullary stenosis, or tumor in this area can be made only by integration of the clinical data, physical findings, and at least two sequential intraoperative cholangiograms (Fig. 5-9). Papillary edema produces a smooth

FIG. 5-10. Cancer of the pancreas. **A.** A 53-year-old female patient presented with jaundice but was otherwise asymptomatic. She had undergone a cholecystectomy and choledocholithotomy 6 years earlier. This transhepatic cholangiogram performed the day after a barium enema (a bad sequence) shows a markedly dilated duct. There are no calculi. The end tapers to a nipple-like configuration **(arrow)** that is characteristic of carcinoma. **B.** The venous phase of the superior mesenteric arteriogram shows impingement on one division of the middle colic vein **(arrow).** This suggests extracapsular extension of the pancreatic cancer. These were the findings at operation.

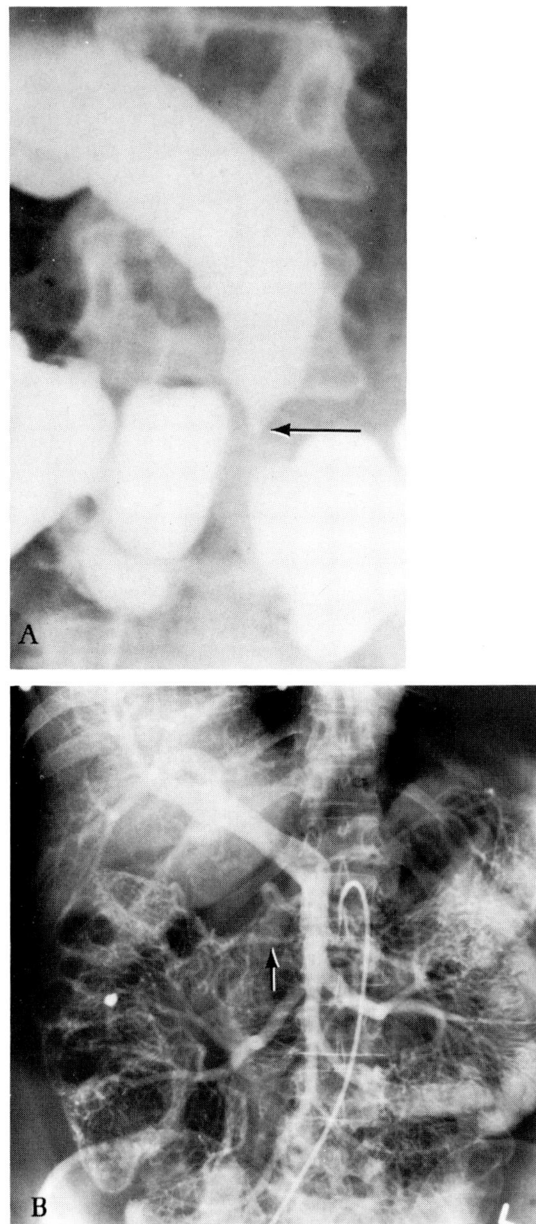

semicircular defect. A stone can almost always be visualized if the contrast material is not too dense. In ampullary stenosis there is never a complete block; some contrast enters the duodenum. Tumors of the ampulla, distal bile duct, or pancreatic head produce a consistent, obstructive, irregular defect (272).

2. One of the major hepatic ducts fails to visualize. This is a significant finding in operative cholangiography, in contrast to intravenous cholangiography. In the latter the anteriorly situated left hepatic duct may not visualize because the study is ordinarily performed in the supine or right anterior oblique position. In the operating room, however, this finding indicates a lesion. The duct proximally should be radiologically defined by direct transhepatic puncture. With this approach, both sides of the defect can be defined and a stone or tumor stricture identified.

3. The length of the opacified pancreatic duct is of no clinical significance. In the experience of MHMC, pancreatic duct pathology, aside from ectasia, has never been demonstrated by this route. Cholangiography is no substitute for the preoperative direct ERCP.

4. A segmental stricture is identified, but repeated biopsies fail to offer a positive diagnosis. The cholangiographic criteria for the diagnosis of bile duct cancer are specific (233). One can confidently choose a surgical procedure on the basis of the roentgen pattern alone (Fig. 5-10).

5. There is diffuse ductal ectasia and contrast material enters the duodenum, but there are no calculi. In the past it was sufficient to accept the explanation that a stone had passed. If the duct is wider than 1.4 cm, a manometric evaluation will aid in screening out cases with choledochoduodenal junction stenosis. Choledochoscopy is mandatory to be certain that there is no tumor.

In rare instances a huge distortive dilation in association with anomalous proximal intrahepatic and extrahepatic ducts suggests the diagnosis of a choledochal cyst. This has been encountered in three secondary cases, in which previous unmonitored cholecystectomy had failed to define that choledochal anomaly.

6. A long segment of cystic duct is retained. This is often merely a radiologic demonstration of those cystic ducts that pass parallel to the choledochus or spiral about to its left side. Ten to fifteen percent of ducts have this configuration. If that segment is open (*i.e.*, drains freely) and contains no calculi, it is of no pathologic significance. The spiral variety of cystic duct may go completely unappreciated, even with meticulous dissection at the gallbladder hilus, unles the cystic duct is viewed in an oblique or lateral position.

7. The patient is jaundiced but the cholecystocholangiogram is normal. It is more reasonable to assume that the fault is in the liver—even though frozen-section biopsy does not always resolve the problem—than that one is dealing with localized pancreatitis, or a stone that has passed, or a very small tumor not discerned.

6 Biliary Manometry and Debimetry

The MHMC experience with the addition of biliary manometry and debimetry to operative cholangiography was initially obtained in laboratory evaluation of the dynamic aspects of the neurohumoral influences on the biliary sphincter in the dog (533). Subsequently, in the department of diagnostic radiology, it served as a convenient additional method for the study of human choledochal sphincter function and contributed to an understanding of its physiology and its surgical pertinent radiology. The method has also aided observations on the mechanism of pancreatic duct opacification, the common channel concept, the significance of duct size, and a mechanism of biliary pain (532). Certain facets of this technique, applied prophylactically, may help to avoid PCS.

The basic clinical techniques were initially utilized by Mallet-Guy (392, 393, 395) and Caroli (111) in France and were then early espoused by Hess (260, 262) in Switzerland and Brucke (95, 96) and Fritsch (206, 207) in Austria. These investigators regard the method as a valuable approach to the dynamic evaluation and differential diagnosis of disorders in the sphincter area and to the demonstration of nonobstructing stones in normal sized ducts.

Mattig (403) obtained data from 239 German clinics and found a varying spectrum of interest in intraoperative collaborative procedures. Of these, 21.5% used cholangiography and 4.5% used manometry routinely, whereas 25% never used cholangiography and 66.5% never used manometry. No wonder, then, that some institutions can provide a wide experience with retained stone disease.

There are significant differences in the evaluation of biliary pressures and the measurements more conventionally obtained in the vascular system and urinary tract (219). The biliary system is a low-pressure, low-flow conduit, in which no peristalsis occurs and a muscular component exists only at the lower end of the conduit. This distal sphincter is influenced by liver function, hepatic secretory pressure, changes in the gallbladder, pancreas, and duodenum, and by the vagus nerves, as well as by hormones elaborated in the upper small bowel. The biliary conduit is significantly vulnerable to all these extraductal influences and they affect the interpretation of the manometric data.

TECHNIQUE OF CHOLANGIOMANOMETRY

The patient is given no morphine or meperidine prior to or during the diagnostic procedure. Atropine in the usual doses has no effect on the sphincter mechanism and is used as needed. In rare instances, patients have inadvertently received 50 mg meperidine 60 min before the determination. There has been no apparent sphincter effect with that dosage after that time interval.

The MHMC experience has been derived from 160 examinations of the common bile duct in patients with biliary lithiasis. Patients with biliary tumors are not included. The portal for study and the technique for intubation is the same as that conventionally employed for cholangiography by the hand-injection or gravity-infusion methods. Previously a simple method was used—introducing a polyethylene tube into the common duct, via the cystic duct stump, and measuring the height of the bile in the column as an index of resting intracholedochal pressure.

Jacobson *et al.* (297, 298, 300) indicated that routine hand delivery cholangiography is attended by pressures of 80–90 cm H_2O. In the septic patient those pressures are enough to cause bacteremia and may be a factor in the genesis of the postcholangiographic chill.

The Caroli manometer was employed for these examinations (Fig. 6-1). This manometer is kept in a sterile pack in the operating room so that it can be readily attached to a portable table covered with a sterile sheet. The determinations of flow volume can also be made with a hand-held graduated syringe (630) (Fig. 6-2). It is simpler than a table manometer and is a routinely available piece of equipment.

Previous experience in the laboratory has

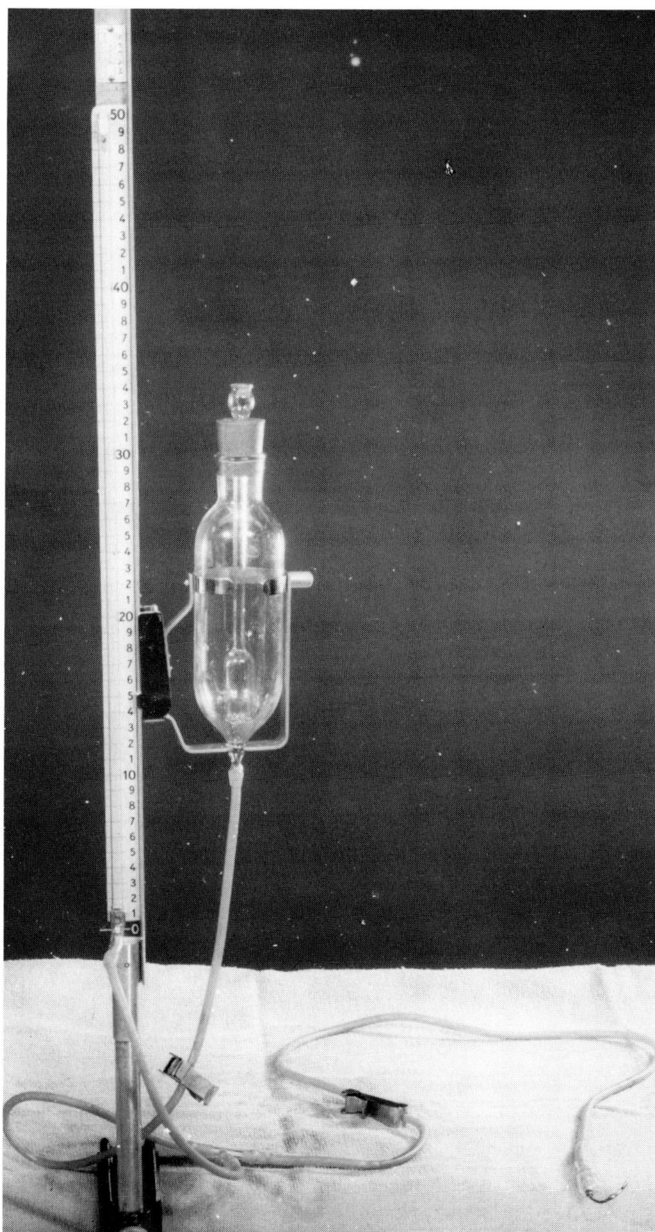

FIG. 6-1. Caroli's manometer: The sterile Caroli manometer is mounted to the edge of a portable table. The saline reservoir is adjusted on the vertically calibrated stand. This is a particularly useful device for determining the passage pressure and residual pressure in the common bile duct.

shown that the initial determinations using saline perfusion and manometric observation alone correlated closely with those obtained by perfusion with contrast material monitored by cinefluoroscopy. Therefore, the initial intraoperative determination is performed with saline, followed by the opacification cholangiogram. This sequence minimizes the possibility of a contrast-provoked sphincter reaction. The sequential use of biliary manometry and cholangiography has been called radiomanometry.

The zero of the manometer is adjusted at the level of the common duct in the midaxillary line and maintained constant for the entire examination. The reservoir, cannulas, and occluding clamps are all manipulated by the surgeon. The rubber tubing is of uniform size, and the male end of the manometer is attached to the duct cannula. The entire system is primed with saline and flushed through. The secure cystic duct cannula or T tube is attached to the manometer only after there is a free outflow of bile. The reservoir is started at the 5-cm mark, then the tubing is occluded at serial 2-cm increments until a rapid fall in the manometer tube indicates that the lowest level for passage pressure has been exceeded. The height at which the column stops is the residual pressure. The reservoir is then raised 1 cm at a time above the residual pressure level to define the passage pressure.

An overshoot approach is an alternate rapid and accurate way of making this determination. The reservoir is raised 5–8 cm above the first passage pressure level and then lowered at 1-cm intervals until the saline level no longer falls. Thus, the passage pressure is determined from alternate and opposing directions.

Brucke (96) designed a manometer (Fig. 6-3) that operates on a different principle: It is adjusted so that the common bile duct is perfused, through the cystic duct, at a constant pressure of 30 cm H_2O. An individually calibrated stopcock lumen is adjusted to maintain flow at that pressure. From the stopcock gauge reading, an accompanying chart permits extrapolation of both the flow rate per minute through the choledochoduodenal junction and the size of the ampulla. Brucke's (95) studies give the normal papilla a caliber of 0.5–1.5 mm, with normal flow rates of 13–60 ml/min.

The cholangiographic component of cholangiomanometry is obtained by replacing the saline with sodium diatrizoate and repeating the perfusion by the same technique. One film is obtained at passage pressure, a second at 5–10 cm above passage pressure with the patient in slight Trendelenburg position. There need be no hurry in obtaining the films, and they are best exposed at 3- to 5-min intervals. When the filming is completed, the reservoir system should be lowered to siphon off the contrast material; it is hyperosmolar, because excessive amounts in the small bowel may provoke diarrhea. The films are developed and interpreted before the cannula is removed.

There are rare technical problems; one must be certain that the system is free-flowing, that bubbles are not introduced, that the connecting tubes do not fall into the unsterile areas, that the connections are secure enough to prevent leaks, and that the zero point is not altered. It is always prudent to check that the solutions are correctly labeled and that the manometer is securely fixed to the mobile accessory table. Pressures below 20 cm H_2O and flow rates greater than 15 ml/min are considered normal. Contrariwise, an elevated pressure and a lower flow rate indicate outflow abnormalities, without indicating the etiologic factor.

CLINICAL EXPERIENCES AND RESULTS

Mattig (403, 404) has emphasized that from a functional viewpoint, the volume of fluid delivered into the duodenum is more significant than the pressure determination. This dynamic approach permits the calibration of the functioning area of the papilla which is the end ostium for the discharge of bile. Others (58, 209) have also reported enthusiastically on this method of calibration. In the one method, the pressure and time are fixed, and the variable is the volume delivered. Normally, 10 cc saline will pass into the duodenum in 1 min at the opening pressure. Another calibrated system fixes the time, and the volume and determines the pressure.

Braasch and McCann (84) used a dilator to calibrate the ostium at the choledochoduodenal junction at the time of common duct exploration. In 95% of instances it is larger

FIG. 6-2. Debimetry. In this readily available technique for manometry and debimetry, the flow rate per minute is measured by stopwatch. A graduated syringe serves as the saline reservoir. The level is adjusted from the base line of the common duct. With this technique the normal conduit allows for the transit of at least 15 ml/min (630).

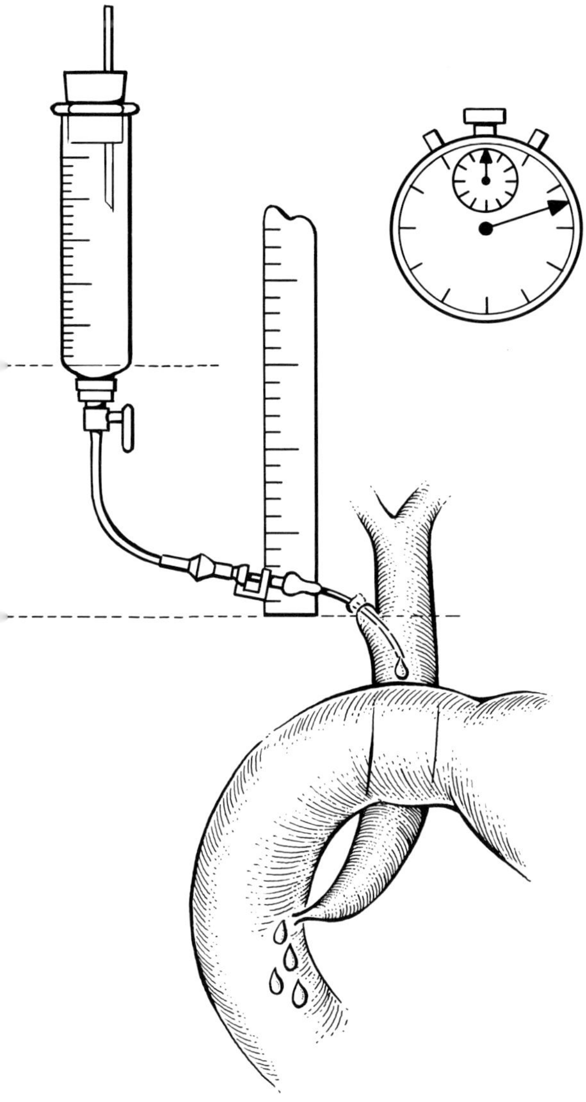

than 3 mm; when it is narrower, the diagnosis of stenosis can be invoked. The probe diameter is two to six times larger than that suggested by Brucke's flow calibration.

The advocates of cholangiomanometry regard it as the most sensitive method of objectively documenting papillary disorders. However, the determinations must be undertaken before the duct is manipulated. It is possible that Vaterian segment cholangitis

FIG. 6-3. Brucke's cholangiomanometer. At a fixed pressure the volume of fluid delivered through the cannula allows for the determination of passage pressure and the volume of flow per minute. This has been termed "debimetry." Because the cannula is calibrated and the flow rate through this system has been predetermined and charted for each instrument, it is possible to extrapolate the diameter of the papilla. A normal papilla is 0.1–0.2 cm and allows for the flow of at least 15 ml/min.

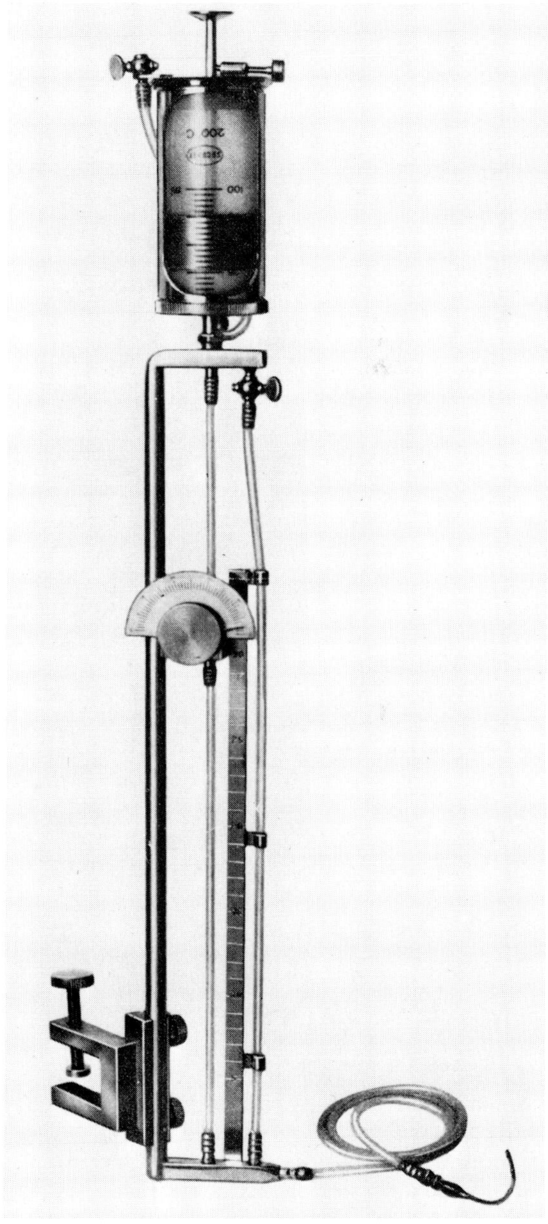

can be functionally evaluated by this method (9, 408, 477, 513, 636).

The results of biliary debimetry as it indicates volume flow must be carefully and rigidly interpreted. In the presence of calculi, an abnormal reading does not necessarily mean choledochoduodenal junction stenosis. On the other hand, normal rates of timed flow in the presence of calculi suggest functional integrity of the Vaterian segment. The obverse need not be valid. Fuchsig and Hartman (209) indicate that the latter combination of findings can lead to the false diagnosis of stenosis in about 60% of instances.

The patients are of two types: those whose common duct was evaluated as an adjunct to cholecystectomy; and those having secondary biliary tract operations for symptoms suggesting ampullary obstructions both with and without stones.

Most of the patients in the second group had also been evaluated by preoperative intravenous cholangiography as part of the PCS study.

The addition of manometry to cholangiography has not adversely altered the incidence of wound infections. There have been no instances of iodism, of an allergic reaction to the contrast material, or of chemical cholangitis. Jaundiced patients in whom ductal exploration was obviously required were excluded from this study.

Among 160 patients, elevated passage pressures were encountered in 62 (39%). Twenty-four percent of the latter patients had choledochal lithiasis. Of the 160 patients studied, 14% had calculi in the ducts. Of those with calculi, 65% had an elevated passage pressure and 35% had normal passage pressure.

There were no specific characteristics of duct size, number, or type of stones in the eight patients with choledochal calculi who had normal dynamics. Although an elevated passage pressure in itself is an indication of partial obstruction in the 62 patients in whom this was encountered, it was not associated with calculi in 75% of instances. The surgeon has to consider the significance of this manometric finding in terms of its specific etiologic and therapeutic implications. In conventional cholangiography one simply notes the absence of stones, and the duct is regarded as "normal." This conclusion is not always wholly satisfactory. The documentation of noncalculous choledochal hypertension must be considered a factor in determining the choice of preoperative procedure (155).

White *et al.* (630) summarized their experiences in 1972 with the statement that the 92% accuracy of cholangiography had been increased to 99.1% when pressure and flow determinations were added to that study. This finding was based on the premise that decreased flow rates (normal 23.0 ± 7.3 cc/min) and elevated resting pressure indicate an abnormality. Their report also stresses this facility for demonstrating small stones and papillary stenosis that otherwise go undiagnosed.

Bohmig and Fritsch (76) do not do this study if the direct intraoperative evaluation reveals an obviously diseased common bile duct. Nevertheless 10% of their patients with choledocholithiasis had a papillary stenosis that could be defined by this method. It is the only method of calibrating and documenting papillary stenosis without stones, an entity that they encountered in 7.5% of their cases.

This diagnosis is reported much more frequently in the European literature than in the United States; either the criteria are more liberal or others are missing the disorder by failing to search for it. Certainly the procedure is so simple and harmless that it is worth using prior to routine cystic duct opacification. The problems have been in the interpretation of the data. Decreased flow rate and increased pressure can antecede the hyperbilirubinemia.

Bourke and Ritchie (78) have evaluated the pressure profile of the sphincter of Oddi area by the pull-through technique similar to that used in the esophagus. In the bile duct normal pressure difference between the duodenum and common duct was about 7 cm saline; the pressure change was abrupt and occurred in the region of the ampulla. In 11 patients with abnormal common bile ducts, this pressure profile was of the normal pattern. In four there was no pressure difference. In three others the intracholedochal pressure was actually lower than that in the duodenum.

In acute cholecystitis, transcystic duct manometric cholangiography at MHMC demonstrated elevated pressures ranging from 26–35 cm H_2O in 7 of 12 patients, none of whom had choledocholithiasis. In three of five patients the pressure returned to normal 7–12 days later, in association with the roentgen observation that the ampullary reaction was less prominent. We assume that these patients had cholangitis, a component of which is ampullary edema, and that this edematous reaction resolved with cholecystectomy and transcystic duct choledochal drainage. The clinical event can be completely unrecognized and an elevated alkaline phosphatase level and exaggerated pain pattern can be less clearly understood in the absence of this manometric information. Two patients continued to have persistently elevated passage pressures. It remains to be established whether this delayed resolution of the ampullary affection is the precursor of ampullary stenosis and whether this is associated with persistent complaints.

The most clearly relevant data derived from the manometric determinations has been in the 35 patients with ampullary stenosis. These patients had already had a cholecystectomy and were being investigated for recurrent bouts of biliary colic and/or cholangitis. All had had preoperative screening by intravenous cholangiography, and in each instance the duct was dilated and the time-density relationship was prolonged.

A single manometric study will not differentiate between reversible edematous inflammatory reactions and fixed stenosis. The time-density evaluation can be a physiological approach to the demonstration of choledochal hypertension in the PCS patient in whom the secretory pressure of the liver challenges the outflow resistance of the entire ductal system. Delayed excretion of contrast material under these circumstances is an objective manifestation of obstruction. In each of these patients intraoperative biliary manometry demonstrated passage pressures in the range of 27–39 cm saline.

PRACTICAL APPLICATIONS OF CHOLANGIOMANOMETRY

If there is a value to intraoperative biliary manometry, it will be that the mensuration of the intracholedochal pressure is a clinically valuable addition to unmonitored cholangiography.

Brucke (96) reports on a personal experience with 750 studies. In 20% of these the cholangiomanometric determination was a decisive factor in choosing the surgical procedure, especially in deciding whether the common duct should be explored. In that experience manometry offered more information than cholangiography alone.

Brücke's present evaluation of his method is indicated in this 1976 personal communication:

> If you find a flow rate of at least 12 ml/min at a standard pressure of 30 cm of saline (corresponding to an opening at the papilla of 9.5 mm) *and* a *residual* pressure not exceeding 15 cm of water you have a normally functioning papilla. In my experience the only exception to this are free floating stones in the common duct, which of course do not constitute an obstacle to the bile flow. Small stones usually become impacted in the papilla during the procedure and cause raised pressures and low flow rates. Thus, to my mind, without using x-ray control, you have a 98% probability of a correct intraoperative evaluation.
>
> If you take all operations on the biliary system, I believe that your decision to open the common duct or not to open it will, in 10% of the cases, be influenced for or against by your measuring results. X-ray procedures at uncontrolled pressure rates are to my mind misleading, except if they show complete obstruction of the papilla.
>
> So, in fact, I am more than ever convinced that manometry *and* flow metering constitute a true progress.

The MHMC experience indicates that documentation of pressure is always pertinent in some problems, difficult to interpret in other areas, and of no aid in a third group. From a practical viewpoint, the passage pressure determination as well as the cholangiogram should be only one facet of the intraoperative diagnosis. The physical examination of the disordered area is the background into which this information must be integrated.

Clinical Considerations

Acute Inflammatory Disorders. The problem here relates to the altered indications for common duct exploration and the definition of the cause for the elevated serum bilirubin that is encountered in about 20% of these patients. At MHMC we have found that there are no stones in the common duct when the gallbladder contains a solitary round cholesterol stone or two or three such large faceted stones.

Cholangiomanometry in these instances

often demonstrates an elevated passage pressure and a prominent ampulla—a combination that is diagnostic of acute papillitis or of acute cholangitis manifested in the Vaterian segment. In those instances the pressure decreases and the ampullary sign recedes following cholecystectomy. The advantage of knowing about an elevated pressure (manometrically) without organic obstruction (cholangiography) is that the duct does not require formal exploration and the cause for jaundice is demonstrated. In these instances, there is probably an advantage to retaining the catheter for cystic duct drainage, continued until the pressure findings revert to normal. The reduction in pressure precedes the roentgen evidence of complete resolution of papillary edema.

The demonstration of normal passage pressure and normal opacification obviates the need for exploring the duct and lends security to the attitude that PCS symptoms are not due to changes in this area (528).

Prior Chronic Cholecystitis with a Solitary Stone in the Gallbladder. These patients rarely have calculous common-duct disease and the manifestations of an acute ampullary reaction are lacking. However, if the disease has been long-standing, I have encountered dilated ducts without calculi and have attributed this to ampullary stenosis. Postoperative follow-up of these patients have been associated with good results as far as the colic is concerned. However, some of them in whom the gallbladder opacified before operation continue to have colic and dyspeptic symptoms. Common duct involvement in these instances has also been encountered in association with the small, contracted gallbladder in which the cystic duct has been effaced and the obstructing large stone lies partially in the gallbladder and partially in the common duct. This phenomenon has been eponymically designated as the Mirizzi syndrome (see Fig. 18-18).

Ampullary Disorders. The mechanism of ampullary dysfunction in relation to gallstone disease is poorly understood, difficult to define, and hard to validate.

There is little doubt that there is an ampullary reaction in association with acute inflammatory episodes in the biliary tract. Whether this is a direct transmucosal in-continuity process or is propagated through lymphatics is uncertain. It is assumed that in some patients this inflammatory episode does not undergo complete resolution and results in a partial obstruction to the biliary and possibly pancreatic outflow sufficient to produce a dilated, hypertensive proximal ductal system.

Biopsy studies in this area have not been especially helpful. The histologic patterns have been granulomatous reactions, acute and chronic inflammation, submucosal glandular hyperplasia, or ulcerations. Some investigators have described the dynamic change of ampullary stenosis without confirmatory histologic changes. The definition of the entity, like pyloric stenosis, has to be by techniques other than histology.

All gastrointestinal obstructions have two factors in common: proximal dilatation and delayed transit. This also applies to the common bile duct. To validate a diagnosis of Vaterian segment obstruction, one should be able to demonstrate both anatomic and functional change. Because there has been a direct correlation between prolonged time–density factors and choledochal hypertension, the diagnosis of ampullary stenosis is made when three criteria are fulfilled: 1) a duct wider than 1.4 cm; 2) elevated passage pressure; 3) resistance to passing a number 3 Bakes dilator through the sphincter. In this combination of findings, a decompressing procedure is indicated.

I have now elected to carry out decompression during the primary biliary operation because the criteria and the procedure have proved so effective in the secondary management of similar problems seen in patients who have undergone cholecystectomy. In this regard, the manometric cholangiogram has proved valuable in the primary selection of patients who have the morphologic and pathologic findings frequently associated with postoperative symptoms. This will apply also when there are no calculi in the duct.

When calculi are found in the choledochus, it is difficult to interpret an elevated intraductal pressure. How much is due to stone obturation? To fixed or reversible ampullary reaction? To cholangitis? The guides to this differential diagnosis are not inflexible, but several observations have been clinically serviceable: fixed organic obstructions are not encountered in ducts less than 1.0–1.2 cm in width; a prominent ampulla on cholangiography indicates an acute reaction; a three-film reproducible stenotic ampullary configuration is more suggestive of fixed stenosis than of the systolic phase of ampullary function. Thick, viscid static bile and primary ductal calculi indicate chronic ductal obstruction.

Presumed Functional Disorders. Biliary manometry has been employed as a means of defining functional Vaterian segment changes. There is a broad zone of poorly understood clinical complexes that are designated as biliary hypertonia, dyskinesia, neuromuscular disorders, hypersensitivity of the biliary apparatus, and "sphincter spasms." Some ascribe a variety of biliary, pancreatic, duodenal, and peptic disorders to presumed malfunction in this area.

In the MHMC cinefluororadiographic experience, the subject is unaware of a prolonged sphincter contraction when this is evaluated at the predistention phase of choledochal perfusion. Nor has it been possible to record tetanic contractions or peristalsis that might indicate true muscle spasm as distinct from simple, prolonged muscular contraction. No correlations have been revealed between a low passage pressure and clinical symptoms. Spontaneous or postoperative hypotonicity (4–6 cm H_2O) of the Vaterian segment is very rarely recognized as a clinical disorder (397).

Elevated passage pressure in association with an abnormal cholangiogram is sufficient to establish the differential diagnosis of a stone, tumor, or stricture. Normal passage pressure and a completely normal cholangiogram establish the presence of a normal extrahepatic pathway. Elevated passage pressure alone may be due to reversible cholangitis or to irreversible ampullary stenosis. In some instances the cause for the elevated pressure is not apparent in the ductal system or in the pancreas duodenum, or lymph node areas. These manometric elevations have been regarded by others as evidence of duct spasm, papillitis, functional disorders, or neurogenic imbalance. The therapeutic implication of an elevated passage pressure determination has to be correlated with the width of the common duct, and the demonstration of an obstructive component.

SUMMARY

Manometrically documented choledochal hypertension has not always correlated with the presence of calculi. Calculi have been found in normotensive ducts. Hypertension has been the first intraoperative indication of the presence of calculi in ducts 1.0–1.2 cm wide. Manometry is of no value for the documentation of stones in the hepatic ducts.

At MHMC we have found that manometry cannot replace cholangiography and biliary endoscopy in the demonstration of choledocholithiasis and in the evaluation of the duct after choledocholithotomy. Manometry represents only one approach in the objective evaluation of the distal common duct (110).

The addition of intraoperative manometry to cholangiography has served to monitor the effect of neurogenic procedures and to establish the diagnosis of choledochal hypertension. Manometric values do not reliably indicate that a stone is not present. Passage pressure elevation and stones do not always go hand in hand. A normal passage pressure does not exclude the presence of calculi.

An elevated saline measurement warrants an especially careful investigation for an intrinsic or extrinsic obstruction. In the presence of a significantly dilated duct and a normal opacification study, the documentation of elevated pressure is a strong indication for common duct exploration. Although a dilated duct and elevated pressure warrant formal exploration directed toward identifying a stone, tumor, or ampullary stenosis, a dilated duct with normal opacification and normal manometric results obviates the need for exploration.

7 Choledochoscopy

Intraoperative biliary endoscopy, termed choledochoscopy, has become an integral part of complete intraoperative common duct exploration. The value of the procedure has been confirmed by numerous investigators, and its status in present-day biliary surgery no longer has to be defended (447).

We routinely explore and irrigate the bile ducts; the same procedure is followed in biliary endoscopy. The addition of choledoscopy to the routine operative procedure is simply that one may look directly at what has been accomplished within the bile duct. In this regard, therefore, there are no disadvantages to the procedure, and there is no increased risk with its use beyond what is associated with the routine common duct exploration and intraductal manipulation. In the MHMC experience with 160 choledochoscopic examinations, there has been no incidence of trauma or of a complication which can be ascribed to the instrument's use.

The first report of intraoperative biliary endoscopy was made by Bakes in 1923 (32) at a surgical congress in Berlin. Bakes is far better known for his calibrated dilators (33). It is a strange quirk that these well-known probes have come to have far less significance than his initiation of intraoperative visualization of the interior of the biliary system.

INSTRUMENTAL ARMAMENTARIUM

The original Bakes choledochoscope was a modification of the instrument used for otoscopy. It consists of a funnel-shaped cone which is manipulated into the bile duct, and the light is reflected from a laryngeal type mirror (Fig. 7-1). This contribution to biliary surgery remained largely unnoticed, and in his original report of about 40 cases he presented drawings of a normal and dilated papilla, an area of benign stenosis, and a faceted stone in the duct. Bakes predicted that this examination could be done in 2 min (sic) and might serve as a way "of maintaining biliary continuity without impediments" and that it would be possible "to collect diagnostic reference material."

In 1941 Monroe McIver (415) of the Mary Imogene Hospital in Cooperstown, N.Y., developed an instrument for the same purpose that was made by the American Cystoscope Company of New York. His instrument was essentially a right-angled observation telescope with an optical and irrigating system, reflecting in this regard the improved optics and lighting system. The intraductal portion of his instrument was 7 cm long and 0.5 cm in diameter. His report contains a black and white photograph taken through the choledochoscope, demonstrating a stone in the distal duct. The report was largely uninfluential.

In the intervening period, Babcock (29) reported on the use of the cystoscope for visualizing the interior of the gallbladder via a cholecystostomy fistula, and Hollenberg, Eikner, and Springs (278) "cystoscoped" a gallbladder as a bedside procedure at the time of withdrawing the cholecystostomy tube. They utilized this endoscopic approach for the removal of calculi retained in the gallbladder. DeWeese (170), in 1942, reported on a similar experience with six cases, and Laubersheimer (351), in 1947, commented on a 10-year experience with 30 cases of cholecystic endoscopy performed with a McCarthy panendoscope and resectoscope. These investigators did not visualize the bile ducts.

A really significant advance in biliary endoscopy was made by Hans Wildegans who was 65 years old at the time and Director of Surgery at the Bethanien Krankenhaus in West Berlin. He published the first monograph on this subject (634). To Wildegans must go the credit for having introduced a modern choledochoscope.

The instrument was further modified by Shore, Berci and Morgenstern (559, 560). That instrument incorporates the Hopkins rod lens, and overcomes many of the less optimal features of the Wildegans scope.

Its optical system permits miniaturization so that the 5-cm long exploring horizontal limb incorporates the optical lighting and irrigating system across a diameter that is only 5 mm × 3 mm. This scope is introduced much more easily over the costal arch into the bile duct than was the Wildegans instrument. There is wide-angled viewing (90°) and an excellent resolution and depth of field. The focus is fixed so that there is a good image quality that does not require rotation of the occular for adjustment (Fig. 7-2).

The choledochoscope, as thus conceived, is basically a rigid right-angled instrument that incorporates a lens system for viewing and an irrigation channel that distends the walls of the bile duct to permit good visualization of the lumen. Normal saline compressed by a blood-pressure cuff is perfused through the system. The interior of the common bile duct can be extremely well visualized. In chronic cholangitis, external transillumination from within the foramen of Winslow has occasionally clearly demonstrated alterations in the wall and vascular pattern of the common bile duct. I have made this observation from without, prior to inserting the choledochoscope, simply by inserting the light-bearing horizontal shaft into the foramen of Winslow. This rigid short-angled system is so adequate that I have not employed the flexible scope.

A side channel on the choledochoscope allows insertion of a biopsy forceps and of stone-grasping instruments. It is possible to attach a still camera or moving picture camera to the ocular end of the instrument, and films of the interior of the bile duct have been made (536).

TECHNIQUES

The technique of biliary endoscopy requires only that the instrument be sterilized and be available at the time of the procedure. The equipment is sterilized in an ethylene-oxide gas autoclave. The instrument table with a sterilized pack is kept on the left side of the patient; the pack is opened by the circulating nurse, and the instrument is handed by the scrub nurse to the surgeon standing on the right side. The intensity of the light beam is adjusted and the saline drip started before the instrument is introduced. There is some advantage to dimming the overhead operating-room lights, although this is not always necessary (Fig. 7-3).

The scope is introduced into the choledochotomy opening after the conventional exploration has been completed. It should be understood that choledochoscopy, in my viewpoint, is primarily a diagnostic procedure and therefore one does it at the conclusion of the surgical manipulation in the management of calculi and as a prelude to operative cholangiography (Fig. 7-4).

I prefer to visualize the hepatic ducts first, because I do not want a stone to fall down from those ducts later. The scope is inserted to its full length. With this, one ordinarily observes the carina, which is the vertical spur between the right and left hepatic ducts. The left hepatic duct is the larger of the two in the presence of choledochalectasia and lies slightly more anteriorly. One can view into the left hepatic duct for at least 2 cm and not see any branches. The scope is then withdrawn from the left hepatic duct, the carina identified as the reorienting spur, and the scope introduced into the right hepatic duct. One should see its dorsocaudal and ventrocranial divisions. There is sometimes an ostium in the carinal spur. In looking at the duct, one is concerned primarily with the presence of calculi, but it is also well to note the manifestations of cholangitis, as these are evidenced by excess mucus production, areas of hyperemia and edema, and even minute ulcerations.

The normal mucous membrane of the common bile duct is smooth and pale yellow-red. One can frequently observe the subepithelial reticulum of blood vessels. The relatively flat mucous membrane has grooved pits

FIG. 7-1. The first choledochoscope. **A.** Bakes original choleodochoscope was first described in 1923. That the illustration is purely diagrammatic is suggested by the position of the proximal occluding clip. **B.** Bakes included his dilator **(1)** as part of the armamentarium.

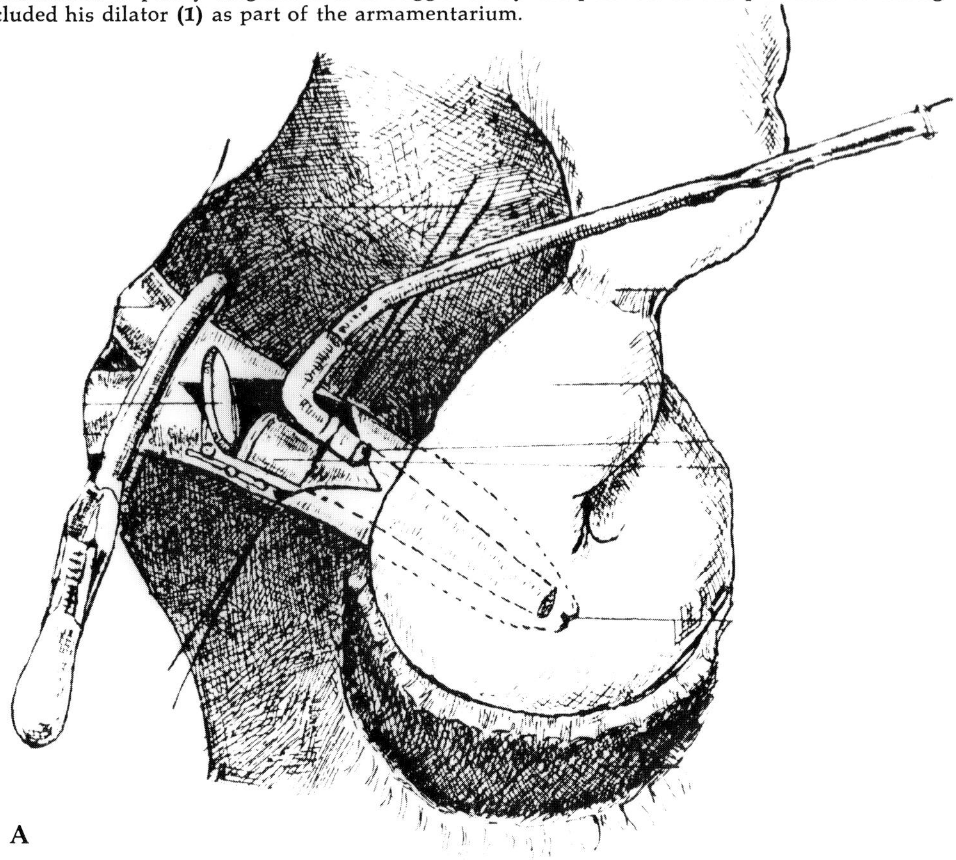

A

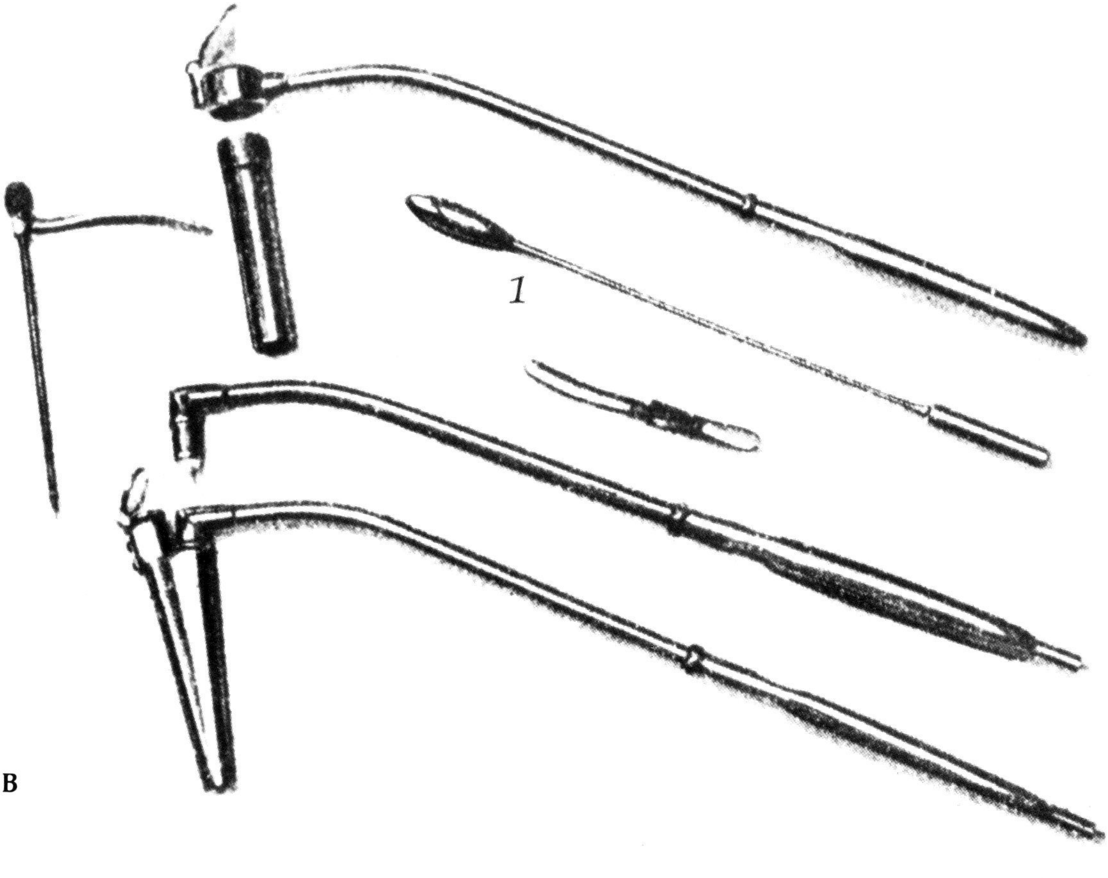

B

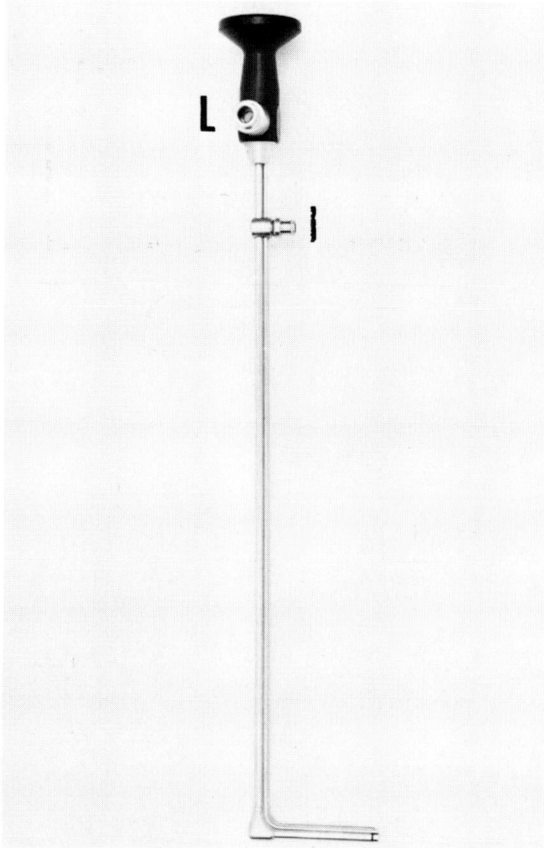

FIG. 7-2. Berci-Shore choledochoscope. This modern choledoscope, as made by the Storz Company with a Hopkins lens, was designed by Berci and Shore. **(L)** Site for connection to the flexible fiber optic cable for light transmission. **(I)** Site for connection to the irrigating system. The instrument is completely rigid, and no adjustment in the ocular is required.

that represent the parietal sacculus. The glandular orifices tend to flatten out and be incorporated into the smooth epithelial lining in the presence of marked ectasia. With this, the proximal hepatic tree has been identified, and the scope is withdrawn. During this manipulation the excess fluid that has distended the duct comes out of the choledochotomy opening, and this is routinely aspirated by a sucker, which is kept in the hepatorenal fossa.

The scope is withdrawn and inserted distally. Again it is well to insert to the depth of the right angle as an initial maneuver under direct viewing. This avoids overlooking a stone between the scope and the duct wall. The choledochoduodenal junction is seen well ahead of the scope head. It is not necessary to enter into the ampulla to visualize the area. There is often a limbus in the duct just before the duodenal orifice is visualized. In the presence of pancreatitis, the manipulation of the duct beyond the first 2 cm should be done under direct vision.

The choledochoduodenal junction can have several shapes. The best view is ordinarily obtained as the instrument is withdrawn. In the vast majority of cases the duodenum has been Kocherized for the exploration. The distal duct can be visualized with the scope in one hand while the second portion of the duodenum is manipulated with the other. The instrument is moved to and fro in a circumferential fashion on withdrawal in order to get a good view of the entire lumen. The ampulla is usually irregularly stellate or quadrilateral, with a rather evident transition from the smooth epithelium of the bile duct to the heaped-up mucosa of the duodenum. The duodenal mucosa may have a polypoid configuration.

The instrument can be reinserted several times during any single examination. One should come away from the examination with a sense of having completely visualized the major hepatic ducts and their divisions and the entire choledochus through the duodenal junction. Occasionally, one sees the opening of the long, parallel, left-sided cystic duct in the supraampullary segment.

The ampullary segment is usually completely flaccid. A former bed for a previously incarcerated or embedded stone may be appreciated as a focal area of congestion and ulceration. Cholangitis is seen much more often than it is clinically suspected, and in its catarrhal form it is rarely suspected, but it is obvious on choledochoscopy. In the more advanced stages there is flagrant ulceration, fibrinous webbing, and a purulent exudate. Brocks (89) reported that half the patients whom he examined had cholangitis. In the MHMC experience, about 60% of the patients with calculi had some variety of cholangitis.

In my experience, if one knows that a stone is there, it is usually possible to extract it in the usual fashion rather than under direct endoscopic vision. However, Shore and Berci (558) have reported on the need to extract

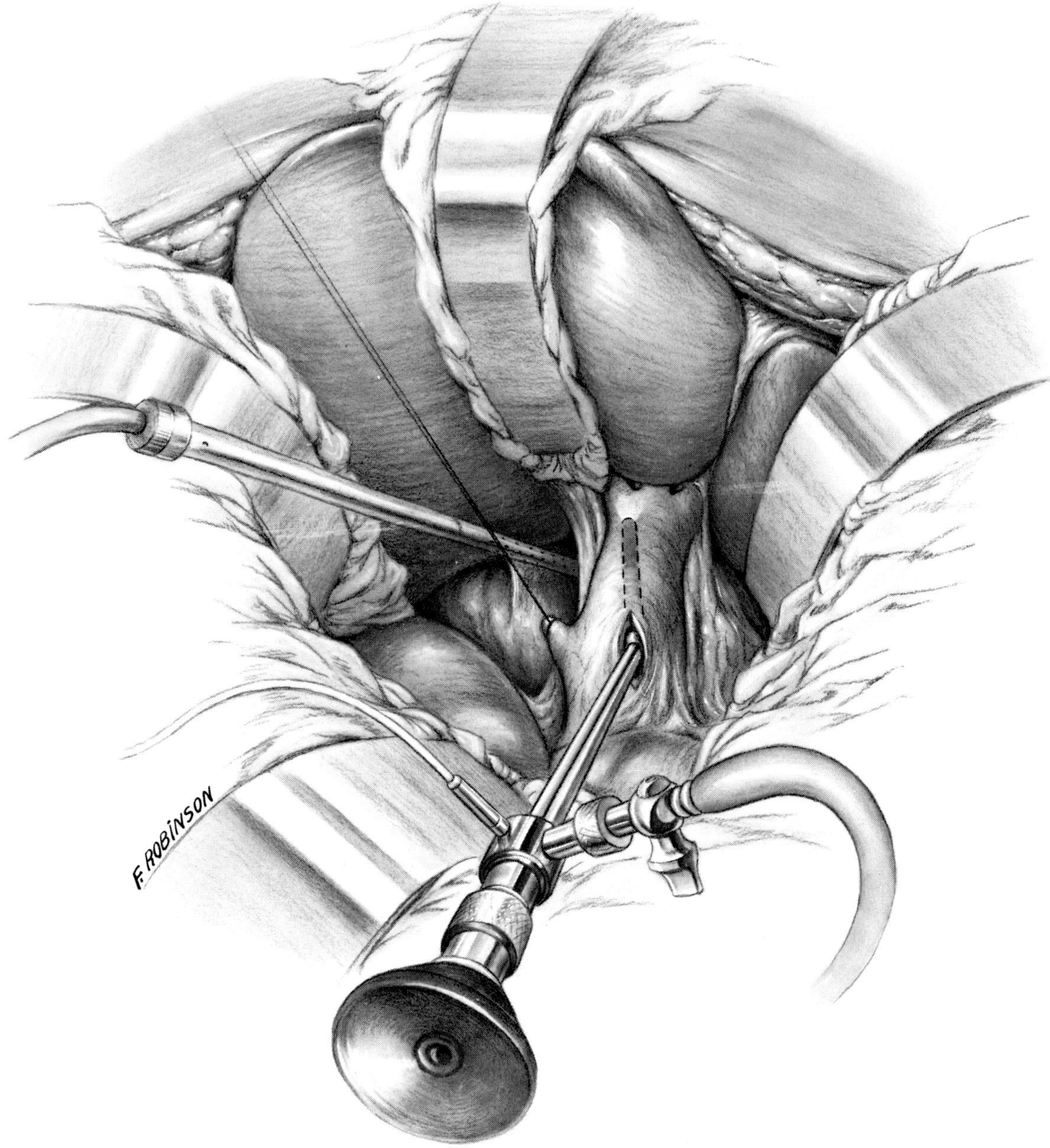

FIG. 7-3. Technique of biliary endoscopy. The choledochoscope in use, showing retractors in place and suction tip positioned to collect the outflow of the saline irrigant. The proximal hepatic ducts are being visualized. (From Schein CJ, Stern WZ, Jacobson HG: The Common Bile Duct. Operative Cholangiography, Biliary Endoscopy and Choledocholithotomy, 1966. Courtesy of Charles C Thomas, Publisher, Springfield, Illinois)

stones under direct endoscopic vision, especially when they are in the hepatic ducts.

When the duct is dilated or I have performed a choledochoduodenostomy, I have frequently taken an elliptical biopsy of the common bile duct mucosa at the site of the choledochotomy.

ENDOSCOPIC INTERPRETATIONS AND RESULTS

One value of endoscopy is in the differential diagnosis of disorders in the Vaterian segment. It permits the differential diagnosis of functional disorders from anatomic (stone,

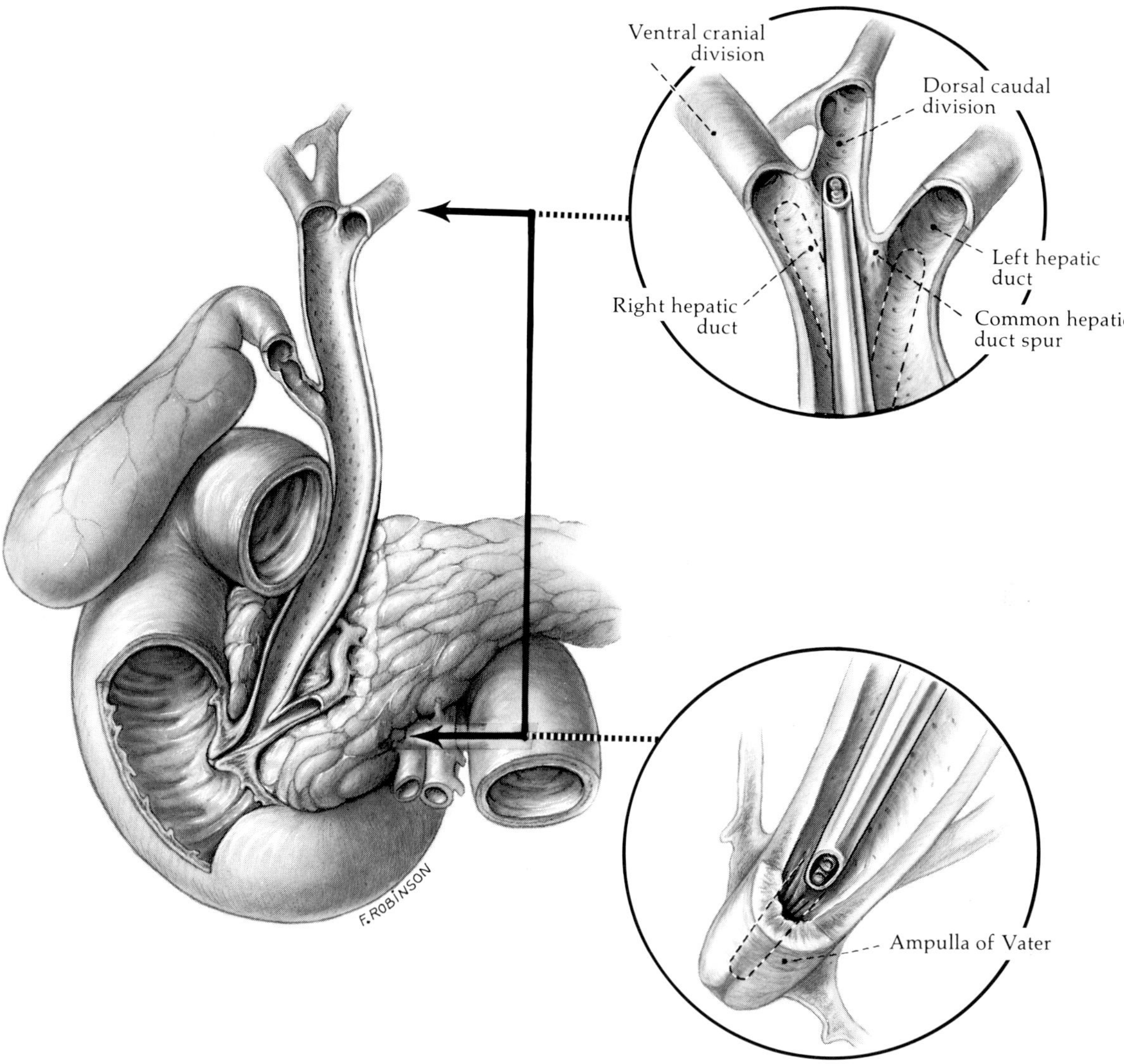

FIG. 7-4. Endoscopic orientation of the common bile duct and its branches in normal conditions. (From Schein CJ, Stern WZ, Jacobson HG: The Common Bile Duct. Operative Cholangiography, Biliary Endoscopy and Choledocholithotomy, 1966. Courtesy of Charles C Thomas, Publisher, Springfield, Illinois)

stricture, tumor) changes at the distal end. It is especially valuable when arrangements for cholangiography have not been made or when cholangiography cannot be performed. It is an interesting historical note that Wildegans regarded choledochoscopy as sufficiently accurate to obviate the need for complementary cholangiography—a point of view that is not supported by my own experience. Normal or inflammatory polypoidal changes can be confused with benign tumors or cancer (18, 92). The earliest carcinoma of the ampulla seen in the MHMC experience was that in a patient with PCS who underwent operation for gallbladder remnant disease; the tumor was found only on endoscopy. Pancreaticoduodenectomy revealed that the cancer involved only the mucosa and submucosa. Whenever the ampullary finding is difficult to interpret by endoscopy, I have not hesitated to do endoscopic biopsy or open duodenal biopsy (517).

Perhaps one of the most valuable aspects of this procedure is determining that the distal bile duct is normal. This knowledge is an aid in interpretating the operative cholangiogram that fails to show passage of contrast material into the duodenum. In the majority of cases in the MHMC experience, this has been associated with the edema consequent to either the inflammatory process in the duct, or to the trauma that goes with intraductal manipulation. If endoscopy shows that the duct is free, needless repetitive cholangiography, duodenotomy, and sphincterotomy are avoided. As experience was gained in this matter, it has not been necessary to open the duodenum for confirmation of the endoscopic findings.

The diagnosis of primary tumors of the pancreas has rarely required choledochoscopic confirmation. I have also found it to be unnecessary and of little value in diagnosing primary hepatic duct cancers.

The value of choledochoscopy in biliary calculous disease has been attested to by numerous other investigators (356, 447, 560). In the MHMC experience with 117 patients who underwent cholecystectomy and common duct exploration, choledochoscopy was routinely performed in all whose ducts were at least 1 cm in diameter. Visualization was accomplished at the final step of the duct exploration but was complemented by post-endoscopic intraoperative cholangiography performed via the T tube. The policy in that series was that when a discrepancy occurred between the endoscopic and cholangiographic findings, it was advisable to reexplore the duct and to repeat both examinations.

In 117 patients, there was a 5.1% potential for retained calculus if the examination had been ended without further investigation. When the common duct exploration was accompanied by endoscopy, the potential for retained stone was 0.9%. When both examinations were done, no retained stones were demonstrated in the postoperative period (Table 7-1).

Similar satisfactory results have been reported in several large series of endoscopies (239, 447, 527, 560).

In the 12% of patients in these series in

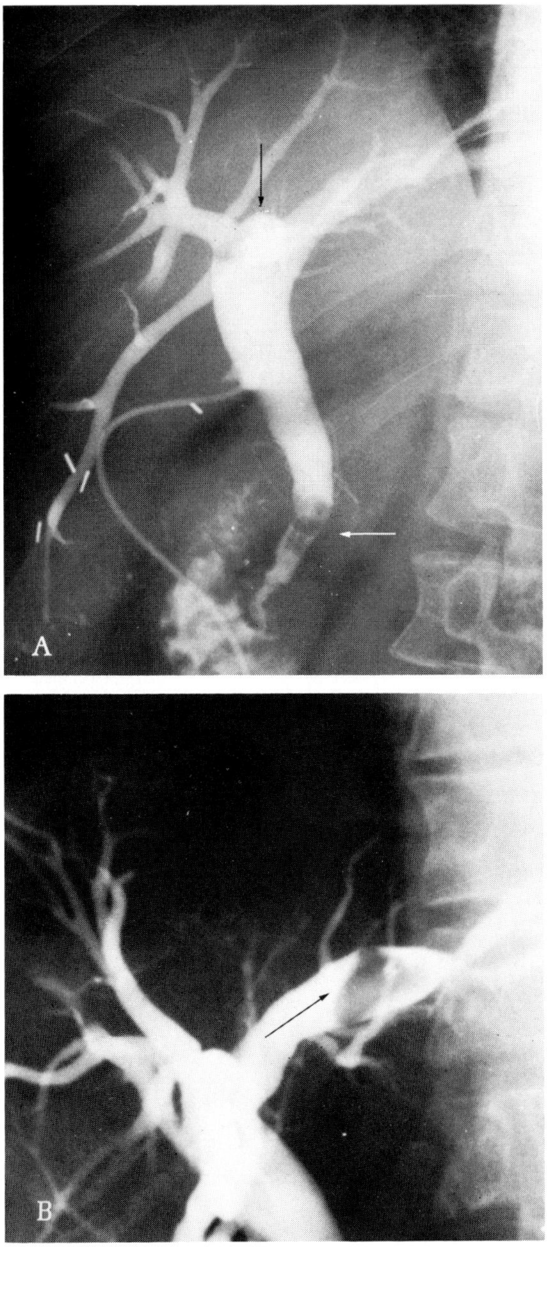

FIG. 7-5. Choledochoscopy complementing cholangiography. **A.** T-tube cholangiogram, obtained in a patient scheduled to have his third procedure for choledocholithiasis, reveals stones **(white arrow)** that were easily recognized. A stone in the confluence of the right and left hepatic ducts **(black arrow)** was not recognized at the time of a second operation and had not been sought for. The error occurred because the medium was too dense and only one view was taken. The error in both instances is fundamentally in the technique and interpretation of the cholangiogram. This is an instance where choledochoscopic policing of the common bile duct can be especially valuable. **B.** This cholangiogram reveals a greatly dilated left hepatic duct with a huge stone **(arrow)**, just proximal to the point where the left hepatic duct divides into superior and inferior branches. The stone had been overlooked at the previous duct exploration. The area is one that is especially suitable for choledochoscopic inspection.

whom the contrast medium failed to enter the duodenum and endoscopy revealed a stone-free duct, the patency of the ampulla was demonstrated on the postoperative cholangiogram. On several of the cholangiograms the endoscopic findings lent security to the interpretation of smooth, round, small, filling defects as air bubbles rather than as small calculi. This obviated the need to reopen the common duct and redo both procedures.

A cooperative study was done in which 155 patients had intraoperative choledochoscopy following primary choledochotomy. Postoperative T-tube cholangiography showed that only two patients of 155 (1.2%) had retained stones. It was known that nine patients had retained stones that could not be removed, and these were treated by some form of internal biliary drainage (447).

Thus, 50 years after the initial description, operative choledochoscopy has been validated as a valuable adjunct to the exploration of the common duct and as a method of reducing retained stones to an incidence below 2% (Fig. 7-5).

In the postcholecystectomy operation performed for recurrent or residual calculi, choledochoscopy is especially necessary so that

FIG. 7-6. Influence of biliary endoscopy on the choice of surgical procedure. **A.** Choledochoscopy and cholangiography can serve as complementary procedures in the diagnosis and management of secondary procedures. A female patient, explored for what was regarded as a cystic duct and gallbladder remnant disease, was found at choledochoscopy to have a tumor at the ampulla **(arrow)**, which was a carcinoma of the ampullary segment. There were no clinical indications that this lesion was present. It is a finding that justifies the viewpoint that choledochoscopy should be a routine part of common bile duct exploration. A pancreaticoduodenectomy was performed. The cancer had not extended beyond the submucosa, and no lymph nodes were involved. **B.** A male patient who had been treated for a presumed carcinoma of the pancreas by cholecystojejunostomy returned 20 months later with symptoms of biliary sepsis. This was related to stricture of the cholecystojejunostomy **(a)** and purulent acute cholecystitis. The patient did not have a cancer of the pancreas; the disorder was chronic pancreatitis **(b)** related to cholecystolithiasis. The anastomosis was dismantled, the gallbladder removed, and the stenosis at the distal end of the common duct bypassed with a wide choledochoduodenostomy. Choledochoscopy confirmed the fact that there was no tumor at the distal end of the common bile duct. (Schein CJ, Stern WZ, Hurwitt ES, Jacobson HG: Am J Roentgenol 89:864, 1963)

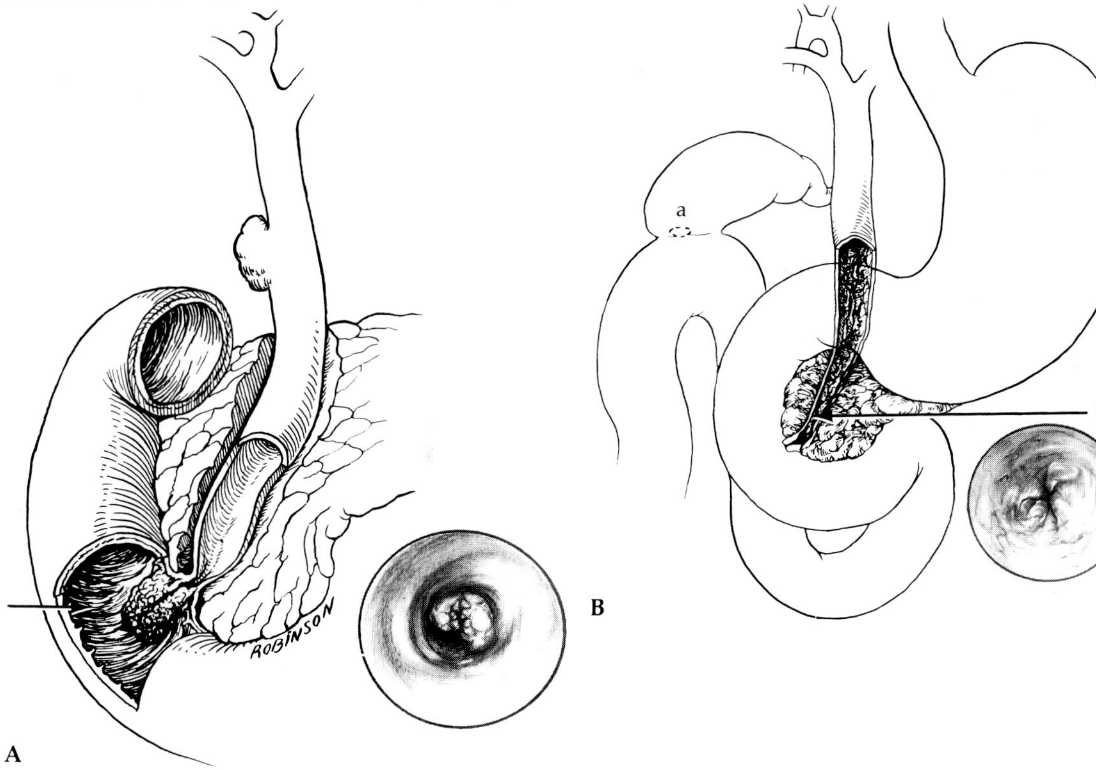

TABLE 7-1. INCIDENCE OF RETAINED CALCULI IN INTRAOPERATIVE MONITORING FOR CHOLEDOCHOLITHIASIS AT MHMC

Procedure*	Retained stone potential† (%)
CDE	5.1
CDE and endoscopy	0.9
CDE and endoscopy and cholangiography	0.0

* The operative procedures appear in the order in which they are carried out during common duct exploration (CDE).

† The potential for retained calculi at each stage of the procedure is calculated for the 117 patients.

the error will not be repeated. I have performed operative choledochoscopy on every secondary choledochlithotomy (Fig. 7-6). There has been some hallway critique that the procedure is no longer required since the dilated duct, especially in secondary or tertiary operations, is now managed by a biliary-intestinal bypass, and if a retained stone were present it would pass through the newly created surgical opening. This may be true, but for the safety of the hundredth man, it is important that no calculi have been left behind. If there are calculi in the hepatic ducts, it is far better to remove them than to await the probability of spontaneous passage through a wide choledochoduodenostomy. In procedures accompanied by biliary enteric bypass, it is also important to know that the blind sac, the distal end of the duct, is empty.

Choledochoscopy should be part of routine common bile duct exploration. Unlike other forms of the endoscopy, the range of pathology in this area is quite small, and basically one looks for stones, cholangitis, or tumors. There are no disadvantages to its performance and the published experience supports its role in diminishing the number of retained calculi.

Biliary endoscopy has its own reason for being. It does not exclude any other means of exploring or evaluating the duct. It does not transfer the responsibility for the interpretation of the findings to the radiologist. When the patient is extremely obese and the x-ray is not satisfactory, choledochoscopy can be. That the examination takes about 5 min and offers information that can be acted on immediately is no small advantage. However, it is no substitute for careful common-duct exploration, for an associated complementary operative cholangiogram, or for the need to manage the obstructed duct by an adjunctive procedure.

III

Specific Problems

8 Gallbladder Remnant Disease

A complete and adequate cholecystectomy requires removal of the entire gallbladder, along with a portion of its cystic duct. The optimum retained duct segment is one long enough to allow for adequate ligature without tenting the choledochus (71, 430). By definition, cholecystectomy implies that the retained segment has no calculi. The retention of portions of gallbladder after presumed cholecystectomy is termed cystic stump syndrome, or cystic duct remnant or gallbladder remnant disease.

In 1936 Beye (61) reported 14 cases of "reformed gallbladder." The earlier term "regenerated gallbladder" has no place—there is no regrowth. Inflammatory changes may enlarge the remnant, but it does not undergo hyperplasia (216, 265).

Larmi (348) from Finland reports that 12% of biliary operations done between 1966 and 1972 were secondary procedures. Twenty percent of these were for cystic duct remnants.

THE IDEAL CYSTIC DUCT REMNANT

The cystic duct's length, width, course, angulation, and relation to accessory ducts determine the optimum site for ligation. Anatomically, the juxtacholecystic segment of the cystic duct is valved by mucosal folds, as originally described by Heister. The juxtacholedochal portion of the duct (pars glabrum) has a smooth inner surface. Particulate matter is more likely to reside on the proximal folds than in the flat distal portion of duct. Therefore, the entire convoluted portion of the duct is preferably excised. It should be demonstrable in the surgical specimen of the original operation.

Some surgeons suggest that the entire length of the cystic duct be removed and that the site of entrance in the common bile duct be directly closed by several interrupted sutures. Though this procedure might have a theoretical advantage, it is not indicated. It can be technically difficult if the common duct is normal, for such suturing may narrow it. Practically, in the completely controlled situation, a 1-cm stone-free stump of cystic duct is consistent with an excellent anatomic cholecystectomy.

An entirely different circumstance exists when the cystic duct has a long or short course parallel to the right side of the common duct, or where it crosses over or under to enter on the left side of the choledochus. It would be unwise to attempt a separation of the two structures in the former instance, or to dissect it out of the pancreas in the latter circumstance. In these situations it is sufficient to ligate the duct at a site distal to the cholecystic ampulla and to verify the absence of a stump calculus by direct visualization, probing, or cholangiography.

In the angular configuration, the stump can safely be 1 cm in length. In the long parallel or left-sided situation, the residual length is of no consequence. A gallbladder remnant containing calculi is diseased regardless of its size or configuration. Any retained segment that is constituted by more than the cystic duct, whether or not it contains stones, is the site of at least chronic cholecystitis and is heir to all of the disease process of the otherwise totally intact, similarly constituted organ. The only exception to this is in the removal of part of a completely normal gallbladder, and the residual segment, the still normal portion, is that innocent viscus.

It is important to know whether the choledochal orifice of the cystic duct is patent, obliterated, or narrowed. The terminal 2–4 mm of the cystic duct lumen is often strictured. This can later be the focus for obstruction and stasis in the proximally retained gallbladder remnant. Complete stenosis of the cystic choledochal junction will have no influence on the proximal stone-free area.

The study of this area has established an anatomic basis for the purposeful retention of at least a certain variety of cystic duct. Flint (201) has indicated that the duct enters the choledochus behind the duodenum in 14% of cases.

There is one especially important reason for retaining a part of the cystic duct. That is when an aberrant hepatic bile duct exists that way. This can only be appreciated when the cystic duct is being dissected down, and the strand—which is the aberrant duct—is determined to have a lumen. If this is not appreciated, then a bile leak, or fistula will eventuate, depending upon the extent of the hepatic area so drained. I have left a cystic duct stump behind in this situation. (Fig. 8-1). I know of an instance in which such a 2-mm duct was inadvertently divided, and the patient remained with a bile leak for 3 months. Then the leak closed spontaneously. In another instance, the situation was recognized and the duct tied off without further incident. The hydrostatic pressure behind this tie, as an indication of the amount of liver parenchyma being drained, was not sufficient to blow the tie off.

REASONS FOR THE RETENTION OF GALLBLADDER REMNANTS

Data on retention of gallbladder remnants are available only by direct information from the first surgeon or by a detailed review of the operative record of the earlier surgical procedure. The reviewer acquires a sensitivity not only about what is in the record but what has been left out of the record as well. Retained gallbladder remnants are the result—for good or for inappropriate reasons—of incomplete definition of the cystic-choledochal junction.

In some instances the anatomic dissection in the area of the cholecystic hilus was regarded as "too edematous for dissection," excessively vascular," the "anatomy anomalous and distorted." Prudence was indeed the better choice and an anatomically safe subtotal resection was accomplished.

In some of these instances the prior operation often appeared to have been a fundectomy or partial cholecystectomy. At the second procedure the unbranched cystic artery and the nerve fibers on the cystic duct are completely intact, suggesting that this area had not been mobilized.

Such a partial cholecystectomy can be the prudent management of a situation that, for that surgeon, could not be otherwise serviced. It is wise, however, to inform the patient that part of the organ has been left behind as being the "safest procedure" at that time and under those circumstances (Fig. 8-2).

The single retained calculus in a short cystic duct remnant is related to tying off the duct on the gallbladder side of an incarcerated stone. The surgeon may not have visualized the duct lumen as it was being transected, or had failed to palpate or probe the duct before delivering the tie. In several instances, the retrieved T-tube cholangiogram of this original cholecystectomy and common duct exploration shows the stone in the distal cystic duct. Stones may remain incarcerated in this remnant and not be passed into the common bile duct because of associated duct junction stenosis. The earlier inflammatory reaction in this area may have been responsible for the difficulty in dissection (Fig. 8-3).

There is anecdotal clinical experience that new stones can be formed in a cystic duct remnant that was objectively free of calculi at the original procedure. In rare instances, it would appear that the surgeon believed he had removed the entire organ and that the amputation at the pouch of Hartmann was regarded as at a level proximal to a dilated common duct. In a still rarer instance, the amputation is done through the waist of an hourglass constriction of the gallbladder.

Retained gallbladder remnants that are not in continuity with the bile flow play a different role. Sometimes portions of the posterior wall, even full-thickness patches, are left attached to the liver when the gallbladder was torn or removed subserosally. These retained, partially avulsed plaques may become devascularized and necrotic, serving as the compost for a subhepatic abscess, or they may be the site for subsequent dystrophic calcification, but they do not cause colic or jaundice (Fig. 8-4).

In most instances the second operation suggests that there was just an incomplete definition and no dissection in the area of Calot's triangle.

PATHOPHYSIOLOGY OF THE GALLBLADDER REMNANT

A gallbladder remnant is diseased in the same way as its parent. When calculi are retained, it is as if no portion of the gall-

FIG. 8-1. Accessory duct. **A.** The problem of the accessory duct in relation to the anatomy of the gallbladder in the region of the cholecystic-hepatic angle **(a).** High ligation of the cystic duct allows the accessory duct to drain adequately **(b).** This is the optimum way of managing this situation. Low ligation of the cystic duct and severance of the accessory hepatic duct **(c)** results in a biliary fistula of varying size and importance, depending upon the area of hepatic segment that is drained. The fate of the ligation of the cystic duct and the accessory duct **(d)** will depend upon the secretory pressure on the liver. If that is low and the duct is satisfactorily occluded, there will be no problem and the situation will go unrecognized. If the pressure is high, it is possible that the tied-off segment will necrose and that a biliary fistula will result. **B.** A simultaneous intravenous cholangiogram **(left arrow)** and fistulogram **(right arrow).** The puddle represents the extravasation from a divided accessory duct that was the source of the bile fistula.

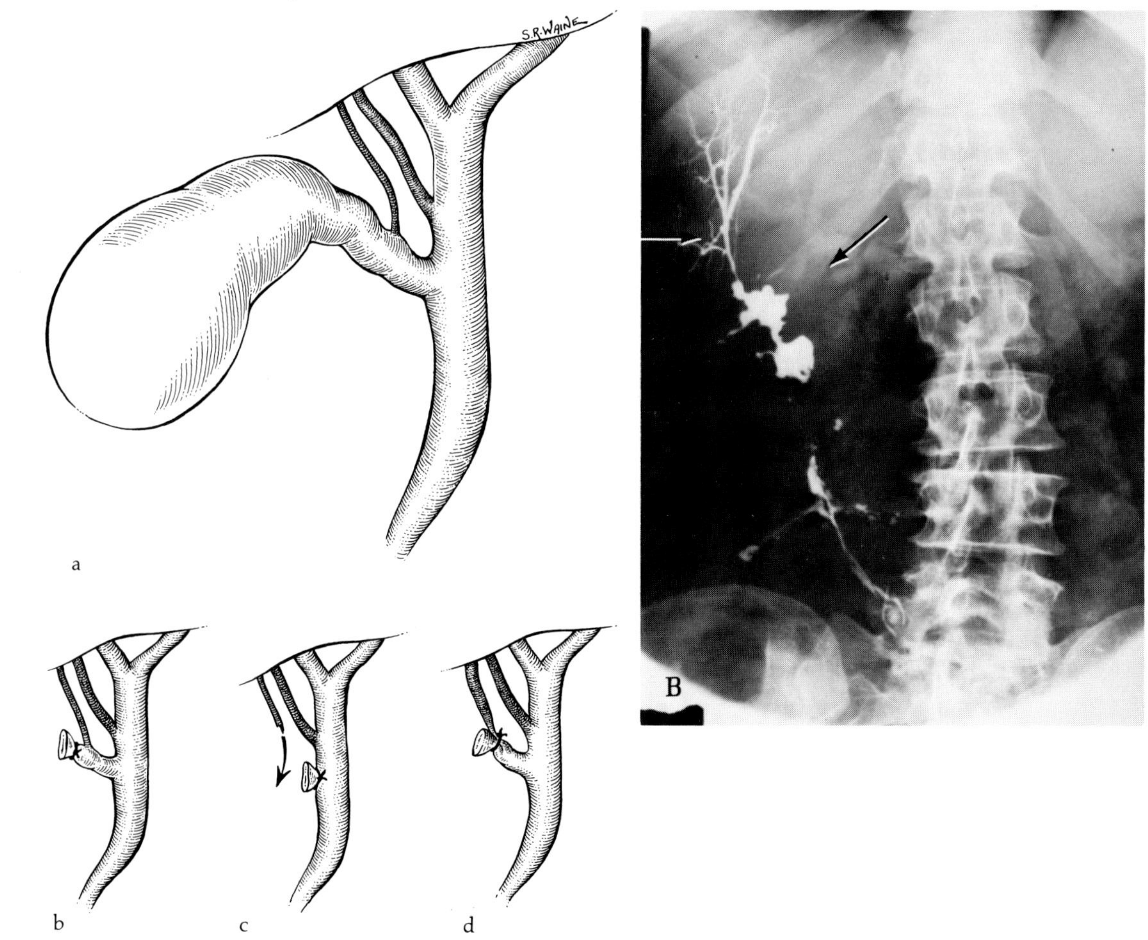

A

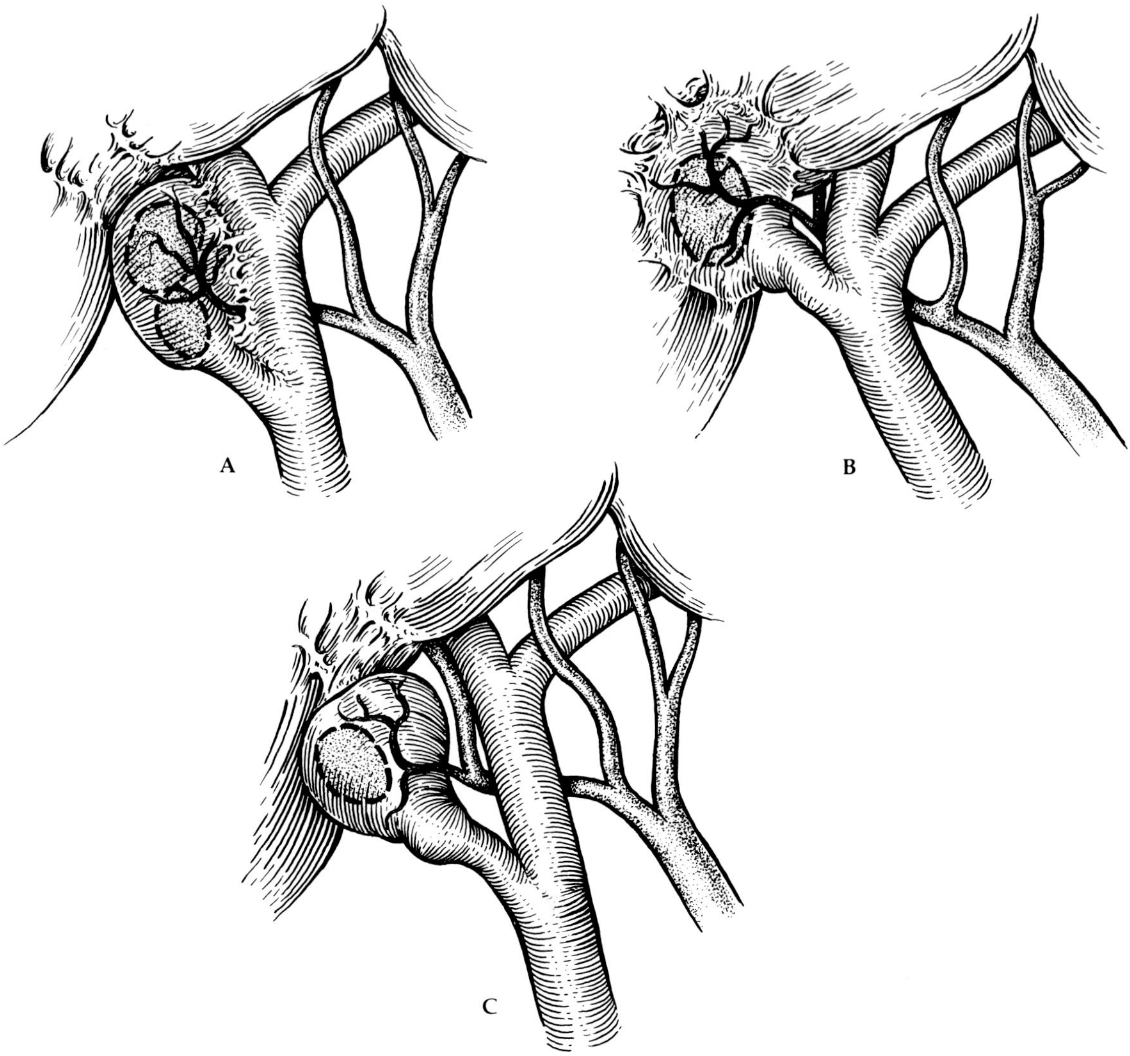

FIG. 8-2. Gallbladder remnants. In each situation there are stones and the cystic duct and artery are intact. **A.** The remnant is adherent to the right lateral wall of the choledochus and the right hepatic duct. There may be an incipient or actual fistula. The plane can be difficult to develop. **B.** The remnant has perforated into the liver. Its posterior wall may have been completely eroded. **C.** The simplest situation with minimal inflammatory reaction and clearly evident planes. The very short cystic artery can be mobilized along with part of the gallbladder wall. (From Schein CJ, Stern WZ, Jacobson HG: The Common Bile Duct. Operative Cholangiography, Biliary Endoscopy and Choledocholithotomy, 1966. Courtesy of Charles C Thomas, Publisher, Springfield, Illinois)

bladder has been removed. The remnant can remain symptomatically and pathologically dormant, or it can be the seat of an acute or chronic (stump) inflammatory process with any event or combination of events seen in previously unmolested acute cholecystitis (93, 134,147).

The remnant can likewise be the quarry from which stones are discharged into the common bile duct. There may be acute suppurative changes, both with and without perforation, localized as well as free, and fistulas between the retained remnant and the duodenum (Fig. 8-5).

In a review of the subject of cystic duct fistula, by Van Houten and Lewicki (601), only three cases are reported: to the duodenum (similar to the one in Figure 8-5), to the

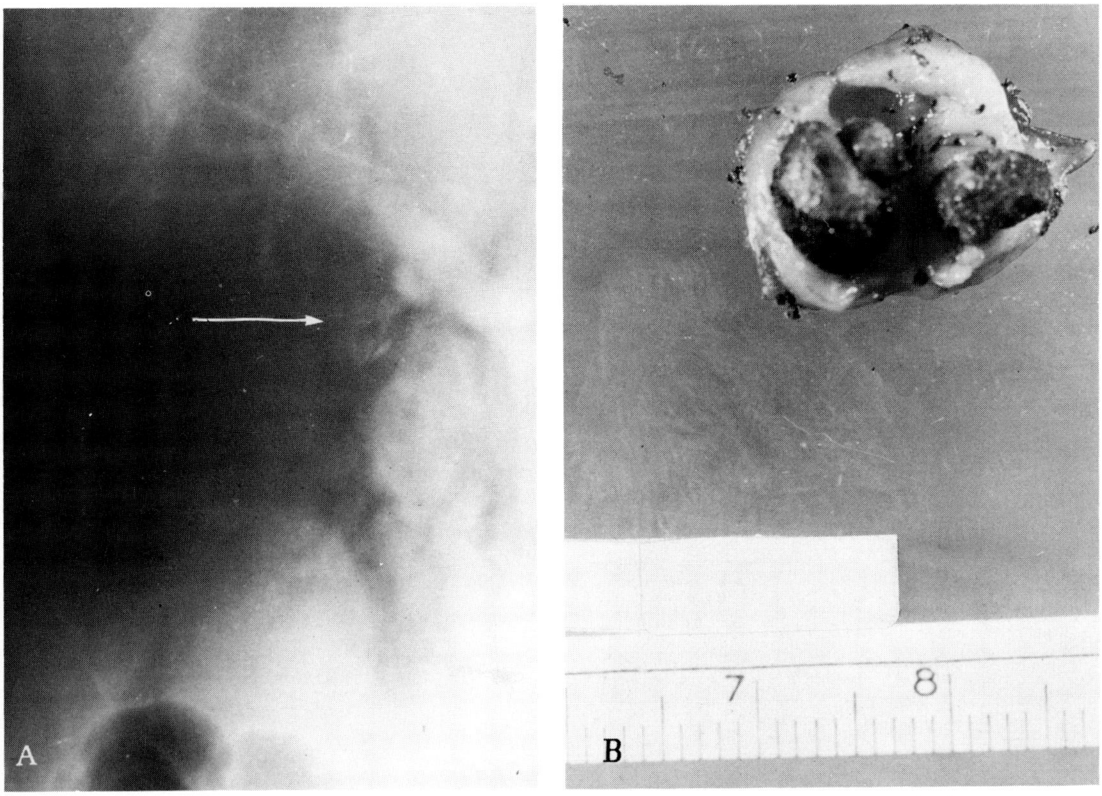

FIG. 8-3. Inflamed gallbladder remnant. **A.** The intravenous cholangiogram shows a calculus-containing gallbladder remnant **(arrow).** Presumably the ampulla of the gallbladder had been divided proximal to this site. **B.** The open specimen shows the acute and chronic inflammatory reaction and several calculi.

colon, and to the stomach. It is my impression that partial resection by fundectomy is more likely to be the source of a subsequent problem than is the viscus treated by either cholecystostomy or by subtotal resection with retained cystic duct (54, 243, 313).

The long cystic duct remnant of the parallel duct type is not to be regarded as a pathologic state if it contains no stones (644). However, it has been suggested that this segment is the trigger mechanism for "infundibulo-cervico-cystic-dyskinesia" (238). The calculus-free gallbladder remnant in its symptomatic pathogenic potential can be therapeutically viewed as noncalculus chronic cholecystitis.

Recurrent episodes of cholecystitis in the remnant, so low-grade clinically as to be asymptomatic, can produce recurrent inflammation in the ampullary area. In some instances their incomplete resolution can lead to stenosis or stricture at the choledochoduodenal junction.

Bodvall and Overgaard's survey (72) of 18 investigators reporting on 452 cases elicited the following data: Average interval to second operation is 4 years (range 1.5–13.5); 32.5% were jaundiced; 19% had associated choledocholithiasis; symptoms of distress presented earlier than infection.

In summary, the entire spectrum of gallbladder disease and its effect on related organ systems and associated anatomic conduits continues to reside in stone-containing retained or subtotally resected segments. The most frequent association is a stone-containing remnant, common-duct stone, periductal neuroma, and choledochal junction stenosis.

The symptoms are specific in the sense that they are the same as those observed in patients who have similarly diseased extrahepatic biliary tracts that have never been surgically approached. Patients who have "biliary" symptoms following a cholecystectomy are sometimes dismissed and told the symptoms are "usual" or functional or unre-

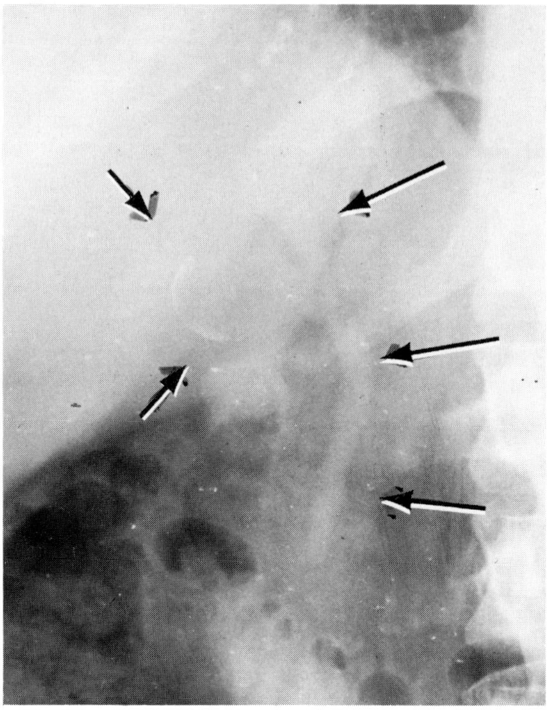

FIG. 8-4. Dystrophic calcification simulating a gallbladder remnant. An intravenous cholangiogram in a patient symptomatic for many years after cholecystectomy reveals a calcified rim density **(two arrows at left)** in the right upper quadrant in association with a normal common bile duct **(three arrows at right)**, which empties satisfactorily. At operation this was found to be an area of dystrophic calcification in the liver bed at the site where silk sutures had been used to peritonealize the area. The patient's condition has not improved with excision of this calcified tissue.

lated because, without adequate investigation, the examiner wrongly assumes that an adequate surgical procedure has been performed.

The interval for the recurrence of symptoms in the MHMC surveyed cases varied from 6 weeks to 20 years, with the majority becoming symptomatic within the first 2 years. It was difficult to separate the symptoms of a diseased retained remnant *per se* from its association with common duct calculi. The retained diseased component frequently manifested itself as a choledochal or pancreatic complication. Only then did it become apparent that the initial procedure had been incomplete. In the treatment of gallbladder remnants, therefore, it is not sufficient to explore just the gallbladder bed; one must be prepared to do the complete choledochal toilet.

CYSTIC DUCT NEUROMAS

In about one-third of the patients with gallbladder remnants of the cystic duct variety, periductal neuromas are identified. These have been cited as an explanation for typical "biliary symptoms" in the presence of a normal extrahepatic biliary tree. The entity was given credence in six cases reported by Womack and Cryder (640) in 1947 in which patients were symptomatically relieved by resection of the neuroma. Since then, the point of view has been that neuromas form in all cases in which the cystic duct is adequately mobilized. It is not a pathologic entity that can be viewed as the cause of PCS. Nevertheless, occasional reports cite patients cured of PCS by resection of the neuroma. Zeff *et al.* (644) state that fewer than 20 cases of amputation neuroma have been reported

FIG. 8-5. Pneumocholangiogram. This patient had had a "difficult" cholecystectomy many years ago and presented again with cholangitis and this film. A coned-down view of the right upper quadrant demonstrates air in the biliary tree outlining the entire common bile duct **(CBD)** and the hepatic radicles—a spontaneous pneumocholangiogram. There are calculi in the left hepatic duct **(arrow)**. At operation there was a fistula between a gallbladder remnant and the duodenum.

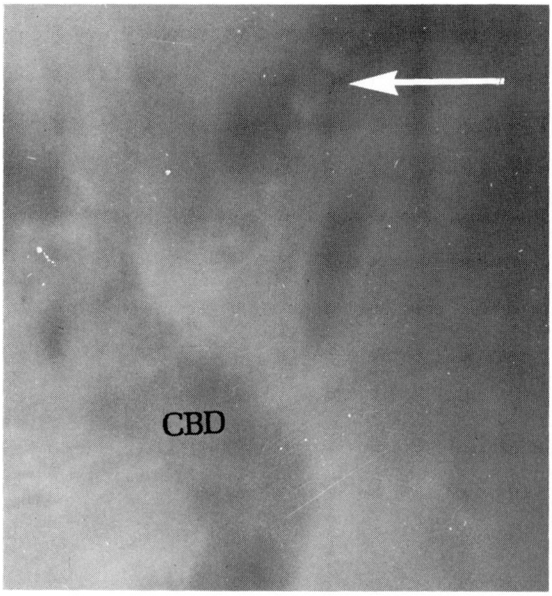

since 1931. In a case reported by Comfort and Walters (140), two neuromas, because of their position, caused common duct obstruction with intermittent jaundice.

In the MHMC experience, only one patient has ever been operated upon for cystic duct neuroma, which occurred in association with a long cystic duct stump containing a calculus. It is likely that improvement of the patient's condition was due more to the revision of the stump and removal of the stone than to resection of the neuroma (Fig. 8-6).

One should not submit symptomatic patients with normal extrahepatic biliary trees to exploration in the hope of being able to find a neuroma that can be amputated to give relief (123). The diagnosis is too uncertain and the supratentorial overlay is often unappreciated. The peri-remnant reaction may be to the suture material, to an inflammatory process, to retained stones, or to all three. Foreign body granulomas caused by silk were found in 11 of the 24 cases reported by Larmi (349). Identical findings have been encountered in patients who are completely asymptomatic. An "amputation stump" neuroma is not, of itself, a cause of symptoms.

CLINICAL ATTITUDES

In the MHMC experience, there were 20 patients with cystic duct remnants, all female; one patient was well for 25 years before be-

FIG. 8-6. Periductal neuroma. **A.** The resected gallbladder remnant exhibits a severe acute and chronic inflammatory reaction. **B.** Microscopic section shows a greatly thickened wall with an acute and chronic inflammatory reaction and deeply situated glands. A neuroma **(arrow)** was incidentally identified.

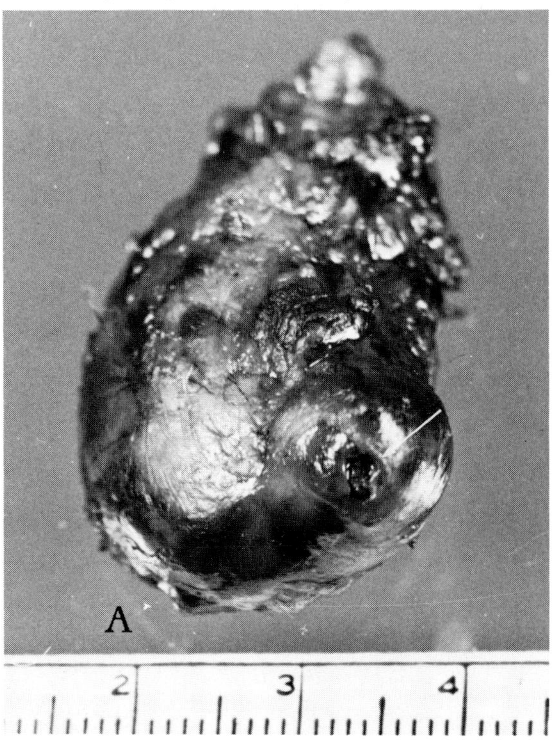

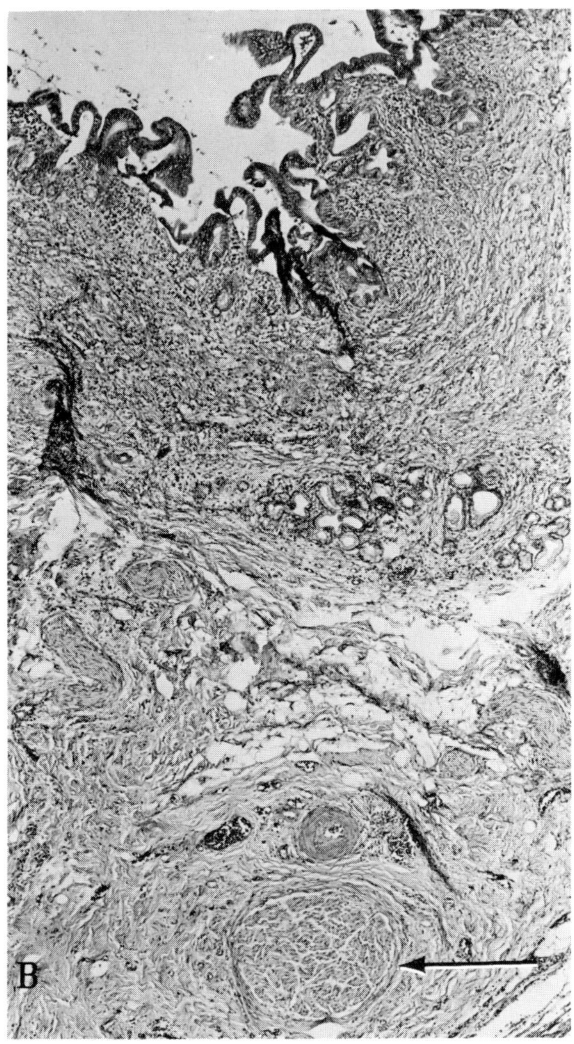

coming jaundiced. Another had never been relieved of symptoms. Although the predominant symptom is pain in 75%, jaundice occurred in 50% and chills and fever in 25%. For those patients whose sole symptom is pain, the diagnosis of noncalculous remnant disease can be adequately, though hesitantly, accepted as the cause of symptoms. However, when the patient has jaundice with chills and fever, there is a strong likelihood that the true cause is a common duct stone, either primary or one that passed from the "quarry" that is the gallbladder remnant.

The practical fact is that the patient with persistent postoperative symptoms should be investigated for the possibility of a correctable anatomic defect. Cholesterol crystals and calcium bilirubinate can be demonstrated on duodenal drainage (Lyons-Meltzer) (M-21) when the source is in the cystic duct remnant harboring a stone.

The roentgen study is best initiated by the

FIG. 8-7. Left-sided duct remnant. **A.** Cholangiogram demonstrates unusual type of cystic duct remnant disease. The huge dilated cystic duct has a left-sided entrance **(arrow).** It is virtually packed with faceted calculi extending along left side of the common bile duct. **B.** T-tube cholangiogram shows a radiopaque stone in the biliary conduit **(arrow).** In the operating room it can be frustrating to the operator to seek such a stone in the common bile duct without finding it, and then to perform an unrewarding duodenotomy and sphincterotomy. He then assumes that the stone has passed. An oblique or lateral view is required to demonstrate that this is in a left-sided cystic duct and not in the common bile duct.

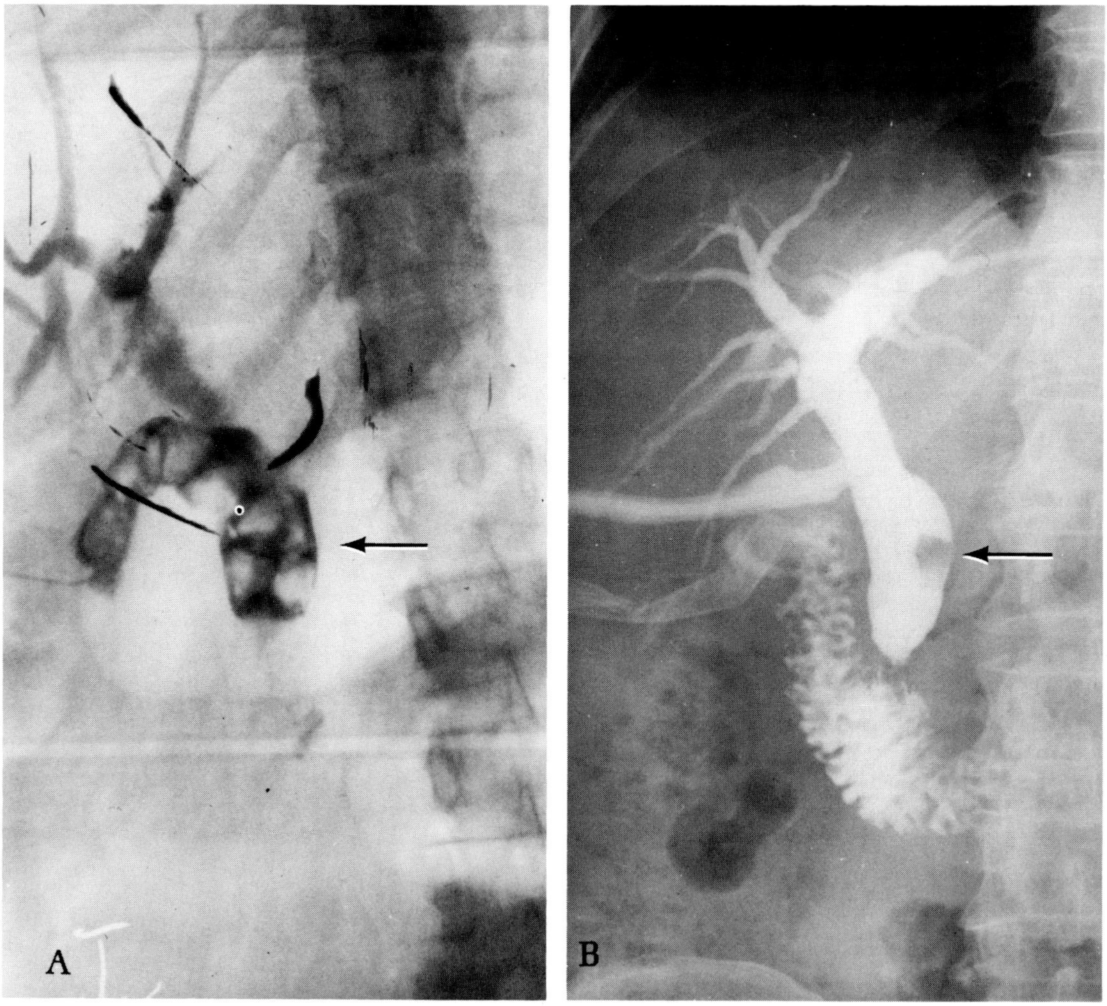

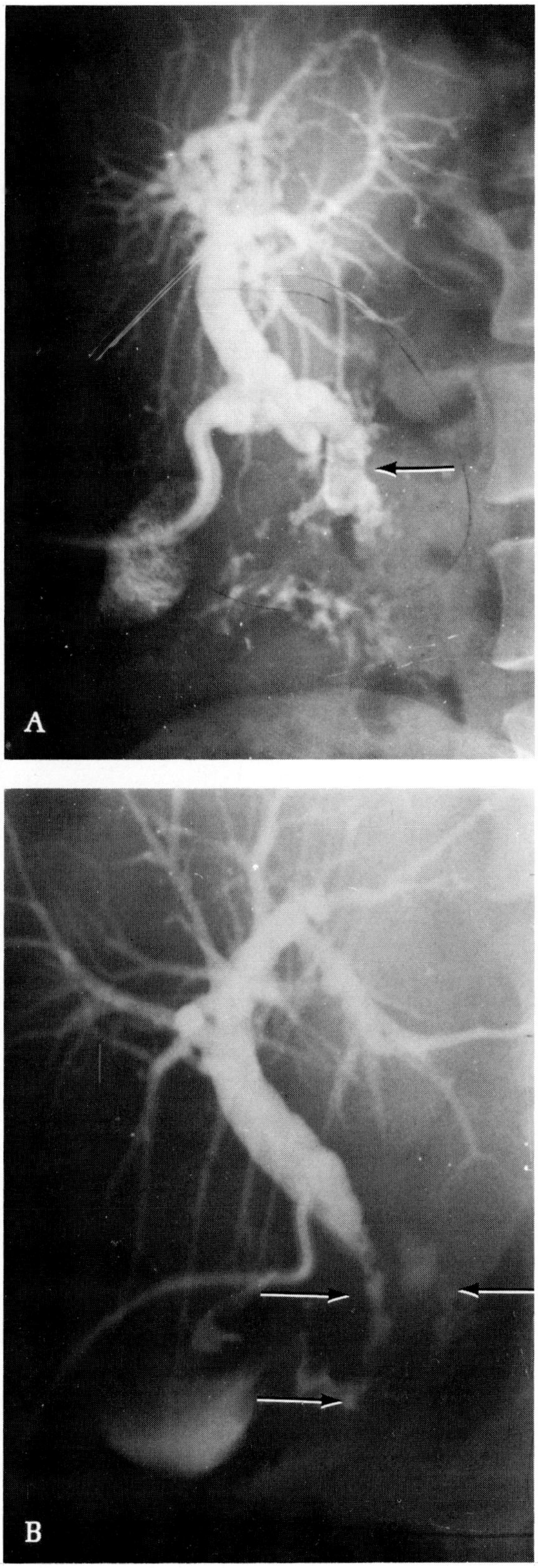

FIG. 8-8. Pseudo-cystic duct calculi. **A.** T-tube cholangiogram of a female patient who was to have a third exploration of the common bile duct for presumed retained stones believed to be in a left-sided gallbladder remnant **(arrow).** She complained of constant severe back pain. **B.** An oblique view shows that the calcifications are in the head of the pancreas **(arrow at right).** The irregularity of the transpancreatic portion of the choledochus **(arrows at left)** is due to the associated chronic alcoholic pancreatitis. There is no biliary calculus disease.

intravenous route because it facilitates mapping the entire ductal system. Only the film that visualizes is of value (509). However, certain contours are specifically required to demonstrate a gallbladder remnant (Fig. 8-7). Oblique and lateral views are necessary to avoid overlapping of the two structures (Fig. 8-8). A false-negative examination results when a stone or cystic duct stricture excludes the contrast from visualizing the proximal segment. This was the finding in slightly fewer than half the cases in the MHMC series. Stones retained in the parallel segment may encroach upon the lumen of the choledochus, which is otherwise normal.

There is no more satisfactory medical regimen for the management of this entity than there is for chronic calculous cholecystitis. The indications for reoperative surgery in the interval situation are identical with those of the primary disorder: pain, infection, obstruction. An asymptomatic remnant does not require excision.

9 Retained and Recurrent Common Duct Stones

Statistically the most frequent indication for surgery in PCS is retained and recurrent common duct stones (40, 182, 225, 227, 283, 370). Five representative clinics, with an experience of 16,700 patients, treated by some of the surgeons who have written extensively on biliary surgery, report that their incidence of retained stones averages 4.3%. This percentage was obtained by those with outstanding surgical expertise. A less sophisticated figure, from a review only of postoperative cholangiograms at three hospitals, showed retained stones in 14% of cases (182,266).

Now that extractional procedures are possible, the number of cases coming to the fore is surprising. With this second-stage confessional available, there is less embarrassment concerning the problem.

Retained and recurrent stones that are producing symptoms are the most clearly definitely correctable entity in the entire symptom complex.

PRIMARY OR SECONDARY CALCULI

All types of stones present after biliary surgery are referred to here as secondary or residual calculi. One must be diagnostically alert to the type of residual stone. The difference between retained and re-formed common duct stones is one of genesis, prognosis, and management. This distinction is of more than purely academic interest.

The residual stone is one that was formed in the gallbladder and passed into the common bile duct and was overlooked at the initial operation. These calculi are distinctly contoured, geometrically well defined, and are often faceted. The majority contain a predominant cholesterol or calcium component.

Re-formed stones arise *de novo* in the ductal system, independent of the gallbladder. They may or may not have been present at the former operation. These primary common duct stones are readily identified because they are amorphous, brittle, ill-defined clumps of mud, silt, or pigmented stasis calculi. They crumble easily and bear a contour relation to the duct. These stones do not contain calcium (Fig. 9-1). Because these primary stones are a response to stagnation in the bile ducts, their removal is not sufficient to manage the problem. The stasis must be corrected at the same procedure (142, 291). This requires the identification and correction of the mechanical block in the biliary outflow tract that is their progenitor. In patients with long-standing disease, the common bile duct is found to harbor calculi of both types. The stasis is initiated by faceted calculi that have obturated the choledochoduodenal junction sufficiently to result in impaired drainage. Madden's review (381) of 107 cases of choledocholithiasis found that in 56.1% the stones were of the primary type alone, and in 6.6%, they were both primary and secondary.

Certain common duct stones developing after operation appear to have their genesis in suture material. Clinical case reports indicate that duct stones can form about a foreign body in 1 week. Fine particulate matter can form in days. One should suspect a foreign body as the nidus of a stone if it has an unusual shape, is situated in an unusual site, or is within an abscess. Turner (594) has encountered catgut embedded in the center of ductal stones. This is unusual.

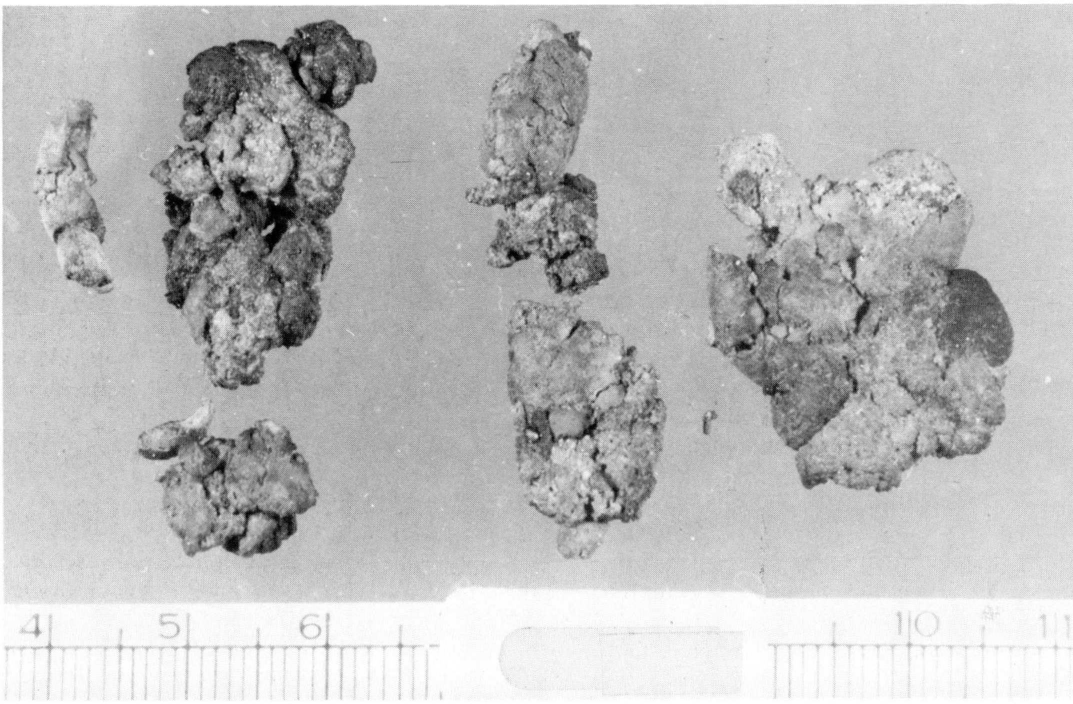

FIG. 9-1. Stasis concretions. Primary common bile duct stones formed in response to stasis have several characteristics: they contain no calcium, crumble easily, and are not faceted.

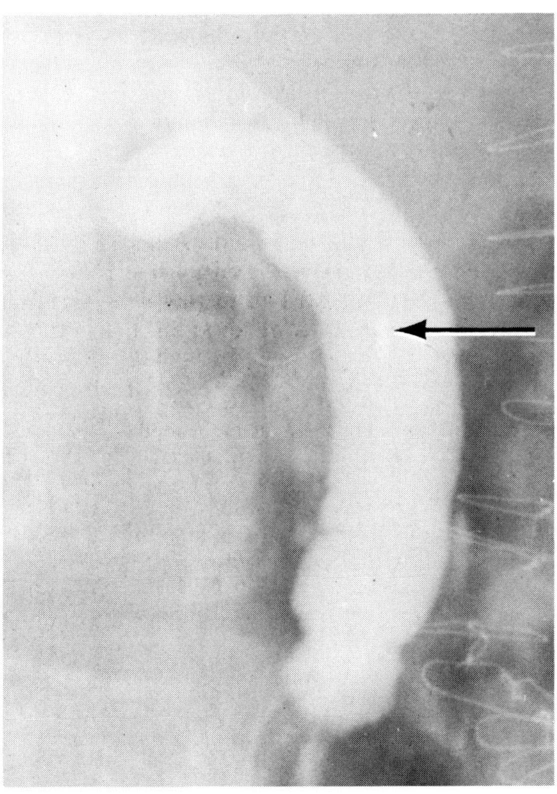

FIG. 9-2. Foreign body in the common bile duct. The use of metallic clips for ligation of deeply placed vessels has greatly facilitated management of hilar structures. They have been used very effectively and in many ways have facilitated this aspect of cholecystectomy. A unique incident was the passage of a clip into the common duct **(arrow).** It has been my policy not to use a clip on the cystic duct for fear that one may sequestrate into the lumen. I do not hesitate to use the clip on the cystic artery.

Ahleberg (8), Silvennoinen and Asp (563), and Millbourn (421) have each reported on these experiences. Larmi (349) has reported finding silk as the nidus of a stone that caused obstructive symptoms in the second postoperative week. He cites references for eight reports of suture-nidus calculi. The precautionary measures called for by these experiences are obvious. There is little advantage to the use of nonabsorbable sutures in cholecystectomy, common duct exploration, or biliary enteric anastomosis (Fig. 9-2).

Residual stones are the consequence of an inadequate biliary cleanout. Insofar as information could be obtained, it appears that the common duct was not opened in about half the cases. When the common duct was explored, no cholangiogram was done in the great majority, and in the remainder various errors in the cholangiographic technique could be retrospectively implicated. In some few cases the stone could not be extracted, and was knowingly left behind.

The commonest error is the failure to investigate the common duct. It is the task of the first operation to identify the common duct and to investigate it in the presence of dilatation, a history of jaundice or cholangitis, or a palpable abnormality. If the indications for direct common duct exploration are borderline, a cystic duct cholangiogram will resolve the intraoperative indecision.

The prior cholangiogram may prove to be a technically poor film, the density of the contrast material may be excessive, or the film may have been misinterpreted because of failure to appreciate a lack of lobar segmental opacification or there has been an erroneous interpretation of the densities in the opacified column.

CLINICAL BEHAVIOR OF RETAINED CALCULI

Stones in the common bile duct have the same pathogenic potental whether or not the gallbladder is present. It is a fact, repeatedly confirmed, that stone disease in the duct may be clinically totally silent, even when there is progressive dilation of the bile radicles and great thickening of the duct wall. Thus, in Weitz's series (621), 50% of cases of residual stone disease had been present for 8 or more years. In this regard the unpredictable temporal factor in ductal stone disease exactly parallels the situation in the gallbladder. There is no way of predicting whether or when the stone harborer will become "sick." One has to distinguish between stones as a pathological fact, and as a disease-provoker (Fig. 9-3).

Monge (429) found that the median period of relief for patients with retained stones was 2 years, with the interval varying from 1 week to 30 years. Such data are of no value for the particular patient except insofar as the range reported means that there are no time limits as to when the problem may present.

Certain of the stones that are left behind after common duct exploration assume positions that result from intraductal manipulation. This pertains to stones in the tertiary radicles, especially on the right. Stones are rarely encountered in this site in the unmanipulated situation. I have assumed that they are thus positioned by flushing and are maintained in areas of cholangitis. For it is probable that they would otherwise be flushed down by the liver.

Best's figure of hepatic duct stones occurring in 7.4% of cases of cholelithiasis (59) is higher than that in the MHMC experience, but one has to differentiate between hepatic duct stones as part of general choledocholithiasis and hepatic duct stasis calculi in intrahepatic duct disease. On the flat film, the differentiation of hepatic calcifications requires a consideration of hemangiomas, the calcified rim of amebic abscess, the laminated cyst wall of hydatid disease, metastatic calcified carcinoma, and calcified gramulomas.

The true liver stone in Western society is the consequence of duct stricture, metabolic disease, or congenital anomalies (388). The patients suffer colic during stone migration. Bove (79) reviewed 20 cases in 1963 and commented on the indication for hepatic lobotomy or lobectomy when the stones cause abscess. In this condition, new hepatic stones form in 3–24 months. Fine bile aggregates, differing from stones only in size, can form in days.

Truly impacted stones producing total obstruction in the sphincter area—as distinct from the suprasphincteric zone—are rarely encountered spontaneously. They have been jammed into this position and are held there by the circular component of the choledochal sphincter. In the imperfectly clarified situation, persistent total obstruction is less commonly due to stone than to a tumor of the periampullary area or head of the pancreas.

A review of previous films makes it apparent that calculi can assume varying positions in the duct. In the MHMC series a distally impacted suprasphincteric stone has been encountered as a cause of obstructive jaundice in cases in which it was the only stone in the common bile duct.

In one-third to one-half of instances, only a single stone is retained. In half those instances it is incarcerated in the suprasphinc-

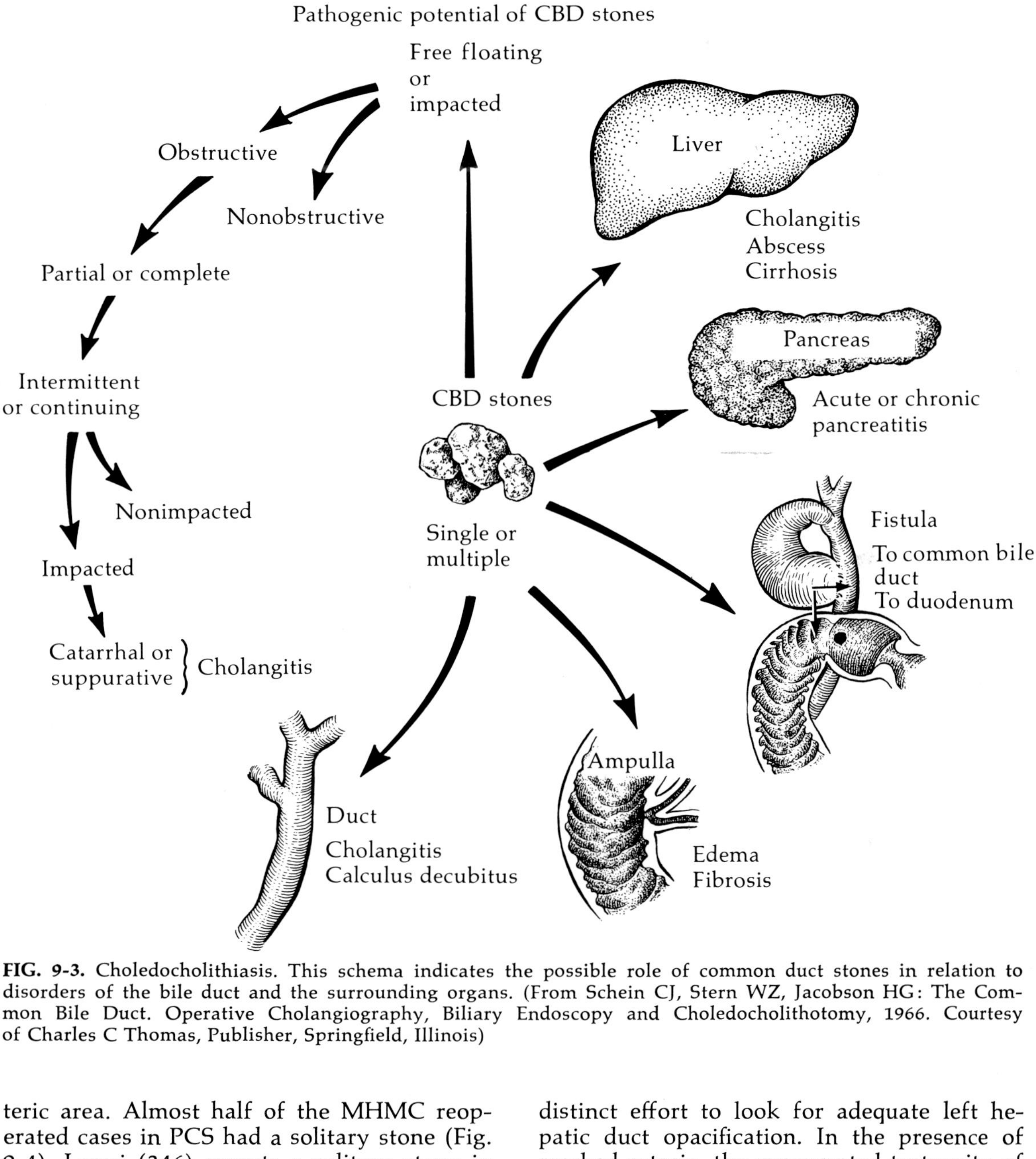

FIG. 9-3. Choledocholithiasis. This schema indicates the possible role of common duct stones in relation to disorders of the bile duct and the surrounding organs. (From Schein CJ, Stern WZ, Jacobson HG: The Common Bile Duct. Operative Cholangiography, Biliary Endoscopy and Choledocholithotomy, 1966. Courtesy of Charles C Thomas, Publisher, Springfield, Illinois)

teric area. Almost half of the MHMC reoperated cases in PCS had a solitary stone (Fig. 9-4). Larmi (346) reports a solitary stone in 6 of 13 residual stone problems. It is possible that, in many instances, an impacted stone is often less a spontaneous pathologic fact than it is an iatrogenic phenomenon that is the sequel to probing and ductal exploration.

The solitary retained stone has also been found incarcerated in the orifice of the left hepatic duct. It can be overlooked on the cholangiogram unless the viewer makes a distinct effort to look for adequate left hepatic duct opacification. In the presence of marked ectasia, the exaggerated tortuosity of the right ductal system may obfuscate the fact that the left hepatic duct has not been opacified. A solitary round stone is also a common finding in the gallbladder remnant; it frequently fits snugly into the thickened wall and may partially protrude into the common duct lumen (Fig. 9-5).

Patients with secondary stones have presented in these ways:

1. No symptoms. The stone is noted on a postoperative T-tube cholangiogram.

2. Cholangitis. These patients have chills, fever, and later jaundice. The interval between these secondary symptoms and the initial cholecystectomy has often been so long that the diagnosis was made late and then only in the course of the investigation of a fever of obscure origin. Some of these patients present with gram-negative sepsis. Rarely, a patient has been seen with advanced biliary cirrhosis secondary to a forgotten operation. It is amazing that some patients tolerate minor symptoms for many years and present for treatment with the advanced secondary hepatic disorder.

FIG. 9-4. Suprasphincteric choledocholithiasis. Transhepatic cholangiogram obtained in a 73-year-old male patient who had had a cholecystectomy 30 years before. He was admitted for jaundice complicated by cholangitis. The common bile duct is greatly dilated and is partially obstructed by a suprasphincteric round stone **(a)**. There is a large, dilated, left-sided-entrance type of cystic duct **(b)**, which is also obstructed by this stone. The patient was managed by choledocholithotomy and supraduodenal choledochoduodenostomy. Infection and obstruction are indications for prompt, totally corrective surgery.

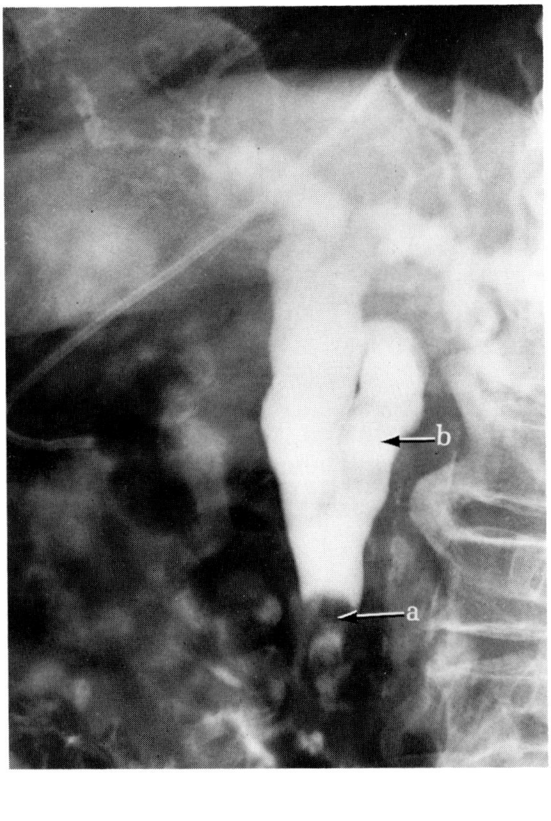

3. Recurrent colic. The patient recognizes that the abdominal pain pattern is similar to what had been the indication for the first procedure.

4. Jaundice. The differential diagnosis often entails a serious consideration of cancer in the biliary–pancreatic tract.

5. Persistent upper abdominal pain and dyspepsia. These patients were previously investigated roentgenographically. Residual stones were present, but they were not always specifically related to the symptoms that stimulated the investigation. The stones can be an incidental finding.

In the series reported by Raymer *et al.* (491), about half the patients with residual stones were jaundiced, 11% had pancreatitis, and 13% had associated gallbladder remnants. These are the usually quoted incidences of complications for patients with previous unoperated choledocholithiasis (41).

This experience has warranted a high degree of suspicion that the patient who has had gallbladder surgery may eventually present again with symptoms originating in an imperfect posthepatic excretory canal. A vigorous diagnostic approach based on this premise has proved rewarding. This has been especially true in those patients with jaundice or sepsis.

These statistics are prejudiced because they do not include the frequency of stone disease in the totally asymptomatic PCS patient. In the absence of symptoms, there would be little reason to investigate this possibility. Such data can only be retrospectively obtained from postmortem statistics.

It is necessary to distinguish choledocholithiasis as a roentgen finding from its role as the cause of clinically definable symptoms. This is simply an analog applied to the ductal system that is recognized as pertinent to the cholelithiasis.

It would be virtually impossible to "sanitize" the nation of all its gallstone-bearers, and it would be quite unnecessary. In the same way 15–20% of common duct stones are silent by the usual clinical diagnostic techniques and go undetected. It appears that common duct stones are less likely to remain silent if the reservoir function of the gallbladder has been eliminated by cholecystectomy or irreversible cystic duct obstruction.

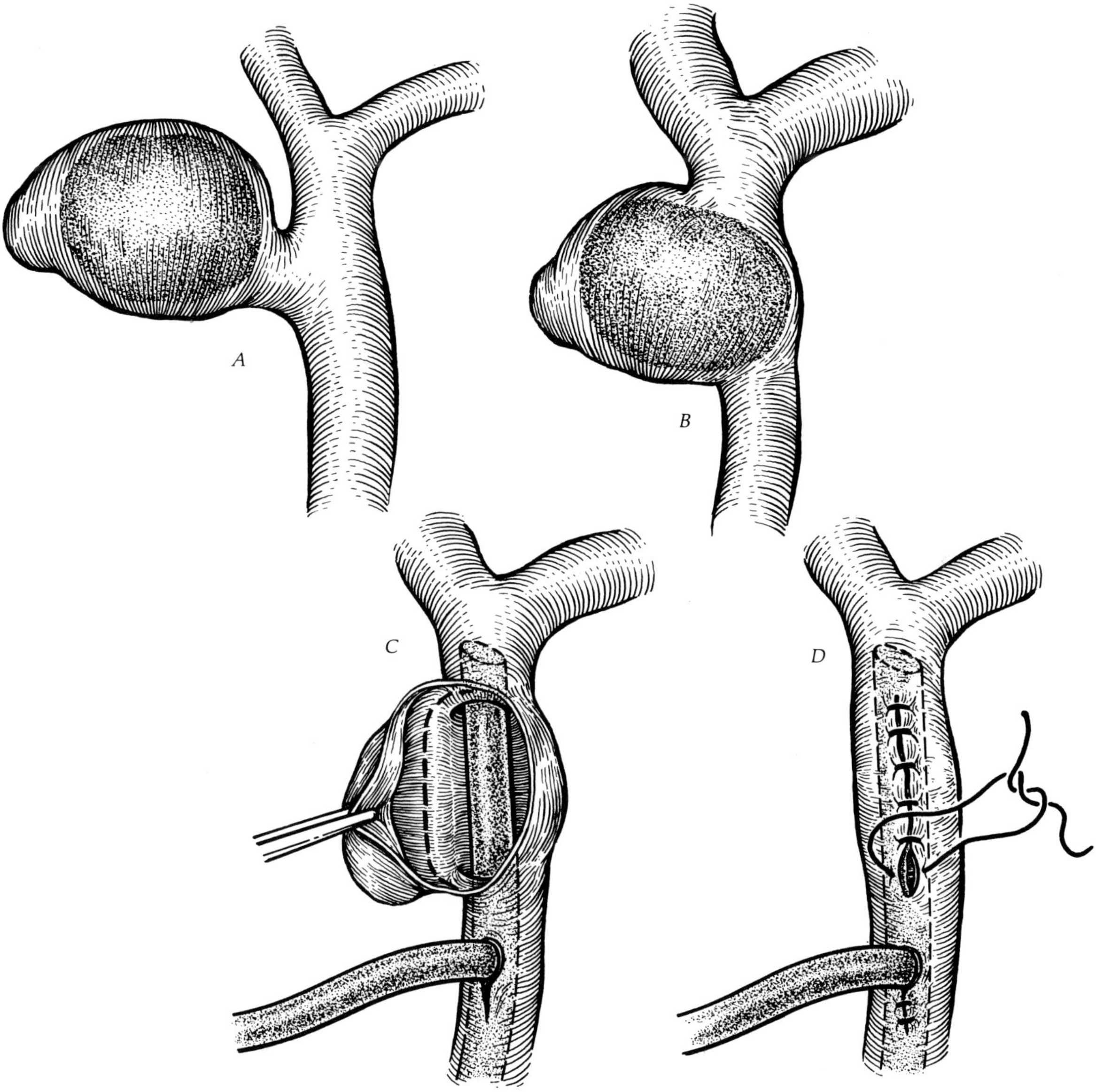

FIG. 9-5. Effaced cystic duct with confluent stone. The example of the confluent stone can be encountered in the previously unoperated situation or as part of gallbladder remnant disease. **A.** The small remnant contracts about the stone and encases it as the shell does an egg. **B.** The cystic duct becomes effaced, and the stone protrudes into and obstructs the common bile duct. This can be a difficult surgical problem. The common bile duct can be divided before the anatomy is clear. **C.** When the situation is suspected, it is safest to open the gallbladder and remove the stone, leaving in a cholecytostomy tube. **D.** It is better if the diseased organ is subtotally resected and a broad diverticulum-like closure of the duct secured over a T tube.

The stones are regarded as likely to be contributing to symptoms if the common duct is wider than 1.4 cm, if the stones are of primary type, if the serum bilirubin or alkaline phosphatase is elevated, or if the liver biopsy demonstrates bile stasis or cholangitis.

A stone can be regarded as innocent when there is no colic, infection, or obstruction. This concept carries the caveat that there is no absolute parallelism there between the morphologic pathology and the clinical syndrome. The former may be subliminally progressive with only minor symptoms and relatively unremarkable changes in the serum hepatic profile. Retrospectively, the two patients in the MHMC series who presented with advanced biliary cirrhosis due to secondary choledocholithiasis where only relatively asymptomatic; they had regarded their symptoms as trivial until they became septic (555).

ANATOMY OF THE RETAINED COMMON DUCT STONE

1. Twenty-two percent were associated with gallbladder remnants that contained stones.

2. Thirty-five percent were considered to be of the primary type.

3. Fifty percent were solitary.

4. In only a rare instance was a stone encountered in a duct smaller than 1 cm in diameter. It was formerly believed that this never occurred, but several recent experiences have demonstrated this association, although it is relatively uncommon.

5. Intrahepatic duct dilatation was present in all instances in which the clinical course suggested that the stone had been present for 3 or more months. This did not apply to instances in which a proximal draining T-tube was *in situ*.

SPONTANEOUS PASSAGE

The most important consideration relating to the retained common duct stone has to do with the possibility of spontaneous passage. Millbourn's studies (426) evaluated spontaneous passage by stool straining. On that examination, stones could be identified in 23% of 284 cases. When that examination was done several times the yield became 36%. On truly diligent search, it gets to be 50%. With the sophisticated methods now in use, this little-employed simple technique has fallen into disuse. Bakes (33) used it in the 1920's to evaluate the effect of dilatation of the papilla, and Acosta *et al.* (2) recently revived it as a way of documenting stone passage in gallstone-associated pancreatitis. Millbourn (427) anticipated the findings of Acosta *et al.* (2) in his observation that patients with pancreatitis passed stones more frequently than did those without this affection. The greatest fecal yield is 4 days after the clinical event of pain, icterus, or hyperamylasemia.

Spontaneous passage can be totally curative. More than half the cases Millbourn followed for 2–13 years remained asymptomatic (427). Spontaneous passage between time of diagnosis and surgery may account for certain negative explorations. It is not possible to document its absolute or even relative frequency (456). In 1941, Millbourn (426) commented that spontaneous passage is much more common than had been assumed. It can be anticipated in about half the patients whose residual stones are less than 7 mm in diameter. Bodvall (70) reports that of 71 patients who left the hospital with the last cholangiogram showing residual stones in the duct, later cholangiography or autopsy showed that these stones had spontaneously disappeared from 32. Bodvall cites the interesting statistic that stones were left behind more frequently during reoperations than in primary choledocholithotomies (70). Silent stones have been found at autopsy in patients known to have had them for 2.5–13 years. Anderson *et al.* (19) noted spontaneous passage in 37% of 80 cases. This supports an alternative to the attitude expressed by Smith *et al.* in 1963 (568) that "once the diagnosis was established with reasonable certainty, reexploration is generally indicated."

The passing of stones has been observed in 14 cases in the MHMC series. The initial diagnosis of residual calculus was made on a postoperative T-tube cholangiogram. X-ray studies done at 3-week intervals demonstrated a stone-free duct. It is assumed that these stones passed into the duodenum (Fig. 9-6). In some instances of stone passage, the exit is not through the normal distal end of the common bile duct, but because of the stone size, it is assumed to have been through a fistula between the suprasphincteric portion of the choledochus and the duodenum.

As early as 1892 Naunyn (441) had noted that the spontaneous disappearance of jaundice in choledocholithiasis could follow the formation of a choledochoduodenal fistula, yet this is rarely seen at autopsy. However, with the introduction of ERCP these choledochal fistulas have been recognized more frequently. Ikeda and Okada (289) have located the orifice of the fistula orad to the duodenal papilla. A large stone was actually observed in one fistula. The fistula formation is due to a stone small enough to enter the intramural portion of the common bile duct but not small enough to pass through the duodenal papilla. It impacts intramurally and ulcerates the choledochal wall into the contiguous duodenum. It is possible that some instances of presumed sphincter ampullary incompetence with a pneumocholangiogram are actually instances of fistulous erosion. The endoscopic recognition of this entity in 20 of 146 patients with cholelithiasis who were subject to duodenal endoscopy has suggested that this type of fistula may be much more common than has been appreciated.

Another type of fistula is caused by a somewhat larger stone—too large to enter the intramural portion of the common bile duct. It can become impacted in the distal portion of extramural portion of the common bile duct. In this position it ulcerates and creates a fistula not on the longitudinal fold of the duodenum, but through that part of the duodenum adjacent to the extraduodenal portion of the common bile duct. Larger stones can pass through it. Ikeda and Okada (289) refer to the former as type I and to the latter as type II fistulas. Stones were not visualized in patients with type II fistula, for it is assumed that calculi as large as $4.2 \times 2.6 \times 2.5$ cm could be passed by this route. In contrast, stones are still visualized endoscopically in patients with type I fistulas.

Spontaneous passage may be realistically anticipated under the following circumstances:

1. The calculi are not larger than 7 mm.

2. The Vaterian segment is open as indicated by manometric demonstration of a passage pressure not greater than 13 cm H_2O.

3. There is no ductal stasis, sharp angulation, or narrowing in the transpancreatic segment.

4. The duct lumen is less than 1.4 cm. Ducts of this size are rarely the seat of choledochoduodenal junction stenosis, such as would not allow for stone passage.

The asymptomatic patient with normal liver chemistry may be managed without operation in these circumstances for as long as the condition remains stationary. These patients have gross anatomic disease without pathologic symptoms.

Contrariwise, spontaneous passage cannot ordinarily be expected in the following circumstances:

1. The calculi are 10 mm in size, especially if they are faceted or multiple.

2. The Vaterian segment is obstructed, as indicated by elevated passage pressure and marked ductal ectasia.

3. The common duct shows the effects of encroaching pancreatic disease.

Patients in this category are unlikely to be or to long remain asymptomatic. They present with the complications of jaundice, sepsis, or colic. In these circumstances, it is best either to correct the ductal toilet prophylactically in anticipation of these complications or to act promptly when they appear.

For clinical situations between these extremes one relies on a comparative evaluation of each of these separate factors. A trial of "labor" can be undertaken in the asymptomatic patient or the one who has a proximally decompressing T-tube.

A calculus sometimes becomes embedded in the duct wall and contours a defect that becomes a diverticulum. This development has been encountered in the MHMC series three times: once at the bifurcation of the major hepatic ducts, where the stone extruded through the septum; and twice in the suprasphincteric area. Kune (340) reported two instances of stones in a diverticulum of the lower common bile duct directly cephalad to its intramural segment.

A basic precaution is required: The pseudocalculus sign in the Vaterian segment is a fact in cholangiography, and its misinterpretation can lead to the erroneous diagnosis of a retained calculus. In a confusing situation, the final differentiation can always be made by repeat timed cholangiography or endoscopy.

In the MHMC series there were two patients who had already undergone a second common-duct exploration for presumed retained stone seen on T-tube cholangiography. One patient died after the operation, of a myocardial infarct. There were no bile duct stones. Both patients had a pseudocalculus sign.

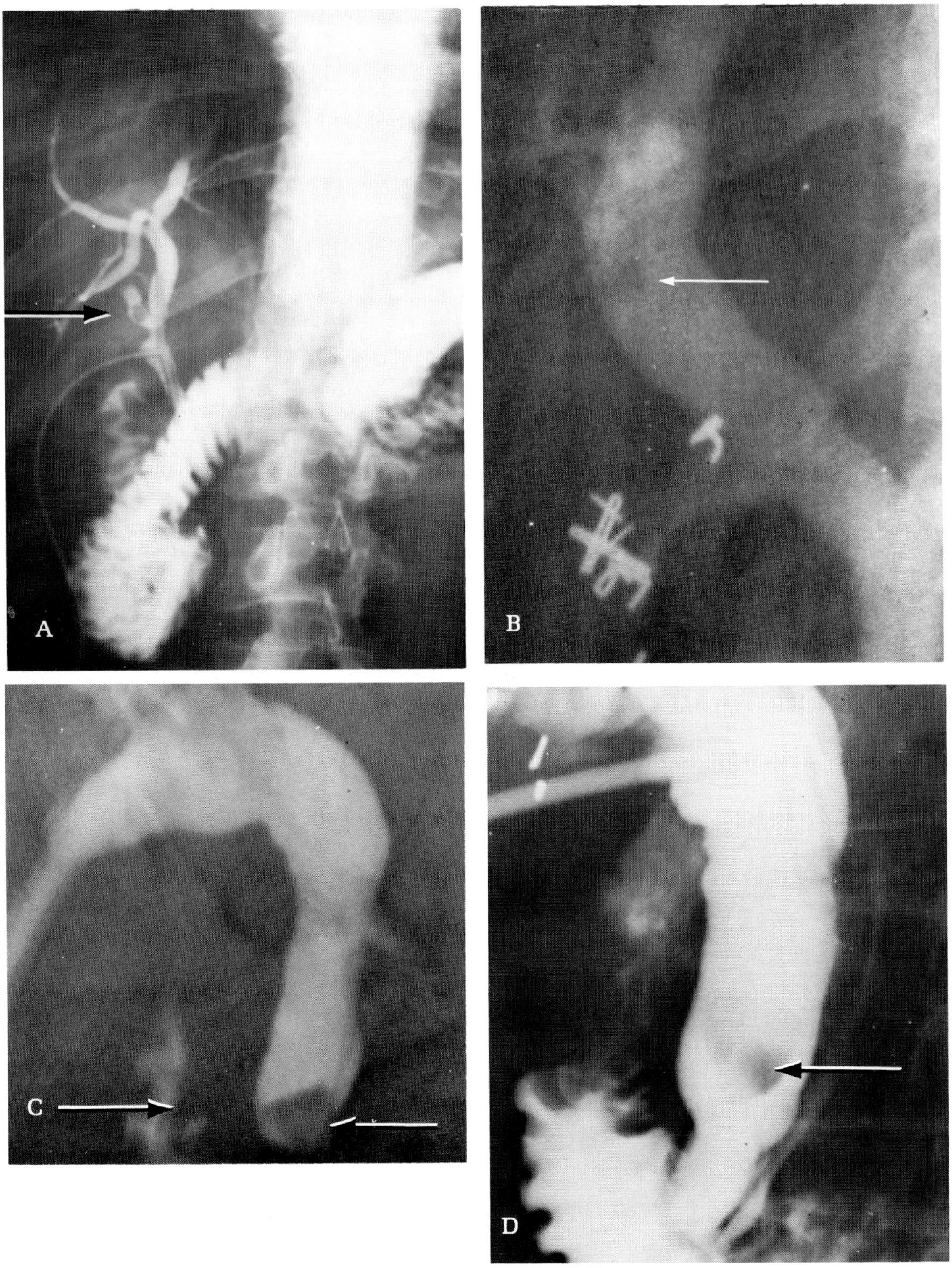
A
B
C
D

◀ **FIG. 9-6.** Spontaneous passage. **A.** Intraoperative T-tube cholangiogram shows a stone in the cystic duct remnant **(arrow)**. The cystic duct had been tied off above this stone. The surgeon had failed to establish that the retained cystic-duct segment was patent. The patient became symptomatic after a bout of colic. A subsequent intravenous cholangiogram was normal, and the stone is assumed to have passed. The size of the stone is a critical factor in determining the possibility of spontaneous passage. **B.** Intravenous cholangiogram of a symptomatic patient reveals a stone in the common bile duct **(arrow)**. It can be assumed that this size stone will pass spontaneously, but the patient may not be relieved of biliary symptoms because the common bile duct is significantly dilated. However, the time–density factor is normal, indicating that there is no choledochoduodenal junctional stenosis. It is assumed that the dilatation observed in this instance is the innocent residuum of antecedent calculus disease. **C.** T-tube cholangiogram shows a retained distal stone **(arrow at left)** in a dilated common bile duct. Note contrast material in the duodenum **(arrow at right)**. The T tube was clamped. Ten days later the stone could not be demonstrated. **D.** Spontaneous passage is unpredictable. In this cholangiogram, a large faceted stone **(arrow)** had been left behind. It was anticipated that basket removal would be required. On the day that the procedure was to be performed, another cholangiogram revealed that the stone was no longer in the duct.

EXPERIMENTAL AND CLINICAL BASIS FOR FACILITATING THE PASSAGE OF COMMON DUCT STONES

1. Sympathetic nerve blocks at the paravertebral level or by spinal or epidural level do not affect the motor activity of the sphincter or its resistance to perfusate.

2. It is established that dog bile will reduce the size of the human gallstones placed in the dog gallbladder.

3. There is no agent that will consistently, permanently, and with total safety dissolve or cause disintegration of *in situ* gallstones in a reasonable length of time. This refers to ox bile, dog bile, sodium taurocholate, caroid, papain, acetic acid and solution G, heparin, and bile acids.

4. Vagotomy at the level of the hepatic plexus will decrease the resistance of the choledochal sphincter. A similar effect has been demonstrated experimentally in the dog with intravenous isoproterenol (159). This beta-adrenergic blocker consistently produced a 35% decrease in resistance and facilitated the passage of experimentally simulated calculi. Simulated stones (metal pellets) in the common bile duct could be made to pass under controlled conditions by a pressure of 280 mm Hg. With beta stimulation this could, on the average, be accomplished at 45% of this pressure.

5. The vapor effect of ether has been employed to produce a gaseous distention within the duct, in the expectation that the stone will then pass through the distended sphincter area. It is not safe.

6. Chemical agents that have been employed have been based on the principle of promoting solubility of the stone's constituents. These include chloroform, alcohol, versine, heparin, and chenodeoxycholic acid.

7. The Vaterian segment may be dilated by passing a catheter through the established T-tube drainage sinus, through the bile duct into the duodenum. This is done with the hope that the stone will pass through the open sphincter.

Each of these methods has been reported to be successful in particular cases. None work consistently.

A decision concerning management of secondary stones with T-tube *in situ* requires the following steps:

1. Confirmation of the diagnosis 3 days after initial demonstration.

2. Determining whether the stone or the sphincter is causing ductal hypertension (a simple spinal tap manometer is adequate to determine the residual pressure in the common duct).

3. Clinical trial of T-tube clamping.

4. Looking for the unfavorable signs of chills, fever, pain, excessive drainage, or elevation of pertinent laboratory values (serum bilirubin, amylase, SGOT, and alkaline phosphatase). Any of these abnormalities suggest that conservative management will not be effective.

If the patient tolerates the clamping, there is no urgency about removing the stone, and the patient can be discharged with the T-tube in. The T-tube can be efficiently plugged with a golf tee.

Depending upon the general status of the patient, one may, after a 4- to 6-week period, redo the T-tube studies. Six alternatives are outlined in the following section.

MANAGEMENT OF RETAINED STONES WITH T TUBE IN SITU

These are the alternatives:

1. Leave the T tube in and reevaluate periodically.

2. Administer solvent instillations and perfusions.

3. Use a catheter for sphincter dilation and weekly perfusion of the duct.

4. Attempt closed extraction by basketing or (duodenoscopic papillotomy).

5. Remove the T tube and a) observe without treatment, or b) administer chenodeoxycholic acid.

6. Reoperate.

With proximal venting there is only a rare indication for urgent surgery; the tube can be left in for months. In this regard, it is wise routinely to use the guttered T tube rather than one with the full cylinder. The latter has no advantage and becomes plugged by bile sludge.

The timing of the secondary procedure can be determined on the basis of the exigencies of the patient's general condition and the specific presence of electrolyte disturbances, wound problems, or ileus. One can effectively medically manage the patient with jaundice or fistula for a few weeks before surgical correction becomes imperative. One has to balance the probability of spontaneous passage or prolonged asymptomatic tolerance against the trial with solvents and perfusion techniques on the one hand, and the risks of secondary surgery on the other. There are extremes: The patient with a wide duct, small stones, and no symptoms needs nothing done. In this case, pull the tube and do intravenous cholangiography or ERCP if the patient becomes symptomatic. There are others who advise that all stones be removed. One can hardly submit to this, on an endemic basis. About 4% of people over 50 years of age in this country have common duct stones. Only some of them are symptomatic and require treatment.

If removal of the stones is deemed advisable, at this time basket extraction of stones via the well-established T-tube tract should be the first interventive approach. The time that it takes for the well-established fistula to mature also allows time for spontaneous passage. I prefer this to perfusion. The high success rate in experienced hands circumvents the need for trial of less certain methods. The practical alternatives in this situation are waiting for spontaneous passage, attempting basket extraction, and then undertaking secondary intervention when the other two approaches are inadvisable or unsuccessful. Nevertheless, there is no advantage to an unrealistic delay in the wishful thinking that the unlikely or unusual will occur to correct the complicated anatomic problem.

Longer intervals of waiting are required for the patient who had had a postoperative myocardial infarct. The corrective procedure, in the absence of obstructive signs and symptoms, can be deferred until the cardiac situation is stable.

THE REMOTE RESIDUAL STONE

On occasion, calculi are demonstrated after cholecystectomy at a time when the incision has healed and all drains have been removed. The difference between the recurrent and residual stone has been commented upon.

A review of 15 reports reveals an incidence range from 2.4% to 28%, with an average of 11.8% (335). These figures, in general, have not changed in recent years. At the Society for the Surgery of the Alimentary Tract in 1972 a review of the experience at three Syracuse hospitals in 1963–1970 revealed that 14% of 302 patients with postoperative cholangiograms had retained stones.

Waugh (614) reported his personal 6-year experience with residual stones at the Mayo Clinic as being 8%. It might parenthetically be stated that those who routinely employ intraoperative cholangiography combined with biliary endoscopy have greatly reduced the residual stone problem (447, 528, 538).

The initial operative findings and the clinical course are often deceptive because biliary fistulas may close though stones remain in the duct and almost 50% of stones produce no serum chemical abnormalities. Half the patients with stones are not and have never been jaundiced. Hicken *et al.* (226, 267) have indicated that 80% of 150 patients with residual stones were able to leave the hospital presumably well.

There is no reason to adopt one attitude toward the symptomatic individual who has had prior biliary surgery and another to the patient whose biliary tract has never been assaulted. Hughes (283) has reported that most patients known to have retained stones reappear with symptoms within 6 months to 3 years and that 50% of these return within 6 months. On the other hand, the other half do well (173). Davidson (162) reported that the asymptomatic common-duct stone played no significant role as a cause of death, but when symptomatic stones were present, they contributed to the cause of death with pancreatitis, cholangitis, abscess, and biliary cirrhosis. Symptomatic disorders require surgical correction.

In clinical practice the asymptomatic state is less common than it is in the autopsy material. The postoperative intravenous cholangiogram is ordinarily undertaken to elucidate symptoms. Hence, the discovery of a common duct stone is hard to disregard in the symptomatic patient. It is possible for a stone to be truly asymptomatic and not pathogenic if there is no duct dilation and serum values for bilirubin, alkaline phosphatase, and the flocculation and transaminase tests are normal. It is also important to evaluate the drainage of the duct by the time-density factor. An asymptomatic common duct stone under these circumstances can be managed by observation if the patient is over 60, not diabetic, and is informed and reliable so that he will seek prompt medical care for an urgent situation: obstruction or infection. Nonoperative management is suggested if there is severe cardiopulmonary or renal disease that makes surgery unusually hazardous or if the patient has a limited life expectancy.

I prefer removing all symptomatic common duct stones in patients who are under 60 because the risk of operation is acceptable and the risk of serious complications increases with age. Diabetic patients should be treated prophylactically on diagnosis because, in this group, the sequelae of the disease can be lethal, and the mortality for emergency surgery is higher than it is with any other metabolic association. In this situation, tolerance is not tempered with time (288).

Understanding residual stone disease rests, in no small part, on the problem of lithogenic bile. This is basic to the genesis of gallstones in general, but it is particularly pertinent here to the not-unreasonable question: "Can it happen again if all the stones are removed now?" The study of Pomare and Heaton (475) suggests that lithogenic bile, as determined by T-tube bile drainage analysis during and after operation, depends upon the presence of the gallbladder. Patients with lithogenic bile profile have reverted to normal after cholecystectomy.

Metzger *et al.* (424) suggest that variations in the composition of hepatic bile are such that random sampling may fail to provide the full spectrum of composition. Small's studies (567) confirm the observation that the coordinates of bile salts, phospholipid, and cholesterol values are so variable that the appearance of lithogenic bile is intermittent rather than continuous. It is, therefore, not always possible with a single determination to screen the lithogenic potential. At this time there are insufficient data regarding the efficacy of chenodeoxycholic acid in choledocholithiasis. Its use in clinical practice has yet to be defined. It appears to have no place in the patient who is already symptomatic.

Recent developments in endoduodenal surgery may alter the approach to the remote residual stone problem. Peroral transduodenal sphincterotomy and stone extraction has been successfully carried out. It remains to be established whether the complications of stricture and pancreatitis are real or theoretical (648).

10 Pancreatitis Linked to Biliary Disorders

It is difficult except in advanced cases to identify the pancreatic affection that is linked to biliary disorders as the cause of PCS. I vividly recall a visiting professor of surgery who was evaluating an obese woman with this problem. He compared palpation of this abdomen to "feeling on the roof for apples in the cellar." He diagnosed the patient as having "pancreatitis" with the comment that "it's a diagnosis that is hard to disprove, and depending upon which way her clinical course evolves, it is a reasonable way of procastinating."

Kourias and Papacharalampous (336) report that 94.2% of their cases of chronic pancreatitis are linked to biliary problems. The commonest associated causes were common duct stone and stenosing papillitis. However, the entity is uncommon and was recognized in only 4.8% of 117 patients with PCS. These figures are pertinent because alcoholism is rare in Greece, and this association can usually be confidently excluded.

In the MHMC experience with the PCS, only four instances of chronic pancreatitis associated with biliary disease could be documented—an incidence of less than 1%. The chronic pancreatitis seen in this institution is linked to alcoholism in over 98% of cases. Acute pancreatitis linked to gallstone disease has been commonly encountered, often as the presenting feature of choledocholithiasis.

The incidence varies with geography, dietary habits, and the rigidity or laxity with which diagnostic standards are applied. Rousselot *et al.* (512) have indicated that when alcoholism and biliary disease coexist, the major effect on the pancreas will be the former.

ETIOLOGIC MECHANISMS

Common Channel Regurgitation

In 1901 Opie (457) made specific comments with reference to the stone-induced, common-channel origin of acute hemmorhagic pancreatitis: 1) The ampulla (termed diverticulum) must be of adequate size. 2) The stone size must be such as to completely block the duodenal exit, but still allow for continuity of the pancreatic duct to the choledochus (see Fig. 1-5C). A large stone does not do this; it blocks all three orifices. Opie's famous case involved a 3-mm ampullary stone, without stones in the gallbladder. 3) He regarded the contractile force of the gallbladder as the motor mechanism for driving the bile into the pancreatic duct (457).

This anatomic potential is present in about 40% of patients. In the cholangiographic experience at MHMC, pancreatic duct visualization has never been associated with the patient's symptomatic recognition of the phenomenon of duct reflux. This observation suggests that instances of bile regurgitation under physiologic conditions is completely innocuous. I know of no report in which bile has actually been seen in the pancreatic duct.

The clinical situation is not analogous to the experimental induction of canine pancreatitis by the forceful injection of bile into the pancreatic duct with or without concomitant ligation of the pancreatic duct. In no single instance of pancreatic opacification during cholangiography have I observed extravasation of the contrast material into small ductules or into a pancreatic cyst, although transitory hyperamylasemia in association with pancreatic duct opacification is reported.

It has been postulated that choledochoduodenal junctional obstruction, often of an ill-defined nature, can be the equivalent of the Opie common-channel obstructing calculus and be the cause of acute and chronic pancreatitis. Such a mechanism is hard to validate, and the anatomic anlage for its possibility is less frequent than the incidence of the acute complication (193) (Fig. 10-1).

It is possible that part of the variation in the nature and incidence of the pancreatic complication is related to the anatomy of the duct of Santorini. Normally the ducts of Wirsung and Santorini communicate. Therefore, if the major pancreatic duct is blocked in the Vaterian segment, it is still possible for the patent minor duct to serve as the channel for pancreatic drainage. This minor duct is assumed to be the major channel for pancreatic drainage in about 10% of people.

Since both ducts participate in drainage of the pancreatic body, is it not possible that the induration so often encountered in the head of the pancreas is the manifestation of impaired flow through one of these drainage channels? It is not far afield to suggest that blockage of the orifice of the duct of Santorini at the minor papilla, with closure of the duodenal stump in gastrectomy is one mechanism of postgastrectomy pancreatitis.

Pancreatitis ensues if pancreatic duct obstruction precedes a potential stimulus to exocrine secretion. The obstruction at the Vaterian segment need only be inflammatory congestion and edema.

In the MHMC series, three patients with acute pancreatitis, as evidenced by obvious fat necrosis, presented after cholecystostomy in which virtually all of the bile had been fistulized. In one patient there were residual gallstones, and in the other two there were common duct stones. Bile drainage alone did not prevent acute pancreatic inflammatory disease.

FIG. 10-1. Pancreatic duct lithiasis with suppurative cholangitis. This T-tube cholangiogram was obtained in a 74-year-old male diabetic who had had no exposure to alcohol and who presented with sepsis. At operation he was found to have an emphysematous, gangrenous cholangitis with a huge intracholedochal abscess. There were numerous small primary and secondary stones in the common duct. Gas bubbled in the purulent exudate. There was diffuse hemorrhagic pancreatitis. The T-tube cholangiogram reveals **(a)** stricture of the transpancreatic portion of the common bile duct; **(b)** dilatation of the proximal choledochus and intrahepatic ducts; and **(c)** several stones in the pancreatic duct. The presence of biliary calculi in the pancreatic duct has been encountered only once in the MHMC experience. Because of the focal gangrenous changes in the common bile duct, T-tube drainage was deemed sufficient and anastomosis was regarded as hazardous. A third operative procedure—a choledochoduodenostomy—was performed when the acute episode subsided.

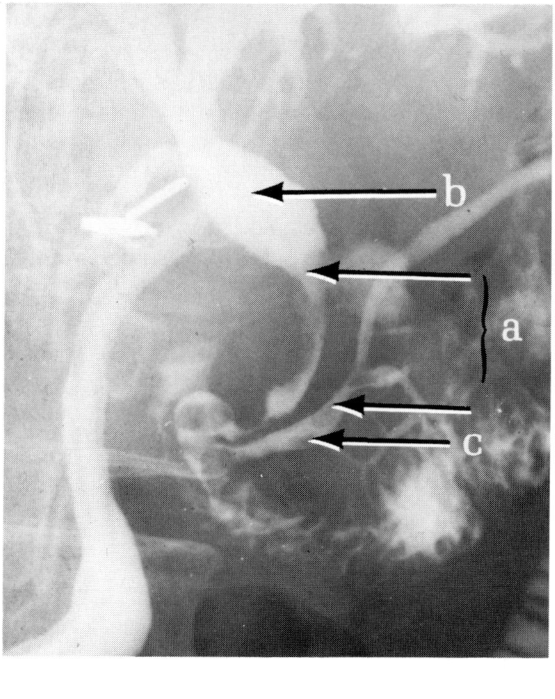

Stone Migration

The report by Acosta and Ledesma (2) is one of the few modern studies documenting the spontaneous passage of stones by stool examinations. A prior study of stool screening had been done by Bakes (33), who documented spontaneous passage of stones following ampullary dilitation. The study by Acosta and Ledesma was carried out in 36 consecutive patients with acute pancreatitis and gallstones. Feces were collected for 10 days and filtered through a metal screen. Stones were found in the stools of 34 patients with acute pancreatitis. When they were not found, it was assumed that ampullary stenosis (choledochoduodenal junctional stenosis [CDJS]) caused the pancreatitis and constituted the obturation that prevented the spontaneous passage of the calculi. In all their cases the pancreatitis was documented by subsequent surgery.

Acosta and Ledesma (2) have thus demonstrated choledochal stone migration as one cause of acute pancreatitis. The size of calculi ranged from 1 to 15 mm. It is the migrating stone that transiently blocks the ampulla. One of the corollaries is that in the patient who presents with acute pancreatitis—in which instance the biliary tract does not visualize by x-ray for a period of as long as 3–4 weeks—it might be advisable to filter the stools for calculi and in that way confirm the diagnosis of gallstone-linked pancreatitis. This procedure is especially advisable in patients who have no history of alcoholism, prior surgery, hyperparathyroidism or hyperlipidemia.

The patient with a documented attack of pancreatitis should be considered as having a diseased common bile duct.

Lymphogenous Disorders

The cystic duct lymph node is hyperplastic in cholecystitis and is often firmly adherent to the cystic artery; the pericholedochal and choledochoduodenal nodes exhibit an acute reactive hyperplastic lymphadenitis in association with inflammatory disorders of the bile ducts (619).

Postoperative pancreatitis can be attributed to operative injury and ischemia (586). This mechanism is probably more often a factor in surgery for difficult duodenal ulcer than it is in biliary disease. In the biliary tract operation, the pancreas may have been injured during the choledochal manipulation and instrumentation. This manifestation of focal traumatic pancreatitis may be completely obscured by the occurrence of an intraabdominal abscess or ileus. The etiologic link may go completely unrecognized.

Traumatic pancreatitis induced by handling and palpation of the organ is certainly a fact in the experimental animal. In the dog, especially, it is an easy way to provoke subcapsular hemmorhage and hemmorhagic pancreatitis. Most of these animals do not get sick.

It is hard to document ischemic postoperative pancreatitis due to intraoperative or postoperative "shock" postulating decreased visceral blood flow to the pancreas as the causative factor.

Effect of Pancreatitis on the Choledochus

The influence of the pancreatic affection on the common duct depends in part upon the duct's course through the pancreatic parenchyma. The variation in incidence and type of pancreatic response can be a function of this congenital anatomic variant. If the common duct passes through the pancreatic parenchyma, it can be partially and circumferentially blocked by acute pancreatic edema or irreversibly occluded by periductal fibrosis. This anatomic situation pertains in about 80% of patients. This is the mechanism for tubular stenosis of the distal common bile duct (3).

If the pancreatic duct is partially or completely extravisceral, it can be pushed aside or displaced away from the vertebral column. In these instances the duct is angulated into a scythe or sickle configuration. The clue to whether this deformity has functional significance depends upon the demonstration of proximal dilatation in the supraduodenal segment, delayed emptying of the intravenously administered contrast material, and manometrically demonstrable choledochal hypertension. Such abnormalities can impair drainage (Fig. 10-2).

In the acute state, the transpancreatic segment of the duct is often seen to bow to the left, later to return to a normal curvilinear configuration. In other instances the deformed position is maintained but has no symptomatic significance (Fig. 10-3). If the contour deformity persists, it has been postulated that the acute pancreatic inflammatory process never resolved completely because the biliary disease was not totally corrected with the initial surgical procedure. The focal inflammatory process, by a combination of edema and scarring, continues to compress or to angulate the transpancreatic portion of the common bile duct and to distort or block smaller pancreatic ductules. This latter circumstance produces the parenchymal retention cysts.

These cysts can be recognized by barium meal opacification of the duodenum. Serial films show variations in size over a period of weeks or months. Enlargement has usually been associated with aggravation of pain. Two cases in the MHMC experience showed a marked decrease in cyst size after secondary choledocholithotomy. The cysts were multi-

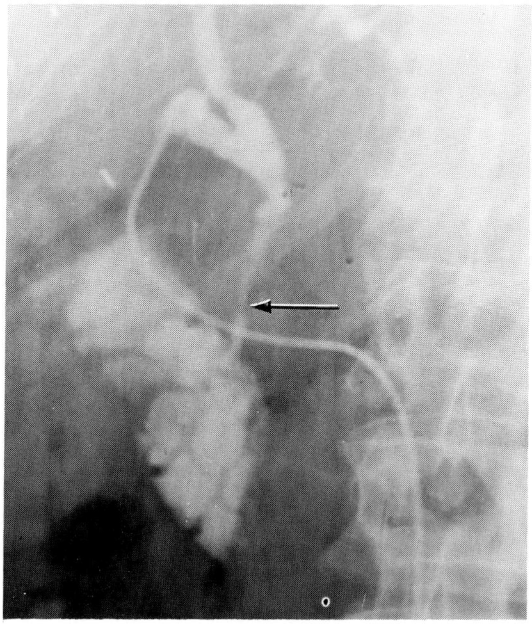

FIG. 10-2. Transpancreatic displacement and stenosis of the common duct. This cystic duct cholangiogram reveals a long tubular stricture of the transpancreatic portion of the common bile duct **(arrow).** There is no proximal dilatation. Manometry showed a normal residual pressure and normal passage pressure. This stricture is not dynamically significant.

FIG. 10-3. Cholangiographic evidence of pancreatitis. The cholangiographic changes that occur in the transpancreatic portion of the common bile duct in association with gallstone-linked pancreatitis are diagramed as follows: **A.** The primary reaction is in the distal section of the common duct where an edematous reaction in the descending duodenum effects a narrowing in the choledochal sphincter area. **B.** There is an exaggerated displacement to the left of the distal portion of the common bile duct. **C.** The most marked reaction in the distal portion of the common bile duct that is affected by pancreatitis is tubular stricture of the intraparenchymal transpancreatic segment. This is in contrast to **A** and **B,** in which the position of the duct is assumed to be partially extraparenchymal. These tubular strictures of the common duct are not always manometrically significant. In this illustration the proximal dilatation suggests that it produces a truly obstructive choledochopathy.

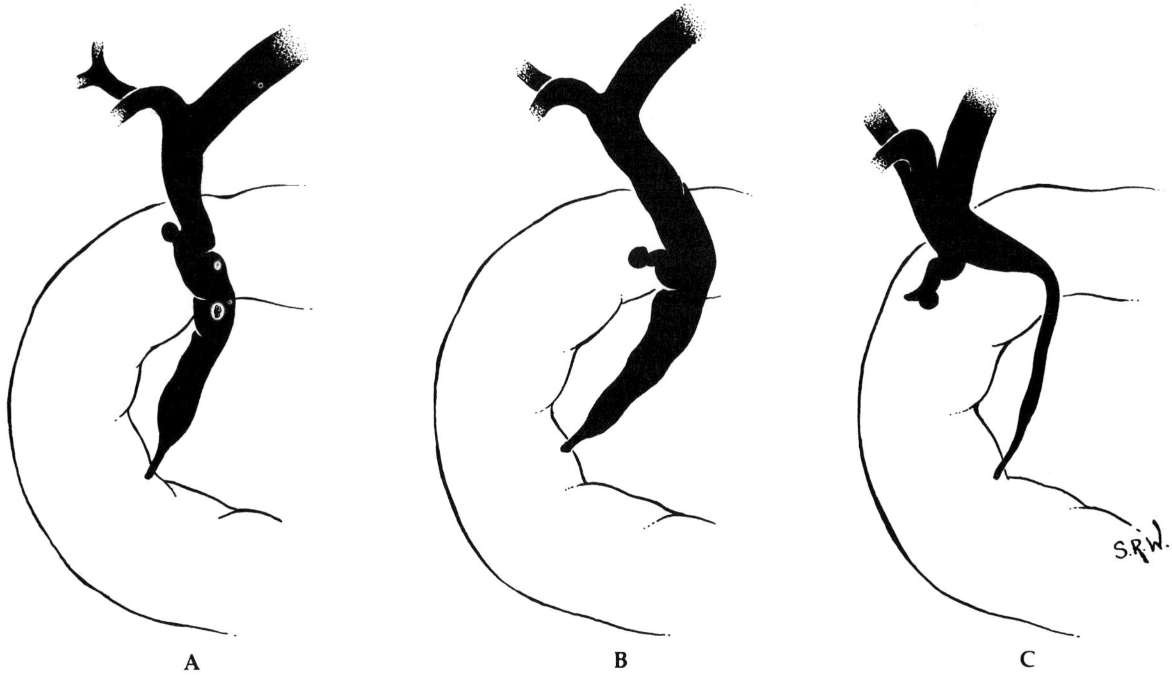

ple, unilocular, and subcapsular; they ranged between 1 and 6 cm in diameter.

Unresolved pancreatitis has been implicated as the cause of CDJS and as the factor responsible for tubular stenosis of the transhepatic segment of the common duct.

Clinical Features of PCS Pancreatitis

1. The vast majority of cases of pancreatitis associated with biliary disorders resolve with a complete corrective biliary toilet. When pancreatitis persists or is recurrent, there is usually persistent biliary tract disease (Fig. 10-4).

2. Pancreatitis that is linked solely to biliary disease is not usually associated with pancreatic calcification, pancreaticoductal lithiasis, portal vein occlusion, pancreatic insufficiency, or portal hypertension. When these complications are encountered, there is associated alcoholism or cancer (213). When the causes coexist, the alcoholic effect on the pancreas is dominant. Pirola and Davis (471) have indicated that alcohol has the systemic effect of contracting the Odditic sphincter and of increasing duodenal motility. This is, in part, the physiological basis for the avoidance of alcohol in the PCS (472).

3. There is no exact clinical parallelism between roentgen pancreas-related deformity of the common duct and clinical symptoms.

4. Suppurative pancreatitis, pancreatic abscesses or lesser sac abscess, and hemorrhagic pancreatic apoplexy are rarely the consequence of biliary disease. In Howard and Jordan's experience (280), the biliary link existed in 15% of cases of hemorrhagic pancreatitis. There was only one in the MHMC series when there had been an antecedent cholecystectomy.

5. When the pancreatitis is assumed to be due to a calculus-linked CDJS (ampullary stenosis, ampullary fibrosis, or papillary stenosis are equivalent terms), the pancreatic duct as well as the common duct become ectatic, and there can be a diffuse pancreatic fibrosis. The clinical significance of this pancreatic finding is not clearly defined either in terms of specific symptomatology or the indications for management. Some of the failures of surgical therapy in the treatment of PCS have been ascribed to persistent pancreatic duct obstruction at the entrance into the duodenum. This assumes that although a proximal vent will decompress the bile duct, it will have no specific effect on the pancreatic sphincter unless the latter is separately divided or bypassed.

6. If serum amylase elevations persist, one may suspect that continuing acute pancreatitis, pancreatic pseudocyst, or renal impairment is the reason the enzyme has failed to clear.

Common duct deformity as indicated by tubular stenosis with proximal dilatation is an absolute indication of pancreatic disease. One such patient presented with suppurative cholangitis, which was treated by choledochoduodenostomy. A second patient continues to bear this same cholangiographic deformity without symptoms. These two cases demonstrate the symptomatic extremes of tubular stenosis. The cholangiograhic features were identical. In two cases in the MHMC series there was no evidence of the disorder beyond the anatomic demonstration of it. However, Warshaw *et al.* (611) reported six cases in which tubular stenosis was present in association with painless obstructive jaundice, recurrent cholangitis, secondary biliary cirrhosis, and chronic abdominal pain. Decompression of the biliary tree by anastomosis of either the gallbladder or common duct and small intestines completely relieved the symptoms and allowed liver function to improve significantly. In the asymptomatic state, the mere demonstration of tubular stenosis does not require decompression. The fact that the pancreatitis in these six patients was due to alcohol rather than gallstone-linked disease may account for the difference. Pancreatic calcification was also present in three of the six patients. Tubular stenosis of the common duct appears more likely to be symptomatic when alcoholism, rather than biliary tract disease, is the cause.

Reverse C curve or scythe deformity of the infraduodenal duct may be regarded as being the source of postoperative symptoms only if the proximal common duct is dilated and if there is retention of the intravenous contrast after 2 hours. Four patients in this category have been treated. Each had recurrent colic; three had been jaundiced; and each had demonstrated an elevated serum amylase during at least one colic episode. Three have been completely relieved; the fourth still has

FIG. 10-4. Choledochlithiasis and the pancreas. Diagrammatic representation of the spectrum of changes encountered in the pancreas in association with residual choledocholithiasis and a calculus-containing gallbladder remnant. (**CDJS,** choledochoduodenal junctional stenosis.)

STONE-LINKED PANCREATITIS

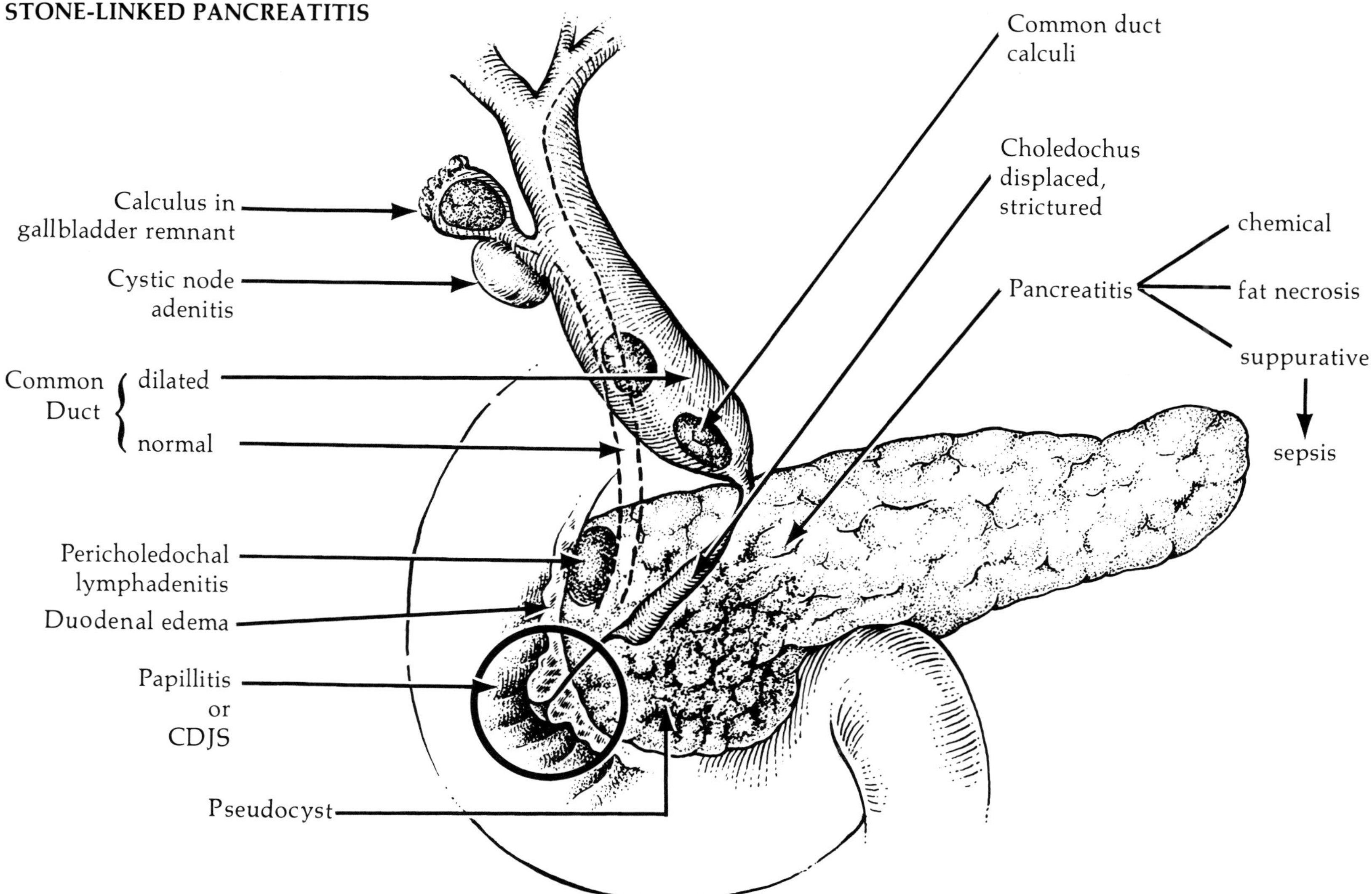

upper abdominal discomfort but less frequently and of lesser intensity than previously.

The healthy pancreas produces the highest serum amylase values. In the disorder linked to biliary disease, both with and without discernible fat necrosis at operation, the serum level can go well above 1000 Somoygi units. There is no good evidence that serum lipase levels remain elevated longer than amylase levels.

There is a good deal of difficulty in correlating the findings of either increased amylase in the blood or in the urine with the clinical symptomatology related to biliary tract disease. There is general agreement that the factor is mechanical obstruction to pancreatic duct outflow. This is less often by an impacted duct stone (the Opie phenomenon) than by some disorder of the Vaterian segment, like stone transit edema. It is the pancreatic secretion against this obstruction, especially following the stimulation of a large meal, that results in injury to the pancreatic cells and allows the amylase to escape, and to be absorbed either directly into the lymphatic or venous circulation or secondarily via the peritoneum. It is in this entity that the so-called spasm of the sphincter of Oddi has been indicted although never proven.

The pathological mechanism is believed to be continuous stimulus to acinar secretion (brought on by the meal) in the face of ductal obstruction. This results in rupture either of acinar cells or of small ductules. Since the pancreas in gallbladder disease (in contrast to the pancreas in alcoholism) is normal, the capacity of this gland to produce large quantities of amylase is retained. There is no correlation between the amylase level and the gross evidence of pancreatitis. Adams *et al.* (5) report that the great majority of patients with amylase levels over 1000 Somoygi units had a surgically correctable lesion, usually acute cholecystitis or choledocholithiasis, or a perforated ulcer or a pseudocyst of the pancreas. The point is that high amylase levels are not related to chronic alcoholic pancreatitis.

Elevated serum amylase levels do not reflect the extent of pancreatitis that will be encountered at surgery. They are to be regarded as simply one other laboratory finding that must be integrated into the total clinical picture.

The urinary amylase determination is more relevant to the evaluation of the acute clinical situation. The normal 1-hour random sample value is 36–364 Somoygi units. In the MHMC series, experience with the 2-hour urine amylase determination has been satisfactory. Values over 700 Somoygi units at 2 hours are abnormal (214).

This laboratory determination is not specific. It is an isolated laboratory value. In the absence of collateral clinical and roentgen findings, no secondary surgical procedure is indicated by this finding alone.

It is possible that these criteria foster underdiagnosis of the pancreatic inflammatory process and that the patient is done an injustice in the adherence to these strict criteria. The correlation of laboratory and roentgen findings suggesting pancreatitis should lead to a search for residual biliary disease.

The intravenous cholangiogram can be of limited value in defining the pancreatic disorder. In the presence of acute cholangitis or acute pancreatitis, the normal duct may not become visualized for periods up to 10 days, even when the subsequent film demonstrates a completely normal extrahepatic ductal system. This is analogous to the failure of the oral route for opacification of the gallbladder in the presence of pancreatitis. The factor of impaired intestinal absorbtion, therefore, is not the only defect. Consequently, a cholangiogram by the venous route is of diagnostic value only if it visualizes; if it fails to do so, it does not indicate organic disease (314, 453, 608). In the MHMC experience the pancreatic duct has never been demonstrated on intravenous cholangiography.

Barium meal visualization can offer collateral evidence of the disease related to the pancreas. One looks for 1) an enlarged common duct as evidenced by a groove on the superior border of the first part of the duodenum; 2) an enlarged papilla in the medial wall of the second portion of the duodenum, as evidence of papillitis; 3) hair-on-end mucosal changes of the second part of the duodenum, as evidence of duodenal edema; 4) motor disturbances; 5) fixed enlargements of the duodenum or fixed contour changes and compression on the second part of the duodenum (these are late signs of cancer); 6) changing contour defects in the duodenal sweep (these are evidence of pancreatic inflammatory disease) (Fig. 10-5).

FIG. 10-5. Duodenal manifestations of pancreatitis. Barium studies in two patients with the pancreatic complications of choledocholithiasis. **A.** An intrapancreatic cystic swelling compresses the descending limb of the duodenum **(arrows).** The process regressed completely after choledocholithotomy and choledochoduodenostomy. **B.** The distortion of the duodenal loop in the C curve area **(arrows)** is evidence of pancreatitis. **C.** The progression of gallstone-linked pancreatitis **(arrows)** to this degree is not common. This patient required drainage of a lesser sac abscess and choledocholithotomy as a second procedure.

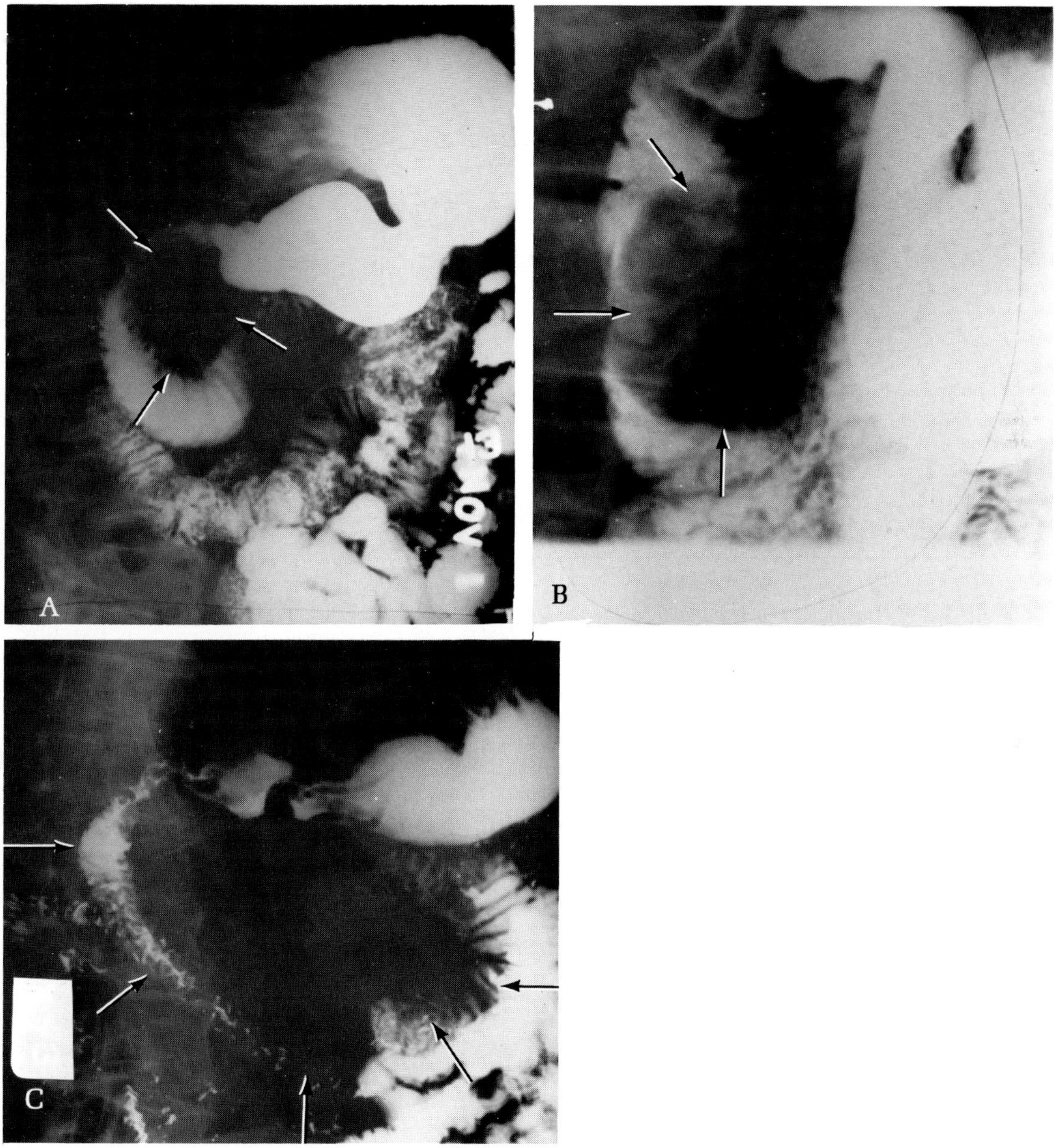

The diagnosis of chronic pancreatic disease has been made by the secretin test. In this procedure an indwelling duodenal tube is used to collect pancreatic juice that is free of gastric contents. The pancreatic juice is analyzed for volume, bicarbonate, and amylase content. The volume of pancreatic fluid is a function of where and how completely the duct is obstructed. The bicarbonate and amylase values depend upon the extent of glandular destruction. A cytologic examination of the fluid may reveal exfoliated cancer cells or chronic inflammatory cells. With minimal disease, the findings are rarely diagnostic or specific. In the normal patient, the post-stimulatory aspirate volume is between 100 and 300 ml at 90 min, the bicarbonate concentration is 90–140 mEq/100 ml (average 109 mEq/100 ml), and amylase, 6 units/kg body weight. The secretin test of pancreatic function requires an experienced laboratory, if the values are to be sufficiently accurate and reproducible as to the basis for decision. The Jorpes unit of activity for secretin is more potent than the Boots. Dreiling *et al.* (179) reported 5% false positive and 5% false negative laboratory values. Dreiling's investigation (178) of 96 patients with PCS showed that only 2% had a demonstrable pancreatic disorder.

In the MHMC series there has been no instance of steatorrhea in association with pancreatitis linked to biliary calculus. That diagnosis is supported when stool examinations show more than ten meat fibers per high-powered field or more than six fat globules stained with Sudan III, or when there is evidence of lipase deficiency (488, 641).

Much of the information about the pancreas that had previously been sought by function tests is now elicited by celiac and superior mesentery angiography and by ERCP (90). The large vessel distortions (both arterial and venous) are associated with advanced disease. The changes in advanced pancreatitis are specific. One of the diagnostic values of angiography is that it may disclose unsuspected carcinoma of the pancreas. Unfortunately, by the time the vascular changes of cuffing, tumor tissue stain, organ displacement, arterial stenosis, splenic vein block, and abnormal vasculature are present, the patient is usually past the already slim chance for curative resection. Angiography is also a valuable asset in the diagnosis of chronic alcoholic pancreatitis. The interstitial pancreatitis of biliary origin is not associated with the angiographic changes seen in cancer (221, 571).

It is not uncommon to see a patient who has recently undergone biliary surgery presenting again with unmistakable evidence of pancreatic cancer. Some of these patients had been jaundiced and the true etiology in the pancreatic head or distal bile duct had been missed. Others were operated upon for presumed biliary colic in the pre-icteric stage, and the tumor in the body of the pancreas had escaped diagnosis.

One of the pertinent problems has been coexistent choledocholithiasis and pancreatic cancer. Considering the age group in which this cancer occurs, it is no surprise that 15–20% of these patients also have stones.

Present techniques with ERCP allow for cytologic examination of pancreatic secretion as an aid to differential diagnosis. This is an extension of the diagnostic validity of cytologic examinations performed by direct needle aspiration of the dilated pancreatic duct during operation (508). A high index of suspicion based on knowledge that a persistent, totally obstructive jaundice is rare in benign disease will alert the surgeon to the problem of cancer. The initial concept of pancreatic cancer as a form of painless jaundice has been proved false; at least 75% of these patients have pain.

It is not true that cholangitis never occurs with cancer; chills and fever do occur in the clinical syndrome of proximal bile duct cancers. Here the surgeon is clued into the problem when a jaundiced patient is found to have a collapsed distal duct system. The intraoperative cholangiogram is diagnostic in almost all instances—the accuracy is in the range of 95–98%.

However, the clinical behavior of cancer of the distal bile duct and ampulla can mimic a stone. Cholangiography, biliary endoscopy, and transductal biopsy with a laryngeal type of forceps help resolve the problem when the clinical suspicion exists.

The surgeon seeing a patient who presents again after having undergone primary procedures for biliary problems should have an aggressive attitude toward the management of this problem. In the absence of absolute contraindications, secondary corrective procedures should be undertaken. In the MHMC experience, there have been two patients with resectable bile duct tumors discovered at second operations done 6 and 9 months after cholecystectomy.

In three others palliative treatment was instituted by intubation across the tumor. No cancer of the body of the pancreas has proved resectable, so that the missed diagnosis is of no therapeutic importance.

INTRAOPERATIVE EVALUATION OF THE PANCREAS

Attempting to evaluate pancreatic disease solely by inspection and palpation has proved notoriously unreliable, particularly with reference to the head of the pancreas. Patterns of consistency, adherence, color changes, and vascularity are influenced by the surgeon's experience and by bruising of the organ during its exposure. It can be difficult to differentiate between nodularity, interstitial fibrosis, peripancreatic lymphadenopathy and cancer induration. A small impacted stone or a small ampullary tumor may induce a degree of pancreatitis behind it, such that only ancillary methods will distinguish the cause from the effect (129) (Fig. 10-6).

Barber (35) has reported the rare instance of pancreatic heterotopia presenting as a tumefaction in the duodenal wall, causing ampullary stenosis. The case was adequately managed by local resection and sphincteroplasty. Barboso (36) has reported ectopic pancreas in the common duct in association with inflammatory changes. Biliary tract disease can be mimicked by pancreatic heterotopia in the duodenum. It has been suggested that certain adenocarcinomas of the duodenum arise in areas of pancreatic heterotopia in the ampulla of Vater or the papilla of Santorini.

The problem of biopsy can be formidable. It may be hazardous to biopsy the representative disease if it is intracapsular—there can be a rapid hematoma, and spreading hemorrhage into the gland can be cumbersome to control. It often requires cauterization or suture ligation that destroys tissue and causes a secondary slough and pancreatitis. Transduodenal biopsy, possibly less hazardous for fistula formation, is often bloody and leaves the organ with an intraparenchymal hemorrhage. Uncomplicated biopsy in this area can be accomplished only when the process has spread beyond the gland and the tissue for diagnosis is obtained from an extracapsular site. In this situation a shave biopsy has proved safe and 90% informative when taken from representative diseased tissue. The tissue is sometimes taken from an area that is more convenient than representative, and the result can be misleading.

Schultz and Sanders (543), reporting on 159 pancreatic biopsies found the accuracy to be 65%, but the mortality from pancreatitis and leak (fistula) was 3.8%. False-negative biopsies were obtained in 35% (this figure would obviously be still higher in the resectable case). The diagnosis of chronic pancreatitis does not rule out a proximal obstructing ductal cancer as the cause of the ductal pancreatitis (587). Although the selection of a suitable biopsy site is essential, it can be difficult to deliver to the pathologist a truly representative piece of tissue without initiating the complications of bleeding, fistula, or fat necrosis (570, 589). In a given case, the surgeon must decide whether the representative area is safely accessible to biopsy (Fig. 10-7).

In my experience the interpretation of the cholangiogram can be positive and accurate. The findings are so specific that one can act on the cholangiographic diagnosis without having to resort to a tissue confirmation. The resectable situation does not require confirmation prior to operation. Desirable, yes; necessary, no.

From a prophylactic viewpoint, it would appear that the incidence of postoperative iatrogenic pancreatitis can be diminished by 1) gentle handling of the duodenum and pancreatic head, 2) the avoidance of the long-arm T tube that goes through the ampulla—which presumedly can obstruct the pancreatic duct orifice, 3) avoiding the use of the Bakes instrument as a dilator (its function as a probe is better performed by a fine urethral whip and follower), 4) gentle common duct exploration with the proper instruments.

It is unfortunate that the term "Bakes dilator" remains in use, for in diameters greater than 3 mm, the instrument can produce submucosal injury. The organization of the ensuing periampullary hematoma then leads to temporary outlet obstruction and subsequently may present as one variety of CDJS.

In the MHMC series intraoperative pancreatography has not been utilized as a diag-

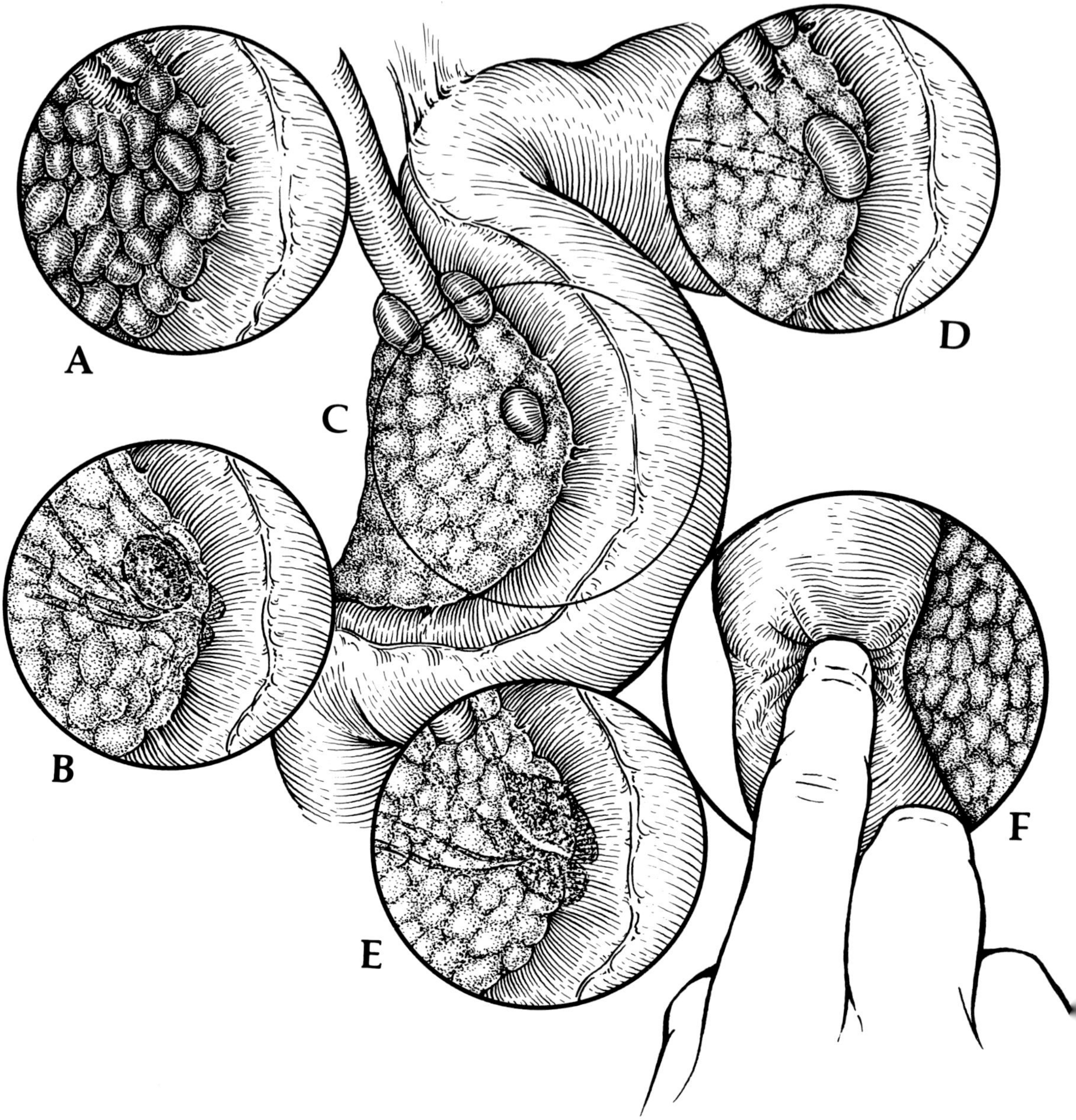

FIG. 10-6. Intraoperative evaluation of the pancreas. Evaluating pancreatic findings by gross inspection and palpation is often difficult, as the diagrams indicate. **A.** Normal pancreas. **B.** Stone in distal end of common bile duct. **C.** Peripancreatic lymphadenopathy. **D.** Lobular pancreatitis. **E.** Carcinoma of head of the pancreas. **F.** Invagination of anterior duodenal wall is the optimum closed method of palpating the changes in the ampulla. (From Schein CJ, Stern WZ, Jacobson HG: The Common Bile Duct. Operative Cholangiography, Biliary Endoscopy and Choledocholithotomy, 1966. Courtesy of Charles C Thomas, Publisher, Springfield, Illinois)

nostic aid. Experiences have been reported by Hess (264) Nardi (438) and Mercadier (423). As an aside, when the pancreatic duct has not been visualized by T-tube cholangiography in the presence of pancreatitis, the visualized segment has never shown an abnormality. Nardi and Acosta (438) made 31 pancreatograms in 50 cases of pancreatitis linked to gallbladder disease. Twenty-one had a dilated duct, three had cyst formation, and seven were normal. A trypsin inhibitor (50,000 units of traysalol) may have been of value as prophylaxis against pancreatitis if given in advance of the disease. A lesser reac-

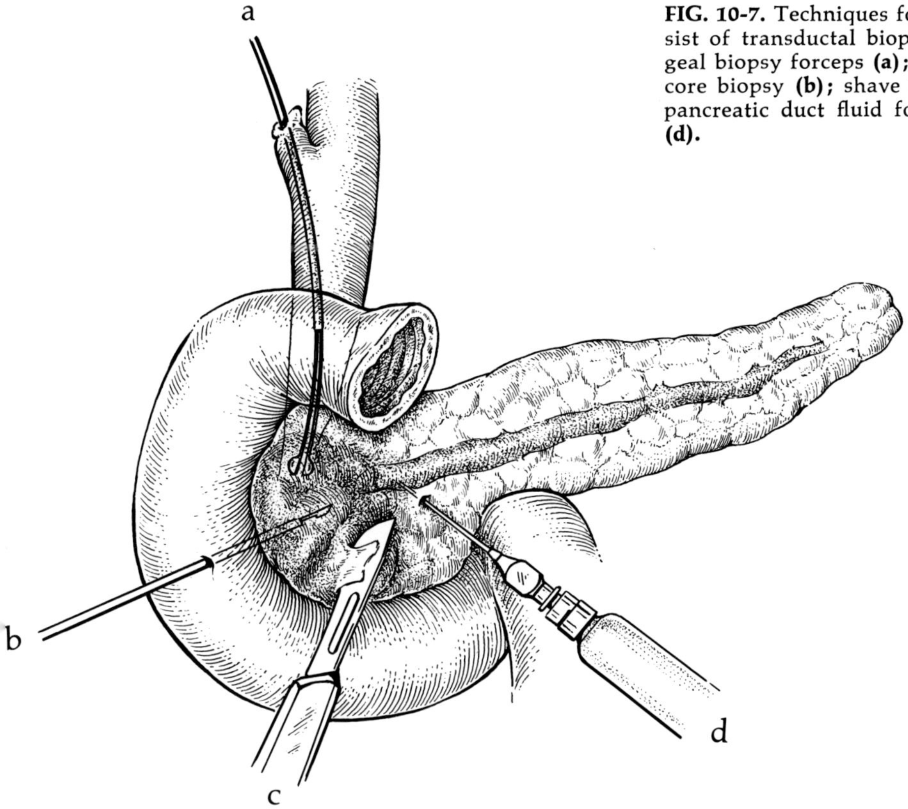

FIG. 10-7. Techniques for pancreatic biopsy consist of transductal biopsy with a flexible laryngeal biopsy forceps **(a)**; transduodenal needle or core biopsy **(b)**; shave biopsy **(c)**; aspiration of pancreatic duct fluid for cytologic examination **(d)**.

tion is to be anticipated in the patient with a chronic fibrotic pancreas (in which this diagnostic modality is not required) than in the normal pancreas, in which rupture of ductules —even with gentle injection of 2-ml bolus— presents a hazardous possibility.

Birnstingl's (61) postmortem studies of the pancreatic duct have indicated that there can be a considerable variation in pancreatic duct width unassociated with disease. Ducts wider than 6 mm have been found in 10% of normal patients; fusiform dilation of the duct and apparent stenosis at the level of the pancreatic neck can be normal variants. Certain of the abnormalities reported by others do not differ from his normals. Interpretations must be made with cautious regard to such normal variants.

The width of the pancreatic duct analyzed on ERCP indicates that in the head, the diameter ranges from 3 to 7 mm, with 70% of the measurements between 4 and 5 mm, with a median of 4.9 mm. In the body of the pancreas, the duct has a maximum width of 2.5–5mm, about 75% of ducts being 3.5 mm. The width of the tail is 1.5–3 mm, with a peak between 2 and 2.5 mm.

The gross findings that suggest pancreatitis linked to biliary disease are a loss of lobular clarity and septation, intraparenchymal retention cysts, shrinkage of the gland with eburnation and increased rounding of the tail as it is visualized in the hilus of the spleen and at its lower edge. In this entity, the pancreatic duct is rarely enlarged beyond 3–4 mm. It is therefore not readily palpable or even aspirable, as in certain instances of alcoholic pancreatitis with a "chain of lakes" configuration of the ducts. Peripancreatitis with marked adhesions to the retroperitoneum is uncommon. This accounts in part for the infrequency of the persistent, narcotic-addicting, backache type of pain (57, 423).

SURGICAL INDICATIONS

It is apparent that the diagnosis of nonacute pancreatitis associated with biliary disorders is hard to confirm. The advanced anatomic changes associated with retention cysts, tubular choledochal stricture, and common-duct displacement are accurately made by radiographic methods (439). Obstructive symptoms may have their source in this entity. There are three indications for surgery here: Jaundice, sepsis, or intermittent colic, together with the preoperative demonstration of residual disease in the biliary tract or significant anatomic distortion of the common duct or pancreas (287, 646).

The use of morphine as a provoking agent is based on the hypothesis that its induced contractions of the Vaterian segment will produce a relative obstruction that will significantly elevate the SGOT, alkaline phosphatase, and lactic acid dehydrogenase. This has been designated as a provocative morphine transaminase test (75).

Nardi and Acosta (438) have used another provocative test to uncover the pancreatitis: 10 mg morphine sulfate and 1 mg neostigmine (Prostigmin) are given intramuscularly. The test is regarded as positive if the pain is reproduced and the serum enzymes are elevated four times above normal. The provocation did not produce acute pancreatitis. Patients with positive responses were found to have pancreatitis linked to biliary disease; all obtained a favorable postoperative result with sphincterotomy; none had a positive response to provocative testing later.

It was Archibald's (23) 1919 experimental observation that the reflux of bile could be produced by sphincter spasm that suggested sphincterotomy as the treatment for recurrent pancreatitis. In 1899 McBurney (407) had employed a transduodenal sphincterotomy—as a type of episiotomy of the ampulla—to deliver a stone caught in the area of the distal bile duct. Kocher (331), in 1895, performed a sphincterotomy with suture of the introduodenal duct to the duodenal wall; he termed this an ampulloduodenostomy. These are the historical antecedents for the procedure that was in great vogue in the 1950's.

For the sake of completeness, other approaches should be mentioned. Mallet-Guy (397) has championed thoracolumbar sympathectomy for the control of pancreatic pain induced by biliary disease. The procedure is anesthetic in effect, eliminating the afferent pain pathway. Some of the earlier literature contained collaborative reports.

At the present time pancreatic resection is preferred for that type of disease. It is a very rare entity in the PCS. Hess (261) has indicated that persistent pancreatic disease may be due to specific stenosis of the pancreatic sphincter, a stenosis that is proximal, and therefore persistent, after the conventional choledochal sphincterotomy or choledochoduodenostomy. In the MHMC series there has been no instance in which this was recognized.

The indication for operation is symptoms associated with anatomic abnormalities. Cleanout procedures are instituted for residual stones or choledochoduodenostomy for dynamically significant tubular stricture. Resectional surgery of the pancreas has not been required for this specific entity.

Medical management in the chronic situation relies on the use of antispasmodics, antacids, or an ulcer type of diet, and on the avoidance of pancreatic insults. The latter requires abstinence from alcohol, avoidance of wide swings between feast and famine, and an adequate vitamin and iron intake. Bile salts and cholegogues play no specific role.

The management of the complicated acute problem of respiratory and renal failure has been particularly well detailed by Gliedman *et al.* (229)

A surgical decision resolves about the timing of the secondary surgical intervention in relation to an episode of presumed acute pancreatitis. If the diagnosis is based solely on hyperamylasemia, then surgery can be performed without considering the laboratory finding. If the patient presents the signs of an associated generalized peritonitis, the condition should be managed by gastric section, intravenous alimentation, nothing by mouth, and antibiotics until there is either complete regression or obvious progression. The surgery is best done as an interval procedure. When the process is progressive, with pancreatic necrosis and lesser sac abscesses, a drainage procedure may have to be the initial approach and corrective biliary surgery undertaken secondarily.

11 Choledochoduodenal Junctional Stenosis

The exact nature of choledochoduodenal junctional stenosis (CDJS) is not yet clearly known. However, this clinical entity may be recognized by its morphologic changes and treated effectively by the correction of a mechanical block, even when the etiologic mechanism is presumptive rather than consistently demonstrable. The disorder was first described by Florcken (202) in 1912. Subsequently Del Valle and Donovan (167) of Brazil and Caroli and Mercadier (112) in France contributed considerably to its documentation and clinical recognition.

Generally, European sensitivity to this diagnosis has been much greater than that in America, as is attested to by the extensive reports by Arianoff (24–26), Kourias (337, 338), and Mallet-Guy (396), among others.

There have been varying attitudes regarding the identification of symptomatic CDJS. On the one hand its very existence has been denied as being a poetic concept. At the other extreme are those who postulate that it is a cause of primary ductal stones, a factor in the genesis of cholecystitis, and an often overlooked cause of postcholecystectomy complaints. The diagnosis is made most frequently by European and South American surgeons, and possibly too infrequently in North America (47, 159, 236, 419, 530, 549, 559, 583, 592).

Choledochoduodenal junctional stenosis is referred to by Arianoff (25, 27) as "papillo-odditis," the stenosing form occurring in 11% of 2576 biliary operations.

The use of other terms for the entity reflects the general ambiguity: ampullary fibrosis, distal stricture, sphincter fibrosis, Vaterian segment obstruction, phimosis of the ampulla, chronic odditis, or chronic papillitis. De Valla and Donovan (167, 168) called it "sclerosing choledocho-odditis," Mallet-Guy (391) referred to it as "maladie du sphincter d'Oddi," Caroli (109) designated it as "papillite icterigeni primitive," and others designated it as "enfermedod del coledocho terminal."

In the European medical literature, especially, it is probably the most frequent indication for sphincterotomy.

DEFINITION OF CDJS

I have elected the term choledochoduodenal junctional stenosis not only because it circumvents the purely anatomic semantic issue of whether there is an ampulla, but also because it avoids a histologic basis for the recognition of the entity and microscopic identification of the site of dysfunction. The term CDJS embraces the entity as a clinical concept with a definable impediment to the free flow of bile into the duodenum in the region of the choledochoduodenal junction.

Information on *in situ* endoscopy of ampullary function has been obtained from the studies of Shore *et al.* (561). Their preparation involved a dog, trained to stand in a frame, whose duodenum had been intubated with a Thomas cannula. Motion-picture filming through this cannula demonstrated a cephalic phase of ejection of bile into the duodenum, contraction of the sphincter with acid, a fixed tonicity between meals, and a continuous leak of bile in response to a fatty meal. This *in vivo* documentation of functional variants makes it possible to accept

TABLE 11-1. DIAGNOSTIC FEATURES DIFFERENTIATING CHOLEDOCHODUODENAL JUNCTION STENOSIS FROM BILIARY DYSKINESIA

	CDJS	Dyskinesia
Duct size	> 1.4 cm	Normal
Probing	Difficult	Easy
Pressure	> 20 cm saline	Inconsistent
IVC	Time–density abnormality	Normal
Cholangitis	Common	Absent
Jaundice	Present in 50%	Absent
Dominant symptom	Obstruction	Pain
Chemical abnormality	Present	None
Stones in duct	Present in about 50%	None

the fact that functional and anatomic disorders in this area can produce alterations in the rate, volume, and periodicity of bile flow.

The disorder CDJS differs from biliary dyskinesia (Table 11-1). The latter is a physiologic dysfunction, whereas CDJS is an anatomic change, albeit of uncertain etiology. Pikula and Dunphy (468) suggested that this type of incomplete stricture may be comparable to megacolon or achalsia.

Data on the frequency of the entity are difficult to obtain. Obviously CDJS is more often found by those who search for it. Thus Paulino and Roselli (464) encountered it in 2.5% of 511 primary procedures and in 12% of 100 secondary operations. Slightly fewer than half of these patients had no choledocholithiasis. Hess (259, 261), employing routine cholangiomanometry, was able to document an ampullary disorder in about 25% of those operated upon for gallbladder disease: in 8–10% of primary cholecystectomies, and in 37% of secondary operations. Kourias (335, 338) considers CDJS the third most frequent indication for reoperative biliary surgery, just behind the retained stone and the retained gallbladder remnant.

Its exact physiological and anatomic obverse is papillary insufficiency, either spontaneous or traumatic, which is demonstrated by barium swallow. In these instances the orally ingested barium regurgitates through the incompetent Vaterian segment and opacifies the extrahepatic system. In no instance has regurgitation of itself been a symptomatic entity. When Vaterian segment regurgitation is a disease, it is due to the associated choledocholithiasis. Fistulization due to spontaneous stone passage may be the etiologic factor in the association.

The evidence of CDJS is a significantly dilated proximal common bile duct and the demonstration of the choledochal hypertension with impaired transit of bile to the duodenum. These are the same criteria that define stenosis in any body conduit—*i.e.*, proximal dilatation and delayed passage with retention.

CDJS may occur as an isolated phenomenon, or it may occur in association with primary common-bile-duct calculi and be the obstructive cause of the stasis that generates these stones. It may also present with faceted calculi in the common bile duct that have their origin in the gallbladder. The specific importance of the entity in the PCS resides in the need to recognize its pathogenic potential. It may be the less obvious cause of a more easily defined stone or obscure cholangitis or of both. If the obstruction is not recognized and corrected, the cholangitis may recur. CDJS may also present as part of the complex within which there is also gallbladder remnant disease (Fig. 11-1).

In my concept of the entity, it is important specifically to delineate what CDJS is not. It is not a histologic lesion, confirmable by biopsy. It is not the reversible edema of the Vaterian segment that is seen in acute biliary tract inflammation, although it may be superimposed on this or result from it. CDJS is a syndrome characterized by obstruction in the region of the choledochoduodenal junction that results in the anatomic change of proximal symmetrical choledochal dilatation. Its physiologic manifestation is choledochal hypertension and choledochal stasis. These anatomic changes may not be symptomatic.

PATHOGENESIS

The precise etiologic mechanism is unknown. The entity is usually encountered collaterally, in association with other biliary abnormalities. It is probable that each of several entities is capable of producing the same end result. The fact that there are these associations does not mandate a cause-and-effect relationship with any single one.

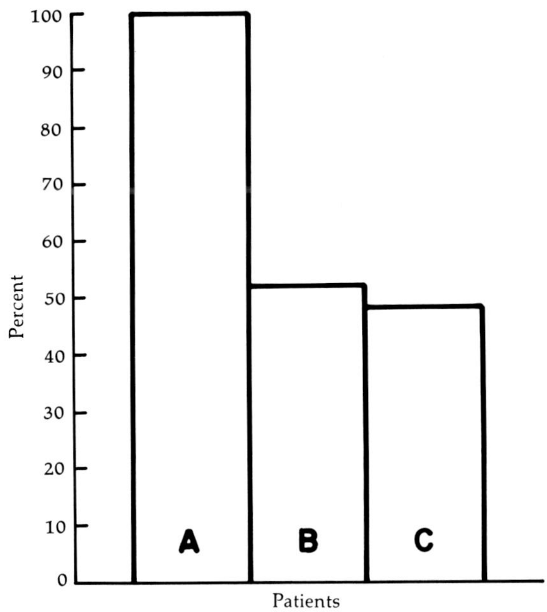

FIG. 11-1. Calculi in CDJS. Almost half the patients with roentgenographically and manometrically demonstrated CDJS were free of choledochal calculi at the time the diagnosis was made. Of 23 patients with ampullary fibrosis **(A)**, 12 (52%) had CBD calculi and ampullary stenosis **(B)**, and 11 (48%) had no calculi **(C)**.

Acute cholecystitis can be associated with cholangitis. The Vaterian segment cholangitic reaction is one of the causes of its concomitant nonobturative jaundice. This serial Vaterian segment reaction is demonstrable on remote cystic-duct cholangiography, where the initially prominent ampullary reaction is seen to resolve with the correction of the gallbladder problem. This can also be demonstrated by a progressive fall in the choledochal residual pressure and a steady increase in flow rates. Incomplete resolution of this inflammatory process in this narrow area can have varying degrees of outlet impediment (CDJS) as its sequel.

Reports suggest that it takes 3–5 years for choledocholithias to generate a significant fibrotic type of CDJS. The duodenal papilla is the narrowest segment of the extrahepatic biliary conduit, it measures 1–3 mm under physiologic conditions. In the MHMC series there has not been, nor am I aware of, a documented instance of papillary phimosis and obstruction linked solely to the duodenal mucosa—the sort of anatomic situation that would require a meatomy (119, 121).

Common duct stones have the potential for traumatizing the common bile duct in one of several ways: direct calculus impaction, mucosal ulceration with focal scarring, or a localized or diffuse cholangitic reaction. The consequence of this choledocholithic reaction in the area of the Vaterian segment can be CDJS.

The inflammatory reaction of gallstone-linked pancreatitis produces an acute ampullary reaction much more often than it does a tubular stenosis in the transpancreatic segment of the common bile duct (476). It is one of the factors responsible for the failure of cholangiographic contrast material to traverse the choledochoduodenal junction. The inflammatory process usually subsides totally when the biliary disease is corrected. When the roentgen sign does not recede in a 7- to 10-day interval, there is often a retained stone or persistent pancreatitis.

It is not possible to support or to negate the suggestion that biliary pancreatitis may have its most important residuum in this Vaterian segment reaction, remote CDJS. The infrequent association with acute pancreatitis is related to the fact that CDJS prevents stones from passing distally, thus altering their potential for producing a transitory pancreatic duct block.

Others have proposed that this variety of outlet obstruction does not exist except as a sequel to operative trauma. Some have suggested that it is a sequel to traumatic choledochal instrumentation, with the creation of a false passage that initiates a periampullary reaction that goes on to peri-orificial fibrosis (643). Reynolds (496) showed that when a Bakes dilator larger than 3 mm is passed through the common duct, it disrupts the ampulla and presumably can result in subsequent fibrosis. This contradicts Bakes's original autopsy study (33) showing that a 13-mm dilator could negotiate through the ampulla without disrupting intrinsic musculature.

The studies in the MHMC laboratory have demonstrated that the passage of a large probe through the junction of the common duct and duodenum can produce a periductal submucosal hemorrhage that is clearly visible in the duodenum. This conceivably could resolve with a scar. Branch *et al.* (87), much earlier, had documented a reaction to dilators characterized by hemorrhage and edema. There is no proof that CDJS follows excessive dilation or abrasive manipulation. That assumption can only apply to some patients because the entity is identified also in patients whose common ducts have never been manipulated.

Coley and Howes (139) were unable to reproduce the entity in the dog by electrocoagulation and the intramural injection of irritating substances into the area. Recent experiences with transduodenal endoscopic coagulation suggest that the potential for postcoagulation stricture can be a function of the type, source, and intensity of the current employed. Proudhomme *et al.* (483) have indicated that excessive stretching, distortion, and bougienage can go on to postoperative fibrosis. In my experience this is a rarity, and the majority of even traumatic intraductal manipulations escape unnoticed.

Biopsy data have not clarified the entity (1, 109, 230, 393, 462, 463). In this area, the mucosae of the bile duct, duodenum, and pancreatic duct converge. The spatial relations can be confusing, and presumed pathologic changes have been ascribed to the method of tissue-sectioning rather than to the disease. The submucosa in this area has numerous tubular and racemose glands rich in goblet cells. Ectopically placed glands extending into the muscular layer, which have been likened to the Rokitansky-Aschoff sinus, have also been encountered in normal persons. De Santis and Tagliaferrai (169) described "adeno connective dysplasia with prevalence of the centrifugal glandular proliferation" as a change associated with age alone.

The incidence of normal biopsy findings has been high in patients regarded as otherwise quite clearly exhibiting the syndrome. A large spectrum of changes have been reported, including hypertrophy, atrophy, erosion, edema, ulceration, submucosal glandular hyperplasia, granulomatous inflammatory change and submucosal fibrosis. Muscular hypertrophy has not been recognized, and I am unaware of a specific study of ganglion cells of the area (38, 137, 237, 325).

Some investigators have found the same histologic changes in the Vaterian segment as they have encountered in normal persons. In this area, with its limitations for full-thickness biopsy, the suitable material is often hard to obtain. Pauline and Calvacanti (462, 463) maintain that there is a histologic specificity to the diagnosis if all layers of the bowel wall are sectioned, and they published representative photomicrographs in 1963. De Santis and Tagliaferrai (169) stressed that the histologic changes are nonspecific and considered their value dubious and irrelevant.

I do not regard a biopsy as necessary to make the diagnosis, and have employed it only when the prominent papilla had to be differentiated from carcinoma of the ampulla (177, 326). Dardinski (160) noted that in 54 of 100 cases, there were changes in the major duodenal papilla with enlargement of folds and thickening of the papillary wall due to hyperplastic mucous glands. Yet this was not associated with dilatation of the duct to indicate obstruction.

DIAGNOSIS

In general CDJS is the sequel of long-standing biliary disease. In Weitz's series (621) of 82 patients, 32 had been symptomatic about 5 years and 50 for 10 years. The associated residual stone is often solitary.

There are no symptoms that are specific to the entity. Pain, infection, and/or obstruction can be the common denominators of choledochopathy regardless of the etiology. These symptoms and signs may accompany residual stones with or without CDJS. One should be alert to the possibility of this entity as the sole or concomitant etiologic factor to be considered in planning a totally corrective operation. The diagnosis may be suggested by preoperative intravenous cholangiography and by intraoperative calibration combined with cholangiomanometry. Choledochoscopy has not been of specific value in this disorder, and I recall a personal communication from Wildegans saying that he had never observed the CDJS endoscopically. Biliary endoscopy is mandatory for the differential diagnosis.

It must be emphasized again that the entire complex of CDJS as diagnosed by roentgen methods may be encountered in the complete absence of symptoms and in the face of a normal profile of liver chemistries (311, 444). In this combination of roentgen abnormality without symptoms or other signs, no treatment is required. It is a curious turn of circumstances in the PCS that there is often the tendency to be forced into aggressive methods of treatment in the face of little objective evidence, whereas these objective signs are not universally recognized as an indication for surgery (Fig. 11-2).

Normal liver chemistries do not rule out this diagnosis. There can be a perplexing disparity between the size of the duct, the manometric determination, and the serum alkaline phosphatase and bilirubin. The latter values may be completely normal. However, one-third of the patients in the group give a history of jaundice; in only 20% was it present at the time of revisional surgery. The serum alkaline phosphatase remains the most sensitive laboratory value (187, 188, 387).

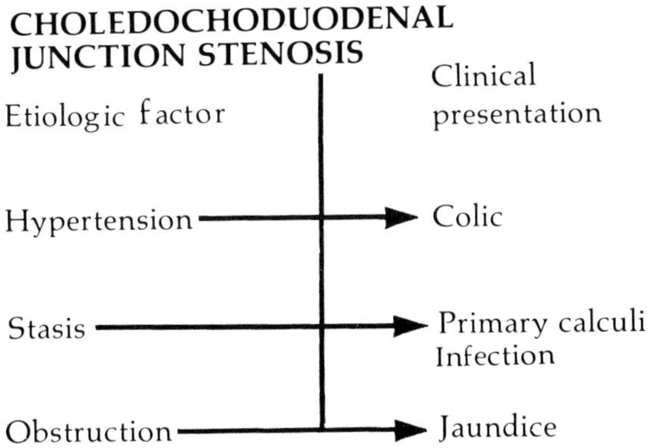

FIG. 11-2. Pathogenesis of clinical CDJS. The diagram presents the clinical manifestations of CDJS as they relate to the pathologic state.

Intravenous cholangiography was performed as part of the investigative study in all patients who were not icteric and whose operations were elective.

Significant dilatation means that the opacified common hepatic duct measures at least 1.4 cm in width. The emptying time is a good physiological means of demonstrating obstruction, for delayed passage into the duodenum beyond 90 min is as diagnostic of obstruction as delayed evacuation of orally administered barium is for the documentation of pyloric obstruction (Fig 11-3).

When calculi are present, however, they may produce the same roentgen findings by obturation alone. In that circumstance the possibility of concomitant CDJS must be judged by other methods (409). Nardi *et al.*

FIG. 11-3. Choledochoduodenal junctional stenosis. **A.** Intravenous cholangiogram made 90 min after injection of contrast material faintly opacifies the extrahepatic biliary system **(arrows)**. **B.** A film 180 minutes after the injection reveals increased density of contrast material in the ductal system, with failure of complete evacuation. (This is an abnormal time–density relationship.) The common hepatic duct and left hepatic duct, the most sensitive areas in this regard, are slightly dilated. In the symptomatic patient this increased opacification of the duct, associated with ductal dilatation and failure of evacuation of all contrast material within 90 minutes, is consistent with a diagnosis of CDJS. The bow to the left is very often encountered in pancreatitis, in which the position of the choledochus is at least partially extraparenchymal. The CDJS can be edematous. The choledochal ectasia is more marked in patients with cicatricial stenosis.

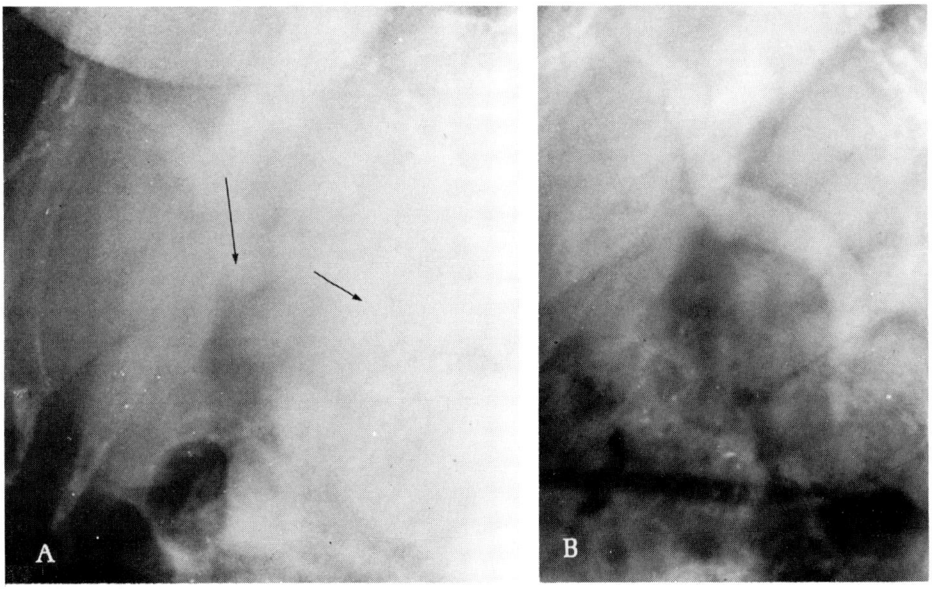

(438) place reliance on a provocative test to help make the diagnosis. Camishion and Goldstein (106) used a similar approach for making the diagnosis of cystic duct obstruction in the presence of a normal routine oral cholecystogram. The patient is given 10 mg morphine and 1 mg neostigmine (Prostigmin) or secretin, and the serum amylase and serum lipase are determined. If the patient experiences pain and these enzymes go up by a factor of four, the test is regarded as positive (431).

INTRAOPERATIVE EVALUATION

The common duct is completely liberated anteriorly and laterally to measure its width. Gentle indentation of its anterior surface with the blunt end of a thumb forceps offers a good indication of its thickness. The normal duct is about 1 mm thick, indents easily, and readily sustains a bile bruise with even gentle palpation. An opaque, thick wall suggests choledochitis.

The epicholedochal blood vessels are distorted with chronic duct disease and do not present as full, freely meandering, obviously pulsatile structures. Instead, the number, prominence, and size of the vessels on the anterior wall of the duct are reduced. Regional lymphadenopathy is usually prominent.

Palpation of the retroduodenal duct and head of the pancreas is notoriously unreliable. By this method, it is difficult to distinguish between stone, focal interstitial pancreatitis, pericholedochal lymphadenopathy, and a hypertrophied Vaterian segment. The assessment of the papillary region by indenting the anterior duodenal wall is difficult, apart from the fact that in about 10% of people the papilla of Vater is not in the midsection of the medial wall of the descending duodenum. Both of these maneuvers are nevertheless worth performing, but the findings must be carefully and differentially interpreted (94) (Fig. 11-4).

In the problem of CDJS there is great advantage to doing the cholangiogram under manometric control. The technique is described in Chapter 6. The critical fact is that

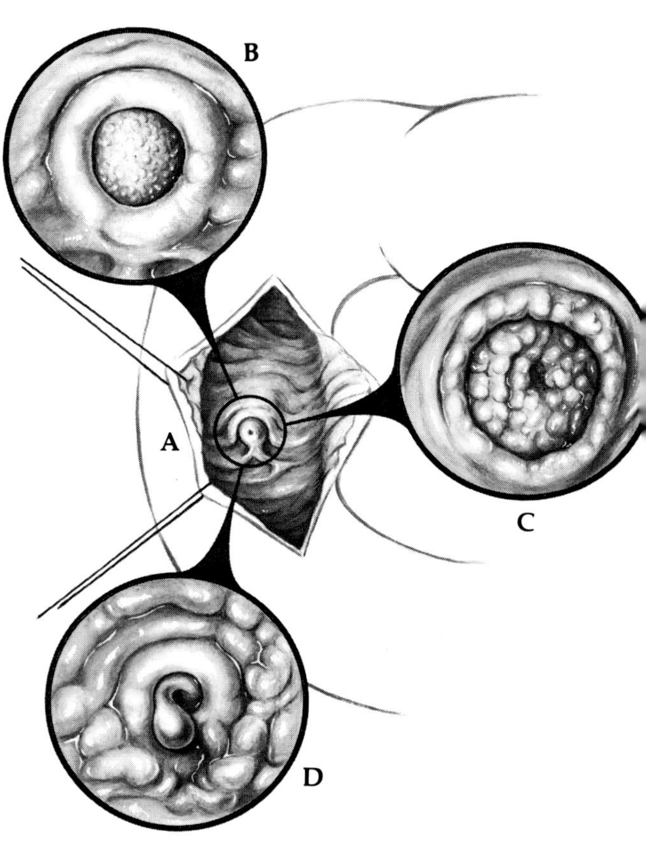

FIG. 11-4. The ampulla in CDJS. Several problems are involved in evaluating the ampullary area: **A.** The ampulla is normal. **B.** There is a crowning stone. **C.** Carcinoma of the ampulla is present. **D.** Benign polypoidal changes may occur. The latter three etiologic factors must be eliminated before a diagnosis of idiopathic CDJS is accepted. Cholangiography and choledochoscopy are mandatory. Duodenostomy is sometimes required. (From Schein CJ, Stern WZ, Jacobson HG: The Common Bile Duct. Operative Cholangiography, Biliary Endoscopy and Choledocholithotomy, 1966. Courtesy of Charles C Thomas, Publisher, Springfield, Illinois)

a diagnosis of CDJS cannot be supported if the passage pressure is less than 20 cm saline. If the manometer is not available, one may measure the resting intraductal pressure by noting the height of a column of bile in a polyethelene tube that is inserted into the duct by means of its wedged-on needle.

In the MHMC experience no specific roentgen configuration of the sphincter segment has been encountered that is pathognomonic of the phenomenon that is CDJS. The unreliability of the single film has already been indicated. The T-tube cine cholangiographic studies of Schein and Beneventano (530) in cases of this disorder have failed to show a rigid fixed configuration of the area. Sequential films can sometimes be superimposed without revealing an alteration of choledochal sphincter function. One may recognize an excessively long sphincter segment (2 cm in length) and the pseudocalculus sign as normal; CDJS may present in association with these signs, but they are not evidence of "stricture."

Direct exploration of the duct is required. In CDJS there is difficulty in negotiating the choledochoduodenal junction with a number 3 Bakes dilator. This has been termed ampullary thrust resistance. The Bakes probe normally passes with just one moment of minor resistance.

The pitfalls in this problem can be either the small ampullary carcinoma or the suprapapillary stone that is pushed ahead of the exploratory probe. Either can mimic CDJS. The distinction is of more than academic significance. Since early, properly treated carcinomas of the ampullary area carry the best prognosis for any cancer in the biliary system, some of these still prove to be resectable 14–36 months after a prior operation. Benign epithelial tumors of the ampulla are uncommon, but in the 30 cases reported on by Anderson and Gregor (18), the presenting symptoms were biliary dysfunction. Cattell and others (118, 120, 122) consider adenomas in this area as precursors to cancer.

The differential diagnosis can be difficult.

TABLE 11-2. MHMC EXPERIENCE WITH CDJS AS AN INDICATION FOR SECONDARY BILIARY TRACT PROCEDURE

Age (yr)*	Sex†	Time after cholecystectomy (yr)	Passage pressure (cm)‡	Duct size (cm)§	Presence of stones in CBD¶
76	F	30	33	2.0	+
65	F	20	29	1.8	0
60	F	22	27	2.0	+
35	F	1	27	1.8	0
70	M	6	27	2.2	+
66	F	15	29	2.2	0
66	F	2	27	1.8	+
55	F	5	27	1.6	0
60	M	5	32	1.4	0
75	F	5	34	2.0	+
68	F	10	39	1.8	0
47	F	2	37	1.4	0
92	F	30	34	2.0	+
55	F	10	37	1.6	+
64	F	13	31	1.6	0
62	F	33	30	2.0	+
73	F	24	27	2.4	0
59	F	4	23	2.0	0
54	F	2	29	1.4	+
30	F	7	27	1.6	0
41	F	9	29	1.6	0

* Range, 30–92
† Ratio, F:M, 19/2
‡ Average, 28.9 cm saline
§ Average, 1.77 cm
¶ Stones in duct, +, 57%; 0, 43%

One patient in the MHMC series required open duodenal biopsy to establish a difficult diagnosis. The patient was found to have an ampullary mass in association with a large cystic duct remnant. The lesion proved to be the earliest carcinoma of the ampulla that this hospital has encountered; it had extended only into the submucosa. When last seen, 7 years after pancreaticoduodenectomy, that patient was free of disease.

In a review of the consultative material it became apparent that some patients have had a truly diseased gallbladder removed when the main problem was, in fact, an ampullary tumor. It can be an easy lesion to miss if not specifically sought for by inspection and revealed by biliary endoscopy or cholangiography. The frequency of this potential problem is evidenced by Baggenstoss (30), who found ampullary polyps in 4 of 100 consecutive autopsies when a distinct effort was made to examine the area. Griffen *et al.* (240) found that four of five cases of ampullary polyps had no associated lithiasis. In the German and Swiss medical literature, a distinct point is made of this possibility and the CDJS that is considered is referred to as the benign type (*gutartiges*) to differentiate it from the cancers in the area. However there is no place for inexperienced meddling; the dangers of biliary and duodenal fistulas are both real and serious.

In summary, the diagnosis of CDJS can be made with the following criteria:

1. Delayed transit of intravenous contrast into the duodenum–more than 90 min.

2. Dilated and thickened common duct.

3. Choledochal hypertension, with passage pressure exceeding 20 cm H_2O.

4. Difficulty in negotiating through the choledochal sphincter with a number 3 Bakes dilator.

CASE EXPERIENCE

The MHMC experience comprises 21 secondary cases (Table 11-2). All other series likewise report the syndrome as more prominent in the female, in range of 2.5/1. When present, the calculi and/or bile sludge in each instance have also been of the primary type, regarded as having arisen in the ductal system. This series specifically excludes patients whose disorder was treated primarily at the time of cholecystectomy or those with a purely faceted stone in the duct.

All patients were treated by removal of calculi and in-continuity choledochoduodenostomy. There was no postoperative mortality and the patients' postoperative courses have been smooth. Four patients developed abdominal wound infections. I believe this is related to contamination from the bile. Each of these patients had choledocholithiasis, in which it has been observed that the frequency of bacterial contamination of the bile is in the range of 90%. The preoperative use of antibiotics appears to have been a factor in reducing the problem in the last half of this

FIG. 11-5. Remote validation of CDJS. Nine years after choledochoduodenostomy for CDJS, a barium swallow examination immediately opacifies the biliary tree and the anastomatic site **(black arrow).** The distal common bile duct **(white arrow)** fails to empty through the normal channels, thus confirming the irreversible nature of the CDJS and the original indication for the procedure.

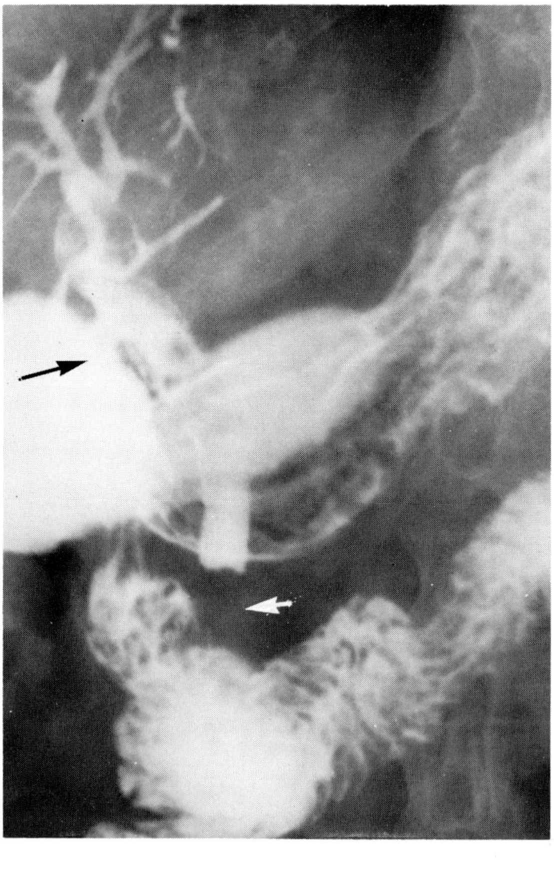

series; in these patients, this infectious complication was not encountered.

The follow-up in the group ranges from 1 to 14 years. There has been no instance of postoperative cholangitis, jaundice, or colic requiring narcotics. All patients were advised to use a choleretic for the first month. No specific medication was otherwise advised, on the principle that if the anastomosis is adequate, nothing else is required, and if the area is stenotic, nothing else really makes a difference. I have cautioned patients against the use of foods with skins that, it has been reported, can get into the anastomosis. I am not certain that it is necessary to avoid raw tomatoes and to peel apples and peaches; but I have advised patients about this report.

The majority of these patients have been remotely studied by barium swallow, and specific demonstrations have been sought in the evaluation. In all instances the following triad was observed: 1) The anastomosis is readily visualized, and barium completely opacifies the ductal system. 2) The barium is spontaneously evacuated from the liver within 3 hours, and in no instance was it present 24 hours later. 3) The area of the choledochoduodenal junction remains obstructed. Examination of one asymptomatic patient by barium swallow 9 years after the procedure showed a well-functioning anastomosis that filled and emptied promptly, but more importantly, there was no transit of contrast material through the distal choledochus. Thus the diagnosis of CDJS is confirmed as to its chronicity and lack of specific anatomic configuration (Fig. 11-5).

In no cases has the barium been observed to empty by the natural route. In no instance has the film demonstrated retained debris or calculi in the distal bypassed segment of the common duct; either this area does not collect or store material, or it evacuates promptly. These roentgen findings of satisfactory anastomotic function parallel the satisfactory clinical response.

12 Congenital Disorders in Adults

Symptomatic congenital disorders of the biliary tract fall into two large groups. Some, such as the biliary atresias, present early in life and require prompt attempts at defining and correcting their manifestations. Another, larger group comprises congenital anomalies and variations that are of no symptomatic importance: the phrygian-capped gallbladder, anomalies of gallbladder position, variations in hepatic attachment, in blood supply, and in duct configuration. These can constitute significant challenges in the intraoperative situation. Mismanagement of such abnormalities can produce a significant postoperative disability. Intermediately, there is a small group of individuals whose congenital anomalies present as symptomatic disease in adult life (253, 302, 612, 645). In the MHMC series several congenital biliary variants have been encountered that were the cause of or part of the PCS.

CONGENITAL DILATATION

Congenital dilatation of the intrahepatic ducts is a rare entity, and at this time only 20 cases (approximately) have been reported —most of them associated with congenital hepatic fibrosis or fibroangioadenomatosis. Only a few "pure" cases have been reported, and one of these patients eventually developed amyloidosis.

Congenital dilatation is a disorder of the segmental intrahepatic bile ducts. The extrahepatic bile ducts need not be dilated although this has been reported. In the pure form the dilated areas become the seat of secondary stasis, cholangitis, lithiasis, and abscess formation. This lesion is frequently not appreciated since the extrahepatic biliary tree appears normal. Therefore, it may first be unmasked on puncture cholangiography or T-tube contrast studies. Oral cholecystography may not reveal the abnormality.

Caroli's disease is a segmental saccular dilatation of the intrahepatic bile ducts, usually with associated cholangitis and liver abscesses and the formation of secondary calculi. It is inherited as a familial mendelian recessive trait (286, 433). The prognosis is serious, with death from liver abscesses and septicemia. The disease has to be differentiated from obstructive biliary tract disease and from the benign form of polycystic liver disease. The latter is asymptomatic and has no communication with the biliary tract and remains complicated unless molested.

CONGENITAL CHOLEDOCHAL CYST

The classic triad of pain, mass, and jaundice is not seen in adults. When the choledochal cyst presents in the adult there is the justifiable query of how this can be differentiated from the grossly enlarged duct that is acquired as a result of obstructive calculus disease (125). The diagnosis of congenital choledochal cyst in the adult can be supported only by the demonstration of a concomitant congenital disordered pattern of the intrahepatic ducts of a type that is not encountered in the purely obstructive choledochopathies (234, 312). This is clearly illlustrated in Figures 12-1 and 12-2, in which the abnormality is characterized by bizarre configuration of the intrahepatic ducts, the absence of an orderly pattern of dilatation (such as would appear proximal to a calculus obstruction) and the corkscrew appearance of some of the minor radicles.

The etiology is unclear. The disorder has been attributed to an achalasia type phenomenon, to an unequal rate of vacuolation of the

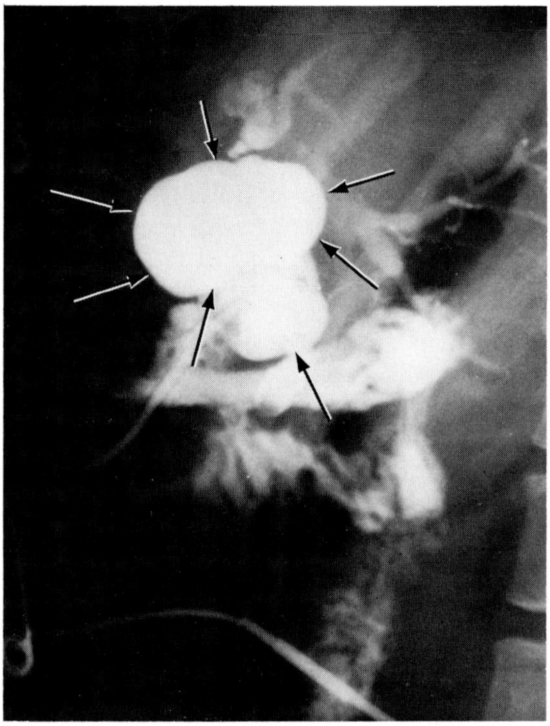

FIG. 12-1. Choledochal cyst. Intraoperative cholangiogram demonstrates a greatly dilated common duct **(arrows).** The intrahepatic radicles have an abnormal configuration and distribution. Contrast material does pass into the duodenum. This patient has formed stasis calculi. The problem here is stasis and sepsis.

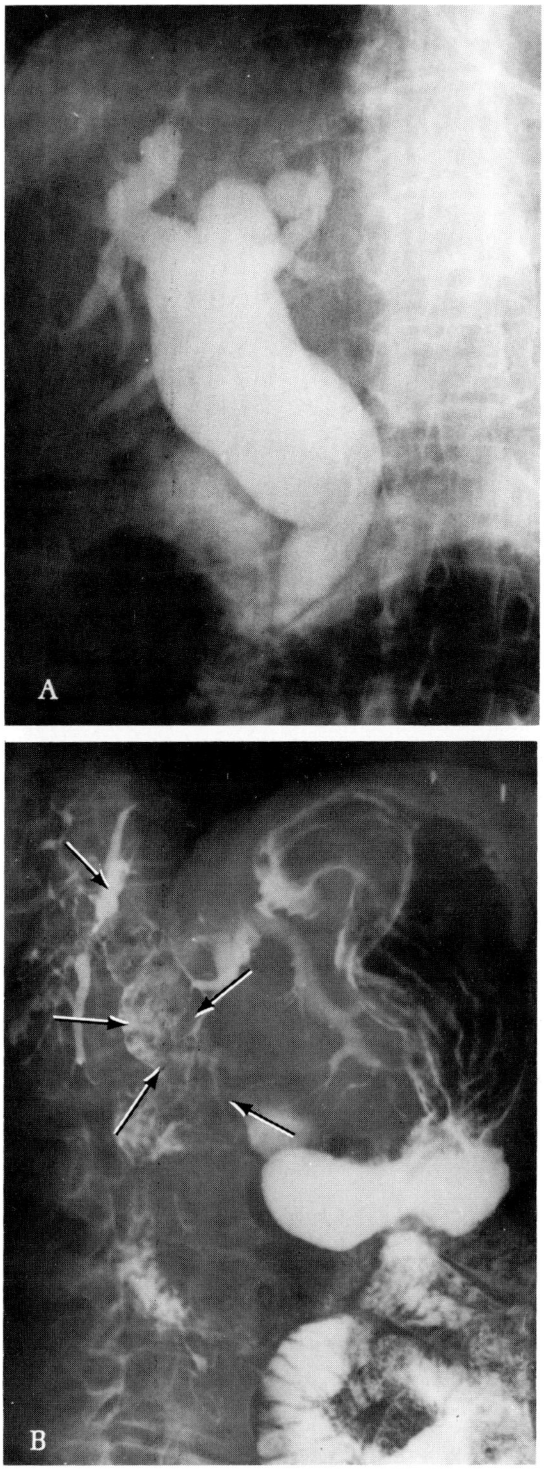

FIG. 12-2. Choledochal Cyst. **A.** Direct-puncture cholangiogram shows a greatly dilated common bile duct emptying into the duodenum. The dilatation is most marked in the supraduodenal portion of the duct. The intrahepatic radicles are distorted and are abnormal not only in their configuration but also in their width. There are no calculi. This is the basis for the diagnosis of choledochal cyst. **B.** Oral barium study after choledochoduodenostomy shows some retained barium on a 24-hour film. The stasis has not been completely relieved by the choledochoduodenostomy. Retention associated with imperfect drainage of the smaller radicles **(arrows)** accounts for the cholangitis that is the complication of this procedure for this specific disorder.

embryonal solid-core common duct, and to a faulty insertion into the duodenum, somewhat akin to the ureteropelvic anomalies encountered in congenital hydronephrosis.

The three patients in the MHMC series were female, ages 28, 64, and 72. The presentation for corrective surgery was for recurrent bouts of cholangitis. One patient had already had a secondary T-tube intubation that had not prevented the recurrence of cholangitis. In contrast to the situation in childhood, none of these patients had a palpable mass, but two had had more than one episode of jaundice.

In these cases, the cyst was a uniform, saccular, unicameral dilation of the supraduodenal segment of the duct, a component of which presented as a large, posterior, dependent sac, which could be appreciated only in the lateral-view cholangiogram. In no instance did this have a short neck coming off a definable normal extrahepatic duct. In none of these cases did the duct contain calculi, though stasis bile was present in all. The readily accessible duct in the hepatoduodenal ligament was the area involved.

The gross configuration of the duct suggested that a satisfactory drainage and decompression of the area could be accomplished by a choledochoduodenostomy, with posterior positioning of the ostium. The cyst and the duodenum were so adherent that no posterior wall suturing was required. Treatment of all three cases was by wide anastomosis in continuity with the duodenum. One patient developed a postoperative complication characterized by fever and anemia. A virulent *Clostridia* organism was recovered from her duodenal bile. This problem resolved with penicillin.

Postoperative oral barium studies have revealed a patent anastomosis and about 90% emptying of the barium in 24 hours in all three patients. However, in each study, some of the barium has been retained in the third, fourth, and fifth order of the intrahepatic ducts. When postoperative symptoms occur, I have come to believe that they are related to the inflammatory process in these abnormal small radicles, which drain imperfectly, and not to disease in the large, anatomically well-drained extrahepatic ductal system. It may well be that no drainage procedure on the extrahepatic cyst can totally and effectively facilitate the drainage of the disordered intrahepatic system. A far better procedure might be resection with the Roux Y hepaticojejunostomy (363, 369).

One of these patients remains asymptomatic; a second has had two bouts of minor cholangitis in 3 years; and the third has had episodes every year for the past 4 years. Each of these has responded to antibiotics. The last two patients are improved but not cured.

There is reported to be a 95% mortality in untreated cases, due to rupture, peritonitis, or cirrhosis. This MHMC series offers an interesting example of how long one can go with the disease without fatal complications.

Lindenauer and Lavanway (363) attribute these postoperative recurrent bouts of cholangitis, which is the problem common to cases with anastomatic stricture, to particulate vegetable matter in the dependent cyst. This is contrary to the two cases described here in which the usual criteria for the evaluation of biliary enteric anastomosis demonstrated satisfactory emptying except of the intrahepatic radicles. Other investigators believe that the best venting is accomplished by the Roux Y choledochojejunostomy, sometimes with resection of the cyst (12, 369). That experience, however, has been in a considerably younger age group. Alonso-Lej *et al.* (12) did a collective review of the problem and found a 31% incidence of cholangitis with cystoduodenostomy and a 10% with the Roux Y jejunal cystostomy.

THE ACCESSORY HEPATIC DUCT

Accessory bile ducts occur in about 14% of people. The majority arise on the right side and represent the drainage of subsegmental areas in the distribution of the dorsocaudal division of the right hepatic duct. In the context of the PCS they assume an importance when the duct has been severed in the belief that this small structure represented a fibrous band; now the patient has a biliary fistula. An accessory duct may have its entrance into the cystic duct (Fig. 12-3), in which case a sufficient segment of that duct must be retained to provide an exit for drainage. This anatomic situation is the best indication for retaining a segment of the cystic duct.

The problem is encountered only rarely

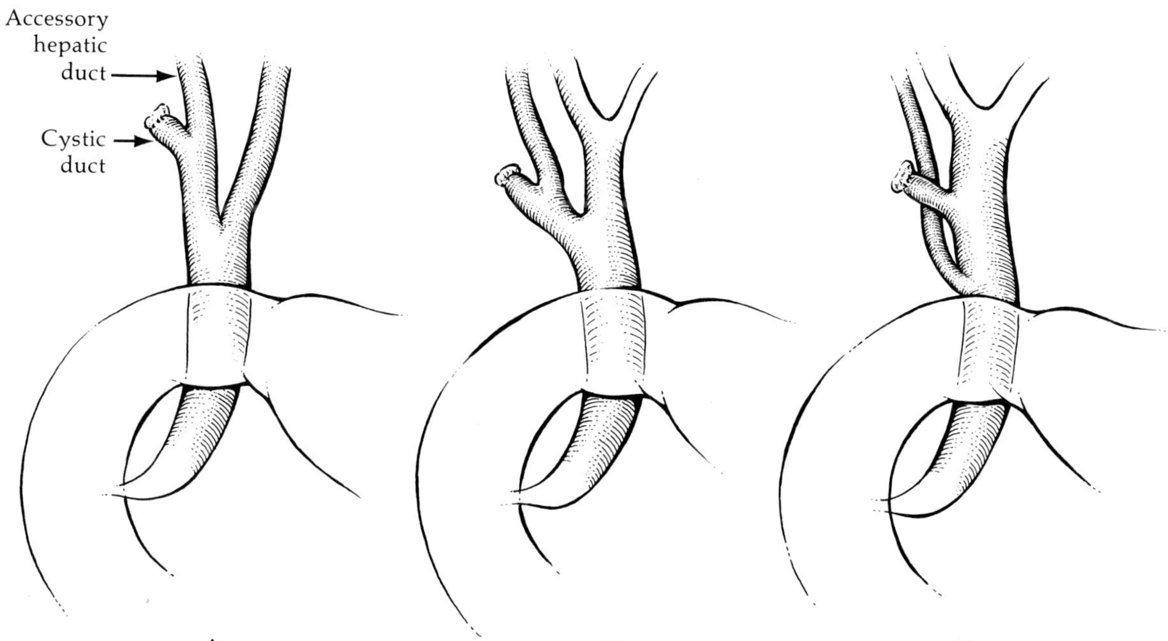

FIG. 12-3. Accessory hepatic ducts. **A.** It is important not to confuse the long right accessory duct with the cystic duct. **B.** The cystic duct must be ligated high enough to allow for outflow from the accessory duct. **C.** This rare anomaly requires cautious definition before any ties are applied or structures divided.

because most accessory right hepatic ducts drain into the choledochus on the hilar side of the gallbladder pedicle. They are rarely visualized. One becomes cognizant of them only on the operative cholangiogram. The fate of the divided accessory duct will depend upon its size, the volume of bile that it conducts, and the presence of the collateral collecting system. Thus the differentiation of an aberrant duct from an accessory duct assumes importance, for in the former instance the conduit is necessary, in the latter it is an accessory.

Whenever I have encountered an accessory hepatic duct 3 mm or more in diameter, I have chosen to anastomose it to the small bowel. I have not regretted the time taken to do this, although there is no way of knowing whether the anastomosis has remained open. I have regarded it as a way of preventing a problem. I am aware of one instance in which a 2-mm accessory hepatic duct was severed and disregarded. The patient drained bile for about 8 weeks and then stopped (232, 359, 474).

In the PCS, I have encountered the problem of the severed accessory duct as the source of a bile fistula that caused a recurrent subhepatic abscess; the abscess failed to respond to several episodes of drainage. The duct was anastomosed to the bowel with a satisfactory result. The diagnosis was made by the instillation of contrast into the fistula, simultaneously with intravenous cholangiography. This is a rare cause of a postcholecystectomy bile fistula. The more common cause is an injury to a major bile duct with proximal slough.

INTRAHEPATIC GALLBLADDER

I have twice treated diabetic patients having obvious biliary sepsis who had been previously operated upon for gallbladder disease. Each of these patients was regarded as having an intrahepatic gallbladder that "it was not safe to try to remove." The indications for reoperative surgery were compelling.

One of these patients presented again with an acute and severe chronic cholecystitis, in which the hepatic flexure and duodenum were densely adherent to the very thick-walled visceral surface of the gallbladder. The lumen contained a solitary large stone that had molded to the contour of the gallbladder and completely perforated through its posterior wall into the liver. This was a posterior intrahepatic perforation by a thick-walled gallbladder. It was not intrahepatic.

The findings in the second case were similar. The body of the gallbladder had perforated into the duodenum as a cholecystoduodenal fistula. The tissue planes were obliterated by a thick scar.

In these cases the declaration of the findings as congenital abnormalities was a misinterpretation of the advanced pathologic state of the disease. The ligneous character of these adhesions and the difficulty in defining planes can also simulate a cancer originating in the gallbladder or colon (452).

These difficult dissections can be worked out very anatomically by the intravesical digital dissection technique (527). One has only to locate the lumen of the gallbladder and evacuate its contents; from there on the procedure is similar to dissecting the adherent structures off an indirect inguinal hernia sac that has been repeatedly contused by a truss.

Another patient had undergone operation for obstructive jaundice in association with chronic cholecystitis. The jaundice recurred 8 months later. At the second procedure a 1.5-cm nodule was present in the wall of the duodenum, alongside the duodenal papilla. It could be nucleated without difficulty. The mass was pancreatic heterotopia. The patient remains asymptomatic.

The septate or hourglass gallbladder presents as a specific aspect of gallbladder rem-

FIG. 12-4. Hourglass gallbladder. **A.** In this typical cholecystogram of an hourglass gallbladder, one may see the upper loculus **(1)**, the lower loculus **(2)**, a normal cystic duct **(3)**, and normal common bile duct **(4)**. Mistakenly, such an organ may be subtotally resected through its waist. **B.** Gross specimen of the hourglass-shaped organ. Only the upper segment has calculi.

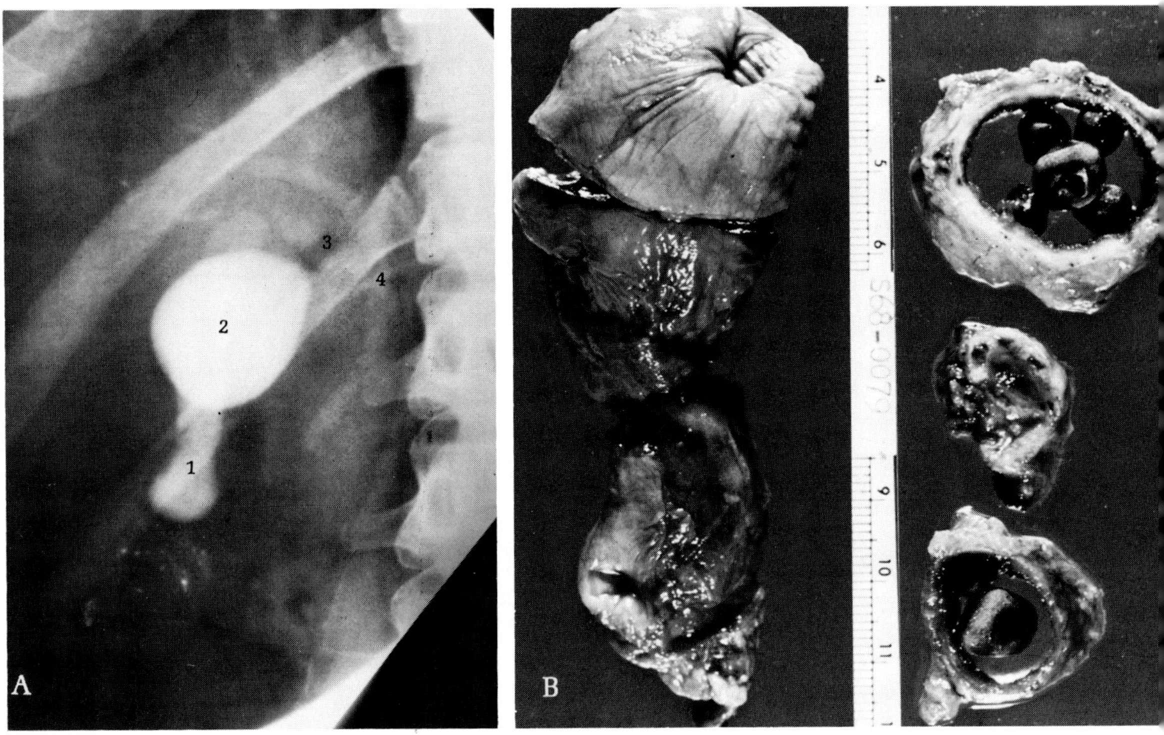

nant disease. This anomaly, upon which inflammatory and calculus disease were imposed, is characterized by a waist-like constriction of the organ, which results in an isthmus dividing the organ into upper and lower loculi (Fig. 12-4).

One patient presented with symptoms and a pathology report on a gallbladder specimen. At the second operation a large gallbladder remnant was encountered. When the problem was reconstructed, it appeared that the first operation had been an amputation through the isthmic stricture and that the lower segment of the "hourglass" had been left behind. It was probably interpreted as a greatly dilated common bile duct.

13 Iatrogenic Disorders

Prior procedures that prove to be incomplete or ill advised often create new problems—iatrogenic pathologic states. Major duct trauma that eventuated in early postoperative stricture or fistula is specifically excluded from this category because this problem is far afield from those under consideration here. Iatrogenic disorders present in seven categories:

1. The misinterpretation of pancreatic disease
2. Inadequate biliary decompression
3. Foreign bodies in the duct
4. Perforative duct trauma
5. Technical complications
6. Cholangiographic misinterpretations
7. Hemobilia

MISINTERPRETATION OF PANCREATIC DISEASE–CHOLECYSTOJEJUNOSTOMY PROBLEMS

The surgeon in each of the four cases reviewed here interpreted the pancreatic disease as a carcinoma and performed a cholecystojejunostomy as a method of relieving the jaundice. No biopsy confirmation was obtained. At intervals of 9–34 months later, the patients presented with chills, fever, and jaundice. These are symptoms of cholangitis or cholecystic inflammation due to a stenosis of the cholecystoenteric anastomosis.

The simple loop type of cholecystoenteric anastomosis ordinarily functions well for a period of about 9–12 months (Fig. 13-1A). It is, therefore, useful for the patient with pancreatic cancer who has definite liver metastases. The valved afferent loop with a distal entero-enterostomy or the Roux-Y procedure is more effective because it shunts the oral intake away from the anastomosis. Tomato and fruit skins have been implicated as producing impaction of the anastomosis, behind which infection can occur.

In each of these patients, detailed studies before re-intervention revealed no evidence of metastatic disease. An inflamed gallbladder and infected common bile duct were evident in each instance (Fig. 13-1). One patient had had a solitary gallstone in a grossly normal gallbladder; in the other two, the gallbladder had been normal at the first operation. In one case, 4 years later, there was a large villous adenoma on the gallbladder side of the cholecystojejunostomy. It had developed since surgery. Such a change has been reported with uretero-enteric anastomosis and is the only such change seen in the MHMC experience.

The indication for secondary surgery was biliary sepsis. The cholecystojejunostomy was dismantled and the revised intestinal wall closed by a series of interrupted silk sutures. The gallbladder was removed.

In two instances cholangiography revealed a patent distal common bile duct and no additional procedure was required. This may represent a complete resolution of the pancreatic inflammatory process. In the other two cases, the ducts measured 2 and 2.4 cm in width; each was decompressed by a suprapancreatic incontinuity choledochoduodenostomy. Each patient has been observed for more than 5 years without recurrence of biliary sepsis.

These cases present the prospective prob-

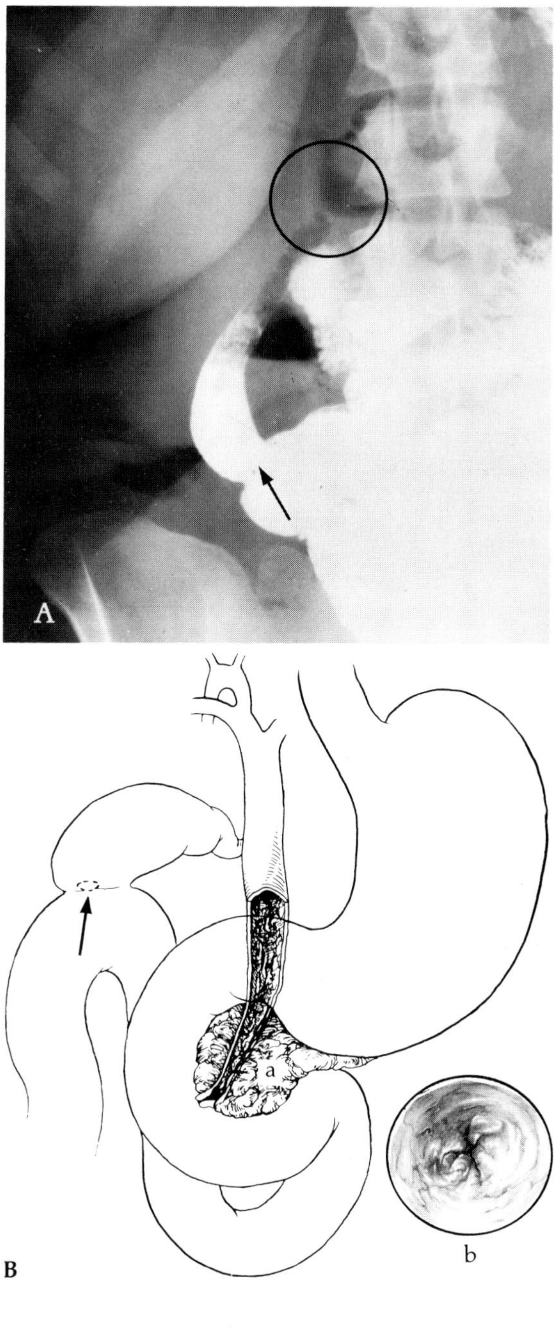

FIG. 13-1. Cholecystojejunostomy. **A.** Barium swallow demonstrates a well-functioning anastomosis **(arrow).** There is a well-outlined pneumocholangiogram in the **encircled** area. **B.** Diagramatic representation of a strictured cholecystojejunostomy **(arrow).** Chronic pancreatitis constricts the common bile duct **(a).** Endoscopic view reveals the tubular stricture **(b).** The anastomosis was dismantled, the jejunum sutured then cholecystectomy and choledochoduodenostomy were undertaken. (Schein CJ, Stern WZ, Hurwitt ES, Jacobson HG: Am J Roentgenol 89:864, 1963)

lem about what to do next time for presumably nonresectable cancer of the pancreatic head with jaundice, in which it is not possible to obtain a satisfactory tissue diagnosis. If absolute gallbladder disease is present (*i.e.*, gallstones or common duct stone), I elect to do a cholecystectomy and choledochojejunostomy. The procedure is somewhat more complicated than loop cholecystojejunostomy, but it has the advantage of being a good decompressive operation for either chronic pancreatitis or pancreatic cancer. I have also employed this approach to the icteric patient with an unproved pancreatic lesion and normal gallbladder. If the patient is not icteric, the lesion unproved and presumed not resectable (for whatever reason), I decompress the biliary tract by a cholecystostomy tube. This permits postoperative cholecystocholangiography and does not alter the area that may have to be surgically explored at another procedure.

The important lesson from this experience is that the patient with biliary sepsis following a biliary enteric anastomosis for unproved cancer should be regarded as having a correctable situation. The initial diagnosis should be questioned when a patient survives beyond the usual time for his presumed disease. A secondary operation does not aggravate the problem in advanced cancer and offers the possibility of salvaging the patient with benign disease.

A complicated diagnostic problem presents when there is a combination of diseases. Ordinarily the surgeon ascribes a benign etiology and course to the pancreatic changes encountered in association with chronic cholecystitis and choledocholithiasis. In the MHMC series were two patients who returned 9 and 13 months after choledochoduodenostomy with obvious liver metastases that were due to pancreatic cancer not recognized at the time of the first procedure. The removal of common duct stones and choledochoduodenostomy at the original procedure had managed the obstructive jaundice and infection in both patients, but the concomitant cancer was not recognized. A third patient had common duct stones, cancer of the ampulla, and alcoholic cirrhosis.

There are those who have little faith in the results of resection for cancer of the head of the pancreas, who would counter that this sort of error in diagnosis makes no difference in patient survival. However, failure to perform such surgery does exclude the possibility of salvage for those with cancer of the distal bile duct or ampulla when the prognosis with excisional surgery is more favorable.

INADEQUATE BILIARY DECOMPRESSION

The enlarged common duct remains with a diseased epithelium that serves as the nidus for further inflammation or new stone formation in some cases. This entity is distinct from recurrent Vaterian segment disease or CDJS, although it may be concomitant.

In this category are included decubitus diverticula of the common duct, segmental intrahepatic ductal ectasia, calculus-induced stricture of the left hepatic duct, and intraductal synechia. These disorders can be identified by cholangiography or choledochoscopy.

The calculus decubitus is the sequel of a solitary impacted stone that has eroded the duct into the pancreatic substances. In that instance the symptoms were biliary colic and transitory jaundice—presumably due to pancreatitis. This problem was satisfactorily managed by choledochoduodenostomy (Fig. 13-2). Another, albeit unusual instance is one in which a residual stone in the hepatoduodenal segment had perforated freely into the peritoneal cavity.

Intrahepatic ductal ectasia of undetermined origin is rare. This has been encountered twice in the MHMC series. It may be congenital, the residuum of an intrahepatic cholangitic abscess, or an area of metaplasia. It can be a cause of symptoms. One of the two patients was treated by direct transhepatic drainage and packing (hepatotomy); the second was managed indirectly by incontinuity bypass. Other investigators have reported hepatic resection for this entity (83, 369, 371).

Postcalculous ulceration with stricture of the left hepatic duct just proximal to the carina has been encountered in a patient in whom the stone ulcerated through the duct. Direct hepatic duct incision, removal of the stone, and T-tube stenting resolved the problem.

Suppurative cholangitis is best evaluated by direct biliary endoscopy before the duct is washed out. Usually the duct is irrigated as part of the toilet of the area, and the cleaning process obscures the pathology before it can be visualized.

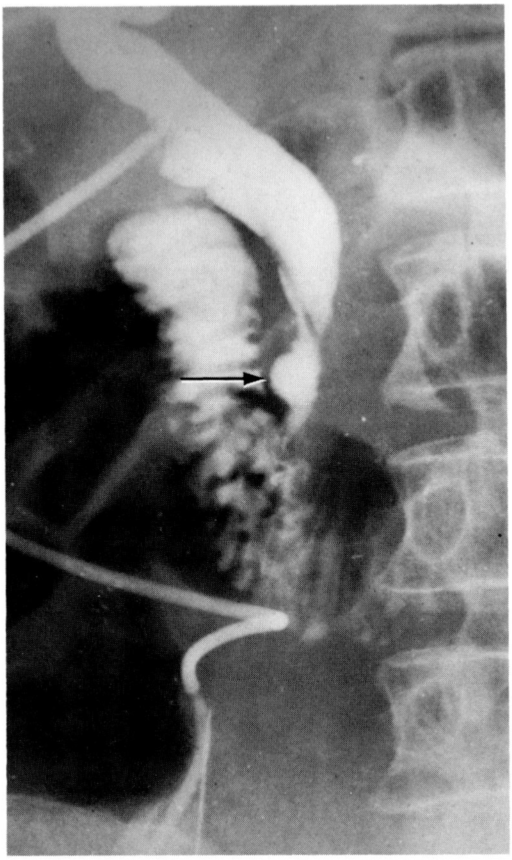

FIG. 13-2. Suprasphincteric diverticulum. T-tube cholangiogram exposed after choledocholithotomy reveals no calculi. The duct is dilated, and a diverticulum arises from the right side of the suprasphincteric choledochus **(arrow).** The T tube was removed and a choledochoduodenostomy performed.

If the duct is visualized directly after the choledochostomy, a spectrum of changes is observed: numerous fibrin adhesions across the duct resemble irregularly arranged clotheslines. This "fishnet" across the duct holds small calculi or bile aggregates within its mesh. If this coagulum is not thoroughly washed out or disrupted by the intraductal manipulations and irrigations, then the calculi or bile aggregates that they enmesh then continue to be an impediment to bile flow, with stasis bile formation. These specific web changes in cholangitis have not been commented upon as a mechanical factor in the genesis of residual cholangitis.

FOREIGN BODIES IN THE DUCT

Foreign bodies are uncommon events in the PCS, but when encountered, they are dramatic and curable. One must be aware of the possibility. It is highly probable that the incidence, like that of ureteral and recurrent nerve injuries, is greater than that reported in the literature—a fact influenced by embarrassment as well as sensitivity to litigation (588).

The surface of the bile ducts is covered by a meandering epicholedochal plexus. In the chronic state it is partially hidden in the epicholedochal reaction but becomes apparent with cuff bleeding at the choledochostomy incision. In most instances the bleeding is controlled by a simple tie or cautery that is reinforced by the through-all-layer closure of the choledochostomy incision. A combination of events can result in minor bleeding into the duct: When control of the cut end of the incision is tenuous, the suture slips and the closure is subepithelial. Bleeding from this cause is not sufficient to produce a systemic reaction or a fall in hematocrit, but it can eventuate in an intraluminal clot that obstructs the flow of bile. However sound theoretically, there is no basis for the practice of subepithelial closure of the choledochostomy incision.

The cholangiographic configuration of the clot is quite characteristic. It presents as a long, nonfaceted, smooth defect in the contrast medium. The single experience in the MHMC series (Fig. 13-3) was satisfactorily managed by heparin irrigation of the duct, which either dissolved the clot or facilitated its passage through the duct (599).

Irrigation of the T tube after it is positioned in the duct serves not only to indicate the adequacy of the choledochostomy closure and the patency of the tube, but also to indicate that there is no intraluminal bleeding. Sloughed cystic duct ligatures can become the nidus of choledochal calculi.

If nonabsorbable material is used to ligate the cystic duct, a foreign-body reaction or stitch abscess may sequestrate the ligature into the bile duct. It then becomes the nidus for the deposition of bile salts. The proof lies

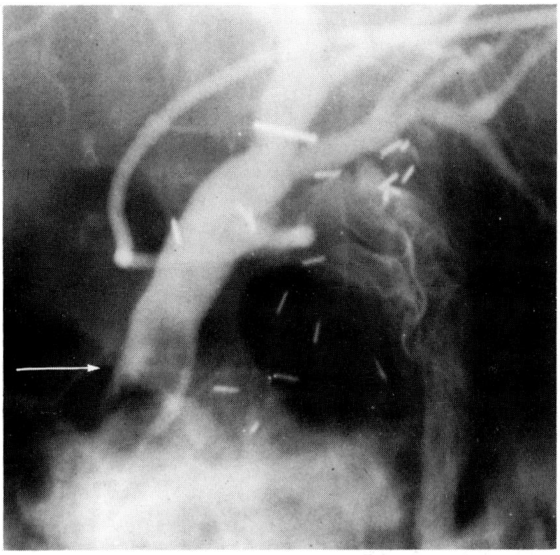

FIG. 13-3. Intracholedochal clot. T-tube study shows a long, elliptical foreign body in the bile duct **(arrow),** a configuration suggesting a blood clot. It either passed or was dissolved with heparin perfusion.

in the demonstration of a piece of silk within the common-duct concretion. There have been numerous cases reported of this entity (6, 34, 105, 562, 625). This complication can be avoided. There is no advantage to silk ligature of the cystic duct or to silk closure of the common duct. In contrast, a small or severely sclerotic cystic artery is better controlled by a silk suture, which can be applied more delicately. I have not seen this slip through into the ductal system, provided the artery and duct are ligated separately. If the duct and artery have been litigated together, the anlage for an arterial-ductal fistula is established (632).

Metal staples are being used to clip hilar structures. They can be confidently delivered deep into uncomfortable sites by means of a long-handled clip-holding forceps. Those who use this method of cystic duct and artery occlusion appreciate the facility with which the clip can be delivered. In only one instance at MHMC was such a clip recovered from within the common duct 3 weeks after it had been used to occlude the cystic duct. In that case, the common duct had not been explored at the original operation.

Remnants of portions of rubber T tubes, encrusted catheters, corroded splint devices and fragments of rubber gloves and Penrose drains have been found within the duct (588).

A much more common problem has been the inadvertently retained sponge, laparotomy pad, or drain. Here the presentation is not with a PCS in the sense of this text but is a residual intraabdominal abscess, a persistent sinus, or intestinal obstruction. The plain film of the abdomen that is part of the roentgen study of the symptomatic patient usually reveals this retained foreign body.

Pfeffermann *et al.* (467) report on *Ascaris* invasions of the common duct, with obstructive symptoms in patients who have had prior biliary surgery and common duct exploration. It is their belief that an incompetent ampulla facilitates the access of the parasite to the extrahepatic biliary tract. The diagnosis may be suspected in patients who have been in the Far East or in the areas where such parasite infections are common. If the diagnosis can be made, a conservative approach with a vermifuge should be used before considering secondary surgery.

PERFORATIVE DUCTAL TRAUMA

It is not possible to evaluate the incidence of perforative ductal trauma (416). It has not been seen at MHMC as a free perforation with a profuse bile leak. I have sometimes suspected that it has been the cause of postoperative pancreatitis, in which case the presence of the T tube has minimized the effect (Fig. 13-4). Smith *et al.* (568) have commented that this complication may be occult and present as an intraabdominal abscess or ileus, or as intestinal obstruction.

One case of obvious perforation was rec-

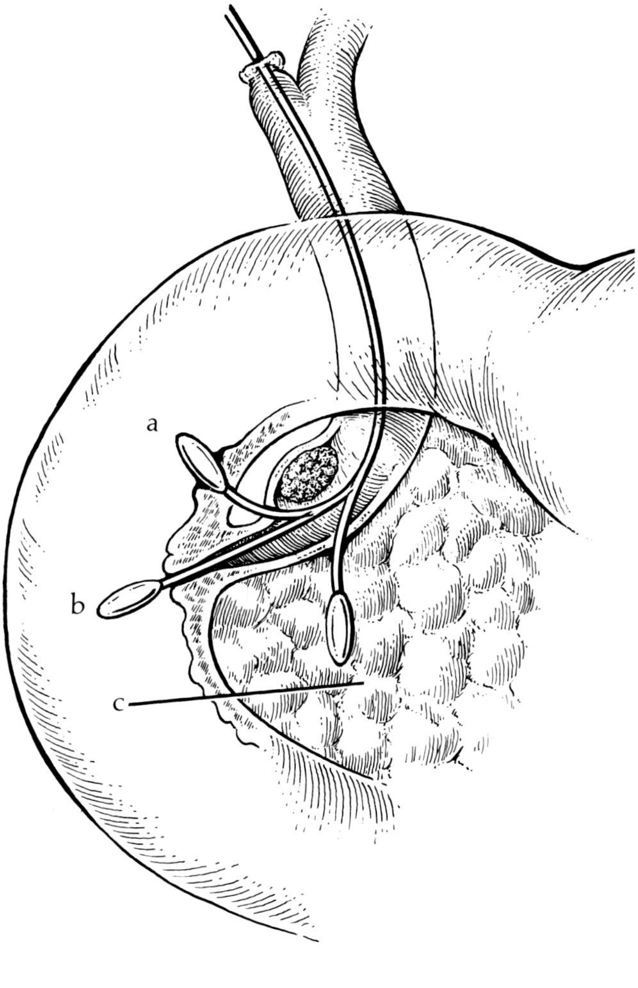

FIG. 13-4. Iatrogenic choledochal perforations. Three types of instrumental duct trauma have been recognized: **(a)** This type results in a suprasphincteric choledochoduodenal fistula. **(b)** This type bruises the ampullary segment with resultant hemorrhage and ecchymosis of the duodenal wall. **(c)** Perforations here produce a true bile leak into the peripancreatic tissues.

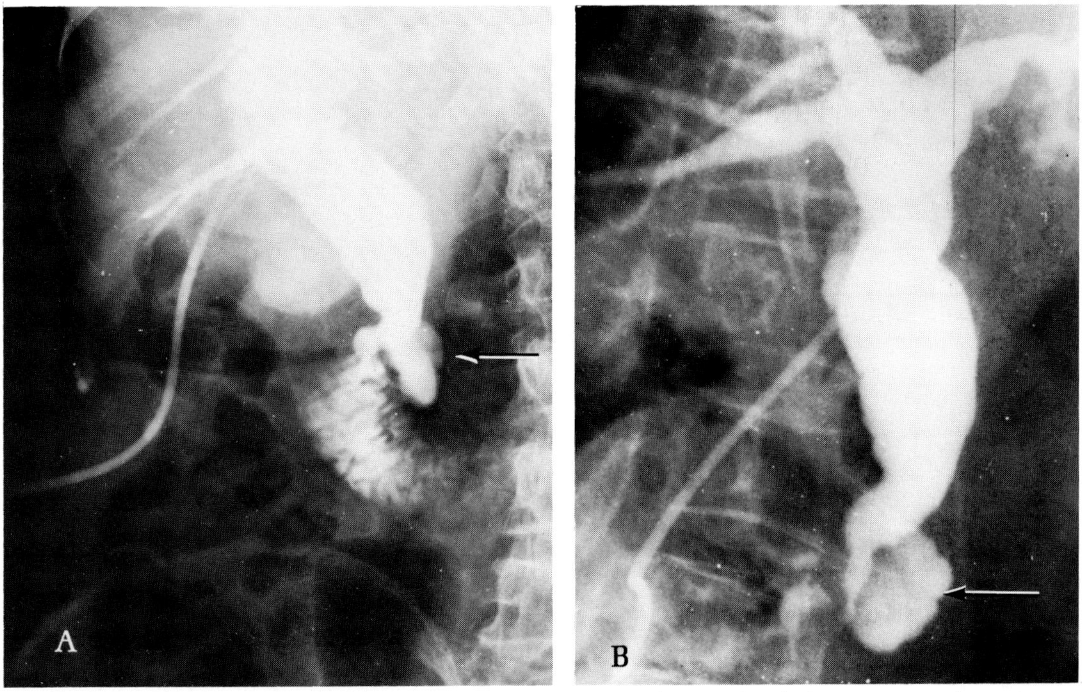

FIG. 13-5. A and B. Iatrogenic duct perforations demonstrated by T-tube cholangiograms, showing extravasation of contrast material in the region of the intramural segment **(arrows).** They are instances of instrumental perforation of the type illustrated in Figure 13-4**(c).** Neither was recognized clinically. The event would have gone unrecognized except for the cholangiogram.

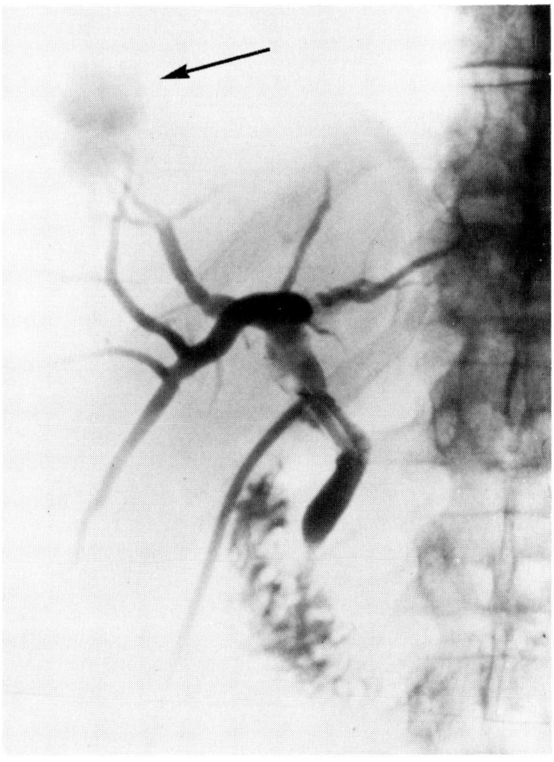

FIG. 13-6. Intrahepatic duct perforation. Intraoperative T-tube cholangiogram shows extravasation into the hepatic parenchyma **(arrow).** The area had been manipulated with a balloon catheter. A 10-day postoperative study was normal.

ognized, not symptomatically, but by the extravasation of contrast material on the remote T-tube cholangiogram. The patient did well but required a secondary choledochoduodenostomy for an ampullary obstruction (related?). It has been suggested that some instances of assumed ampullary fibrosis are actually due to traumatic perforation of the distal common duct, with the creation of a false passage (Fig. 13-5).

Perforations of the proximal duct into the hepatic parenchyma probably go unrecognized. Their presence is suspected only if there is a blood trickle with or after the exploration. However, this experience has been reported with the balloon catheter (20, 103). A presumed example (Fig. 13-6) of this complication appeared only as a roentgen fact. The T tube was removed and the patient has had no problem.

TECHNICAL COMPLICATIONS

The major reviews on choledochoduodenostomy are uniform in reporting that subsequent anastomotic stricture and cholangitis are unusual (197, 258, 382, 537). The MHMC experience with 100 consecutive cases confirms the rarity of such an occurrence. However, special-interest groups do report this experience, and are undoubtedly specially skilled in executing this biliary enteric anastomosis. It is difficult to ascertain the incidence of complications in the surgical experience at large.

In the MHMC experience, each of two patients has had a single transitory episode of fever in addition to hyperbilirubemia. Barium swallow showed an open anastomosis—*i.e.*, the barium moved in and out. Both patients responded to antibiotics, cholegogues, or cathartics. It was assumed that there was a small, radical intrahepatic obstruction. The reasons for this are unclear.

Three patients seen in consultation demonstrated distinct causes for postanastomotic complications. One 84-year-old man presented with portal hypertension secondary to biliary cirrhosis that resulted from a complete anastomotic stricture (Fig. 13-7). He had had a long history of several prior bouts of cholangitis that had been disregarded. This is unfortunate since anastomotic revision by Roux-Y cholangiojejunostomy is a good salvage procedure.

The second patient suffered postanastomotic cholangitis originating in the bypassed segment. This disorder, always a theoretic consideration, has been considered as one of the potential complications of choledochoduodenostomy. Certainly the reported statistics have not borne out this theoretic possibility. In the vast majority of cases, this blind end empties retrograde through the anastomosis, or in the normal pathway if the Vaterian segment remains open. There has been a single case showing significant barium retention, in which this mechanism was presumed to be the cause of the cholangitis and biliary cirrhosis to which this patient's illness progressed. However, the common duct was not dilated, and there was an associated anastomotic stenosis.

The third case was an instance of postsphincterotomy cholangitis. The patient had had cholecystectomy, choledocholithotomy, and sphincterotomy, the latter procedure undertaken because of a past documentation of clinical pancreatitis. At the secondary procedure, 1 year later, the area of the sphincterotomy was not inspected; the 2-cm-wide common bile duct was anatomosed in continuity to the duodenum. There have been no further symptoms, although for a short time the patient's complaints suggested a peptic ulcer. This could not be demonstrated. Three months later she became asymptomatic and has remained free of biliary complaints for 5 years.

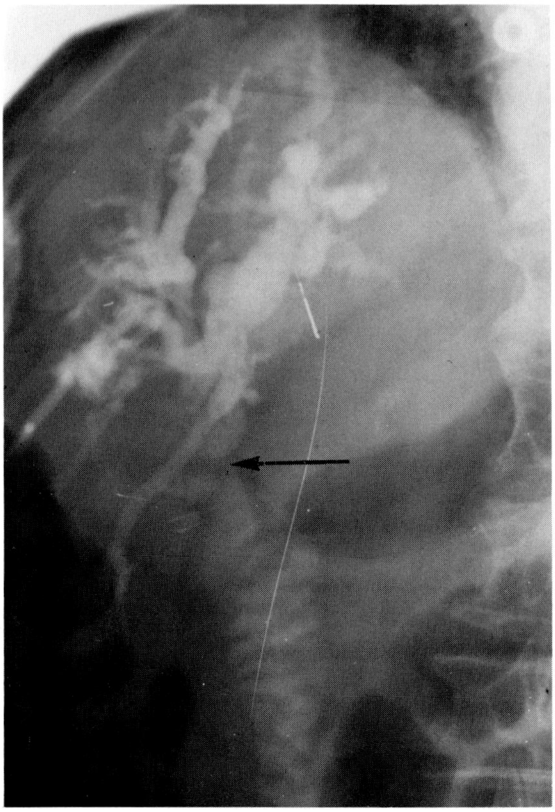

FIG. 13-7. Anastomatic stricture. 84-year-old man admitted with portal hypertension, biliary cirrhosis, and bleeding from esophageal varices. Percutaneous cholangiogram shows a strictured choledochoduodenostomy **(black arrow),** with a proximal sac full of stones and marked intrahepatic ductal ectasia. Some contrast goes through. The patient had completely forgotten about the operation, performed many years before. This is an example of iatrogenic biliary anastomatic stricture running the full course of unrelieved obstruction. It is important to observe not that the biliary radicles fill, but whether they fail to empty satisfactorily. The left hepatic duct and its tributaries are especially dilated.

CHOLANGIOGRAPHIC MISINTERPRETATIONS

Misinterpretation of the cholangiogram is included as an iatrogenic problem because it is often the basis of a consultation. The first experience with this entity occurred at a time before these roentgen phenomena were well understood. A female patient underwent a secondary bile duct exploration for an assumed retained distal stone. At the second operation, common duct exploration and duodenostomy were carried out. No stone could be found. It was assumed that it had passed. She died of an acute myocardial infarct on the fourth postoperative day. At autopsy no residual biliary calculi were found. Only years later was it appreciated that the roentgen finding, which was the sole indication for the second operation, was the systolic phase of choledochal sphincter function—the pseudocalculus sign. Details of this normal radiologic phenomenon have been considered in Chapter 2, in the section on the choledochal sphincter.

The other reasons for the failure to appreciate coexistent ductal disease are related to the inadequate cholangiogram. The errors in this regard are 1) a technically poor film that cannot be correctly interpreted because the position is poor, obfuscations caused by overlying metallic objects, the spine overlies the opacified column, or too much motion; 2) too dense contrast material that hides intraluminal defects; 3) failure to appreciate the fact that one of the hepatic ducts is abnormal or had failed to opacify; 4) misinterpretation of an air bubble, barium fleck, or colon gas as a stone.

These errors in interpretation have been partially responsible for inappropriate surgical measures. In some instances not enough has been done, and in others, unnecessary maneuvers have been carried out (Fig. 13-8).

FIG. 13-8. Opie's common channel suggested. **A.** T-tube cholangiogram appears to be typical for the Opie common-channel regurgitation phenomenon in that both ducts are dilated and fail to empty. This suggests obstruction to the outflow of both systems. The secondary pancreatic duct branches are opacified so that most of the pancreas is outlined. **B.** A second film, a few seconds later, shows free flow from both ducts. Serial films are necessary to avoid misinterpretation, not of the film, but of the apparent changes that they indicate. The pancreatic ducts have emptied completely.

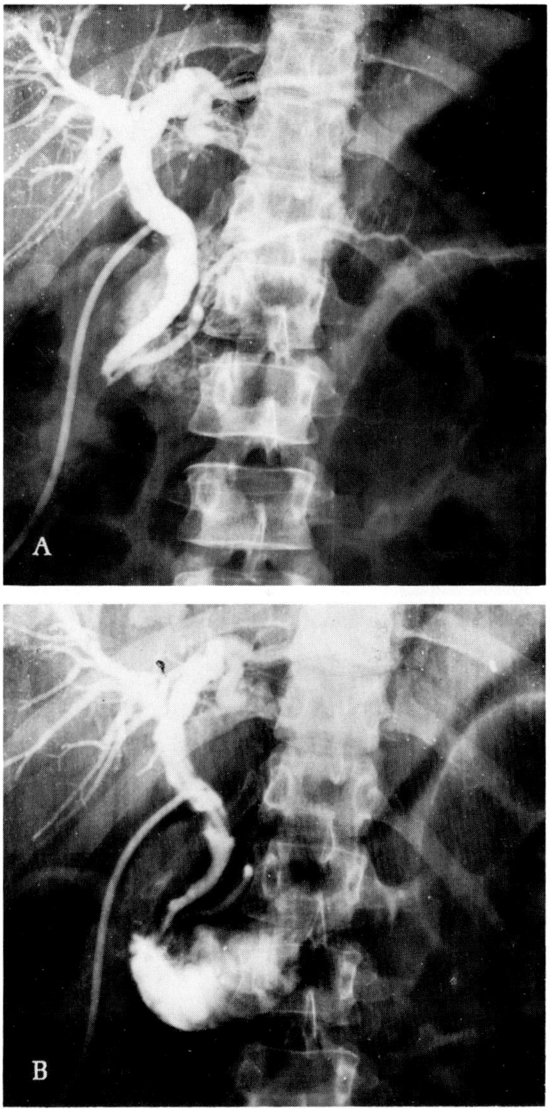

HEMATOBILIA

Instances of upper gastrointestinal bleeding that have their source in the liver or extrahepatic biliary system are best evaluated by arteriography. Instances have been reported which are believed to be directly related to the prior biliary surgery (191, 347, 523, 548).

I have encountered three cases: 1) A false aneurysm of the gastroduodenal artery, with rupture into the common bile duct, resulted from an injury to the arterial wall by a suture placed during a choledocholithotomy 11 days previously (17). 2) Mass ligation of the cystic duct and artery resulted in necrosis with the formation of an arteriocystic duct fistula (632). 3) Intrahepatic injury of a bile duct and vessel occurred in association with transhepatic cholangiography and needle biopsy of the liver.

These occurrences are iatrogenic and apart from the true aneurysms of the hepatic artery that perforate spontaneously into the biliary system (637).

14 Postcholecystostomy Problems

Bobbs's historic first cholecystostomy was performed in Indianapolis in 1868. The patient, Mary Wiggins, was 32 years old at the time. Bobbs knew that he had left stones behind. His patient died at age 77 of an unrelated disease. There is a lesson in that follow-up.

The immediate or late problems of the patient who has had a cholecystostomy are not, semantically, PCS problems. However, they fall within the penumbra of the individual being evaluated for secondary biliary surgery. It is proper, therefore, that these problems be considered. The entity is considered apart from gallbladder remnant disease and subtotal cholecystectomy.

VALUE OF CHOLECYSTOSTOMY

A cholecystostomy is a satisfactory temporary compromise procedure because it allows for decompression of the gallbladder and removal of its stones without much manipulation. It was presumably performed because the local process or the general condition of the patient suggested this less complicated approach in a specific situation. It is dramatically effective in relieving the biliary sepsis of the toxic patient with acute obstructive cholecystitis. It can be anticipated to be of special long-term value in one with a solitary gallstone who is statistically prone to that disease but who rarely has an associated choledocholithiasis. The latter patient is a member of the largest group in 50% of patients who are likely to be symptomatically cured by cholecystostomy.

This statistic is slanted because it obscures the fact that it pertains only to survivors. The statistics, even in recent times, indicate that cholecystostomy in the aged still carries a mortality in the range of 10–15%. The mortality is equally high for those with acalulous acute cholecystitis, which often presents in the postoperative period of another disease. The mortality is not unanticipated, the lesser procedure having been undertaken for the more complicated local problem or the more desperate constitutional situation.

However, cholecystostomy does not correct disease in the ductal system. Recurrent pancreatitis or colic is not prevented, and the vesical itself remains diseased. In the MHMC series, acute cholecystitis and cholelithiasis have recurred within 6 weeks of removal of the cholecystostomy tube. Acute pancreatitis has occurred with a functioning cholecystostomy tube in position. It does happen again.

Problems present in two areas: In the early phase the patient still has the cholecystostomy tube *in situ*, and residual disease is diagnosable by cholecystocholangiography. In the remote phase the patient's symptoms appear after the drainage tube has been removed.

EARLY-PHASE PROBLEMS

Early-phase problems are considered in six major categories, as they are defined in the postoperative cholecystocholangiogram.

1. Stones are shown to be retained in the gallbladder (Fig. 14-1). This is encountered in 20–40% of cholecystectomized patients. There is the potential of repeating the disease

FIG. 14-1. Stone retained after cholecystostomy. **A.** Cholecystogram was obtained after a cholecystostomy for acute cholecystitis. A de Pezzer catheter is *in situ*. Several retained stones in the gallbladder **(arrows)** were removed with an endoscope via the fistulous tract created by the catheter. Postextraction film revealed a normal extrahapetic conduit. **B.** Cholecystocholangiogram obtained by instilling contrast material into the cholecystostomy tube reveals a stone in the distal portion of the gallbladder just above the cystic duct **(arrow).** The common bile duct is of normal width and contains no calculi. This stone was retrieved with a bronchoscope and stone-grasping forceps.

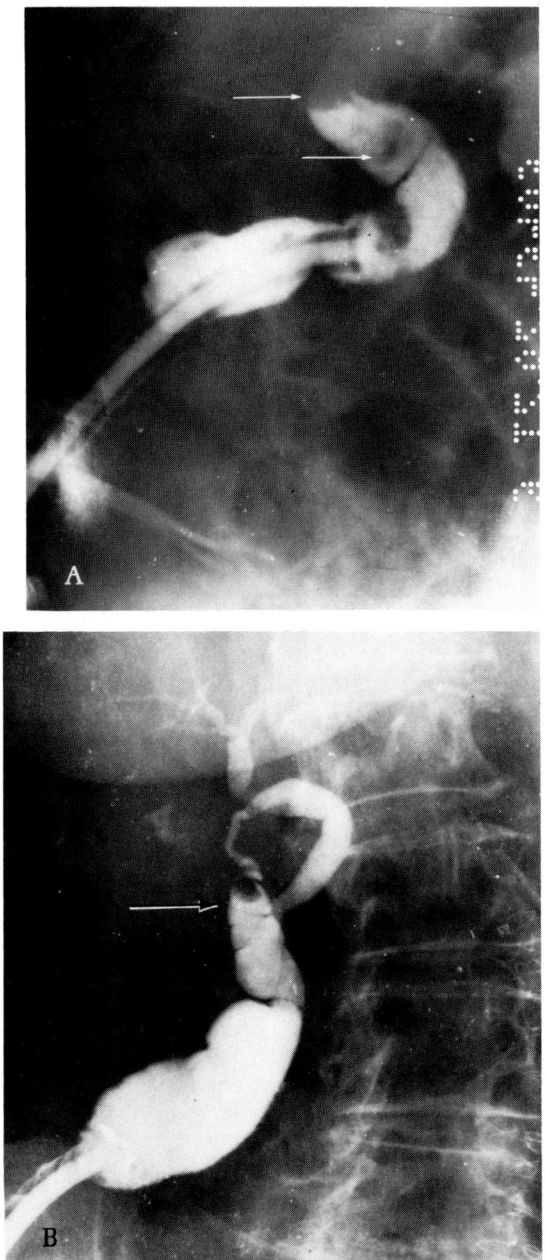

process in the gallbladder. It can be risky to remove the tube.

2. The gallbladder is stone-free, and the cystic duct is open. This is the best circumstance for recovery and restitution to normal. The prognosis for cholecystostomy is not good if the cholecystogram shows that the cystic duct is blocked (Fig. 14-2) (228). Such patients are particularly prone to recurrent cholecystitis because the block persists.

Welch(622)found symptoms present in four out of five such situations, and they required subsequent cholecystectomy. Ross and Dunphy (510) indicated that 50%, and others that as many as 80% of patients remain well. The postoperative cholecystocholangiogram is a guide to the probable prognosis. Only 12% of those with normal cholecystograms who had had cholecystotostomy for primary biliary disease became symptomatic. In similar circumstances Welch (622) indicated that 33% of those with common duct stones and 80% of those with impaired distal choledochal opacification will become symptomatic. The tube can be removed. The patient is advised to return promptly for definitive correction if he becomes symptomatic.

Another acceptable viewpoint is that all patients who have once had sufficient disease to require cholecystostomy should have a cholecystectomy if the contraindication to the definitive procedure on the first occasion can be corrected. However, patients in this anatomic circumstance stand the greatest chance of being among those who will continue to be asymptomatic. This decision is often best judged by observation of symptoms, rather than by adherence to protocol.

3. The gallbladder appears normal but the common duct harbors calculi or is enormously dilated (Fig. 14-3). This situation is the most frequent numerator in the fractions of cholecystostomized patients presenting for elective evaluation of the PCS. They have the symptoms of colic or of transitory cholangitis. The work-up reveals a greatly enlarged common duct with its associated pathology.

In this set of circumstances the gallbladder can be either the innocent vent, or the active lithogenic reservoir. This evidence of disease that has already been symptomatic enough to require surgery is preferably managed by secondary total definitive correction. A cholecystostomy does not protect the patient from

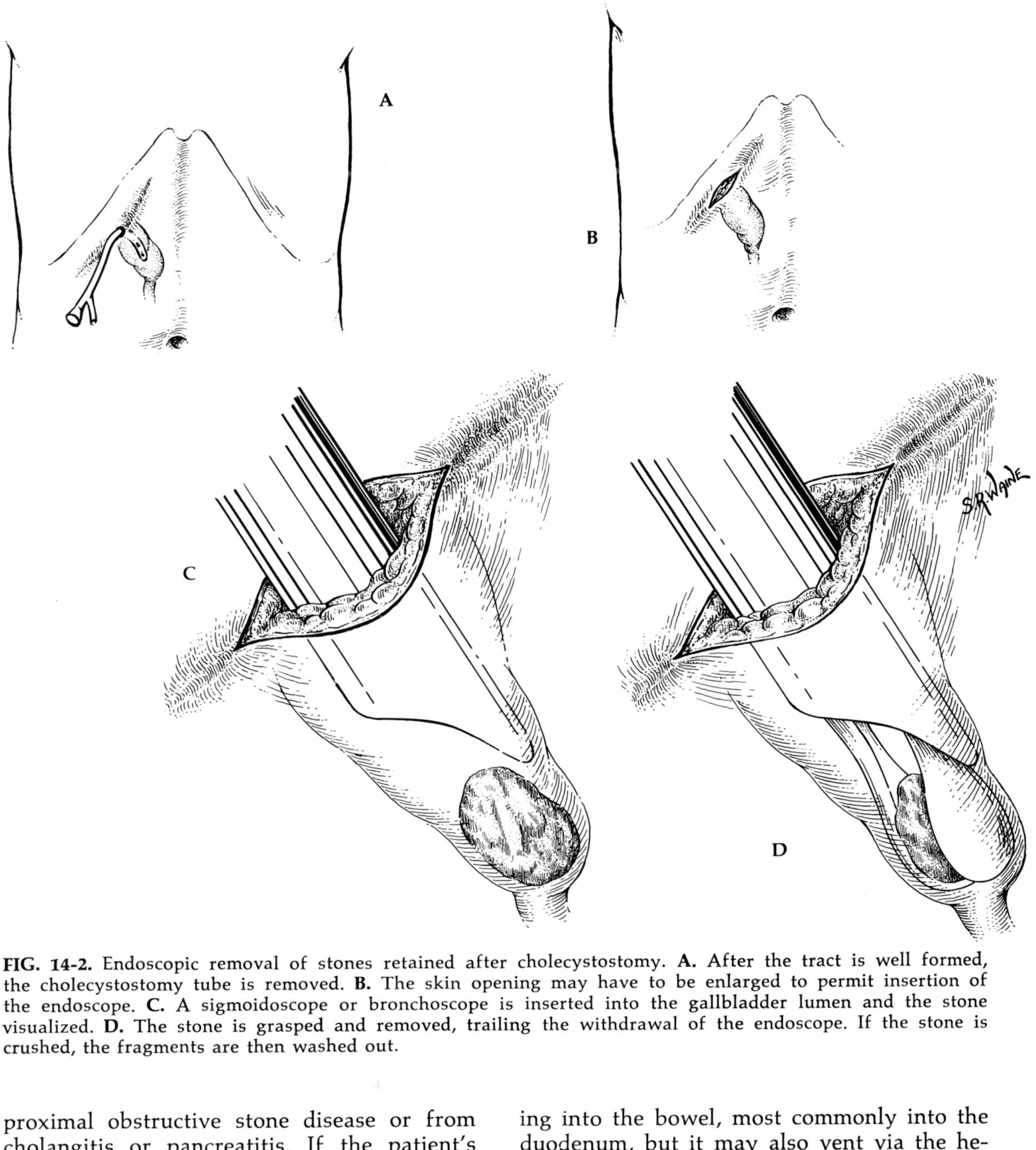

FIG. 14-2. Endoscopic removal of stones retained after cholecystostomy. **A.** After the tract is well formed, the cholecystostomy tube is removed. **B.** The skin opening may have to be enlarged to permit insertion of the endoscope. **C.** A sigmoidoscope or bronchoscope is inserted into the gallbladder lumen and the stone visualized. **D.** The stone is grasped and removed, trailing the withdrawal of the endoscope. If the stone is crushed, the fragments are then washed out.

proximal obstructive stone disease or from cholangitis or pancreatitis. If the patient's condition is too poor for surgery then the tube should be left in. When a septic or obstructed complication is present, the "too sick" patient has no alternative but to undergo a corrective procedure to improve his condition.

4. There is a biliary enteric fistula (Fig. 14-4). The fistula is the result of an acute cholecystitis that has decompressed itself by fistulizing into the bowel, most commonly into the duodenum, but it may also vent via the hepatic flexure or the stomach. There are at least two major problems here: The stone may produce an obturator obstruction of the ileum via the cholecystoduodenal fistula. This stone should be sought by a careful GI series with small-bowel follow-through. The less frequent problem can be recurrent cholecystitis since these fistulas do not always cicatrize and become self-obliterating.

FIG. 14-3. Choledocholithiasis after cholecystostomy. **A.** This patient had had a cholecystostomy and cholecystolithotomy. Postoperative contrast study shows a large stone in the common bile duct **(arrow).** However, contrast material goes around the stone and enters the duodenum. **B.** A repeat cholecystocholangiogram 3 months later shows that the solitary common bile duct stone has moved distally and now obstructs the flow of contrast material **(arrow).** There is more marked proximal duct dilatation, despite the functioning cholecystostomy. A second operation was performed—cholecystectomy, choledocholithotomy, and choledochoduodenostomy.

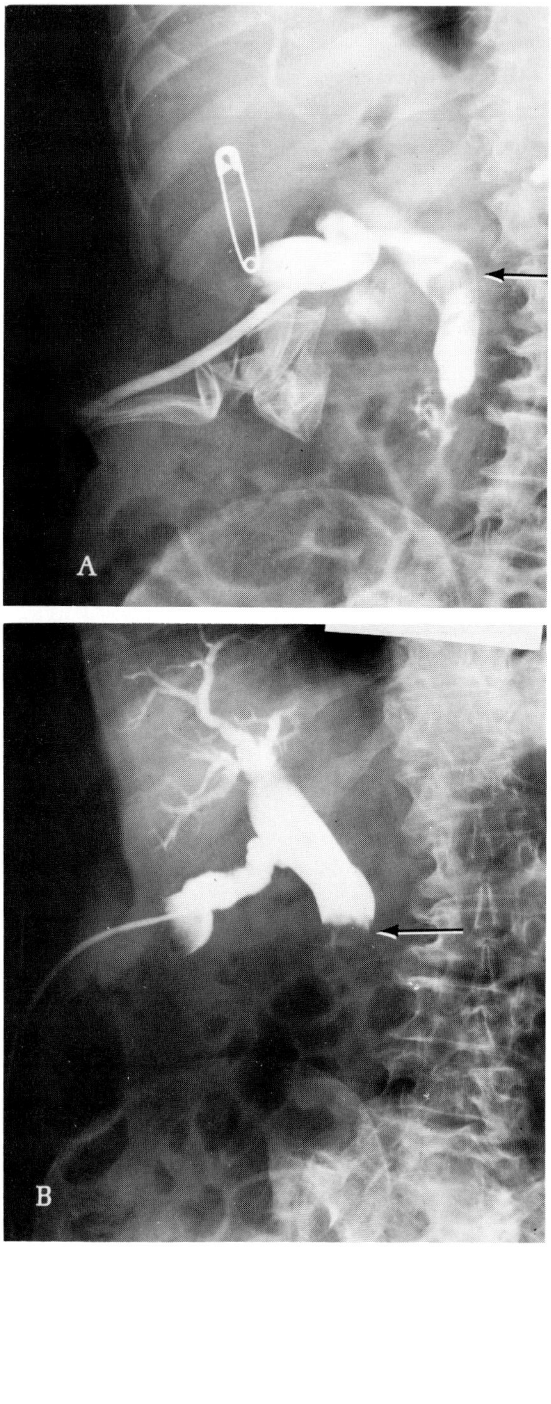

On the other hand, I have encountered completely asymptomatic cholecystoduodenal fistulas in elderly patients unable to recall the original event (141). The general condition of the patient determines whether this pathologic finding requires surgical correction. I tend to conservatism, with the admonition that, should relevant symptoms appear, a prompt reevaluation will be necessary. If the indication for the initial vent procedure still exists, then the asymptomatic patient with anatomic disease should only be observed.

5. The cholecystostomy fistula does not close. If the drainage is only mucous, the cystic duct is probably blocked. In this case, it is usually safe to remove the cholecystostomy tube, and the patient remains with a mucocele of the gallbladder. If the drainage continues to be biliary, then some block in the distal ductal system requires cholangiographic diagnosis.

6. The cholecystostomy fistula does not drain. There is an obstruction (tumor or stone) proximal to the cholecystodochal junction. In rarer instances the tube itself is kinked, blocked, or knotted. Irrigation and manipulation may correct the malposition.

LATE-PHASE CONSIDERATIONS

There is no direct temporal connection between the cholecystostomy and the reappearance of significant symptoms. In the MHMC experience it has varied from 6 weeks to 34 years. The manner of presentation is in no way distinctive except for the patient in whom an acute obstructive calculus cholecystitis spontaneously drains through the previous cholecystostomy scar. The only correlation is in the observation that when a patient with a previous cholecystostomy presents again, there is often extensive disease in the common duct: multiple calculi; thick-walled, greatly dilated ducts; and choledochoduodenal junction stenosis. The markedly advanced pathologic findings are often at variance with the anamnesis.

In the final analysis, the cholecystomized patient must be evaluated for elective cholecystectomy in terms of his operative risk, the persistence or correction of the original indication for the cholecystostomy, the persisting disorder in the biliary tract, and the symptoms it provokes, all balanced against life expectancy (366).

FIG. 14-4. Cholecystic fistula. **A.** Flat film of the abdomen shows a spontaneous pneumocholangiogram **(arrows).** This can be caused by gas-producing organisms, by a fistula to the duodenum, or by an incompetent ampullary segment. The differential diagnosis can be made by opacification studies. **B.** Contrast study performed through a cholecystostomy tube reveals a fistula between the ampulla of the gallbladder (above the cystic duct) and the descending limb of the duodenum **(arrow).** No stones are present. At the time of the second operation, it is important to look for a gallstone in the bowel since this type of fistula is the precursor of an obturator ileus. **C.** This patient has a cholecystostomy tube *in situ,* which had been inserted at an operation performed for acute calculus cholecystitis. The patient is now jaundiced. There is a large solitary round stone in the common bile duct **(white arrow).** The cystic duct is not dilated **(black arrow).** For this stone to have entered the common bile duct, one has to suspect that there is a cholecystocholedochal fistula.

This is a rare variety of the confluent stone problem, which is due to a cholecystocholedochal fistula. In order to manage this safely—the gallbladder remnant should first be opened and the stone removed. The fistula is thus visualized. The gallbladder is amputated leaving enough of the dilated ampulla (Hartmann's Pouch) to permit free flow of bile through the common bile duct. The duct is rarely patulous enough to do a primary closure over a T tube without stricture. The retained normal cystic duct can be pedicled into the choledochal aspect of the fistula with a series of interrupted sutures as a type of "satchel-handle" seal.

D. A technique for the management of this type of fistula **(a)** is indicated. After the fistula is dismantled **(b, c),** the duct is intubated from below with a T tube. The common duct is then either closed by direct approximation **(d),** or by a satchel-handle use of the cystic duct **(e).** (From Schein CJ, Stern WZ, Jacobson HG: The Common Bile Duct. Operative Cholangiography, Biliary Endoscopy and Choledocholithotomy, 1966. Courtesy of Charles C Thomas, Publisher, Springfield, Illinois)

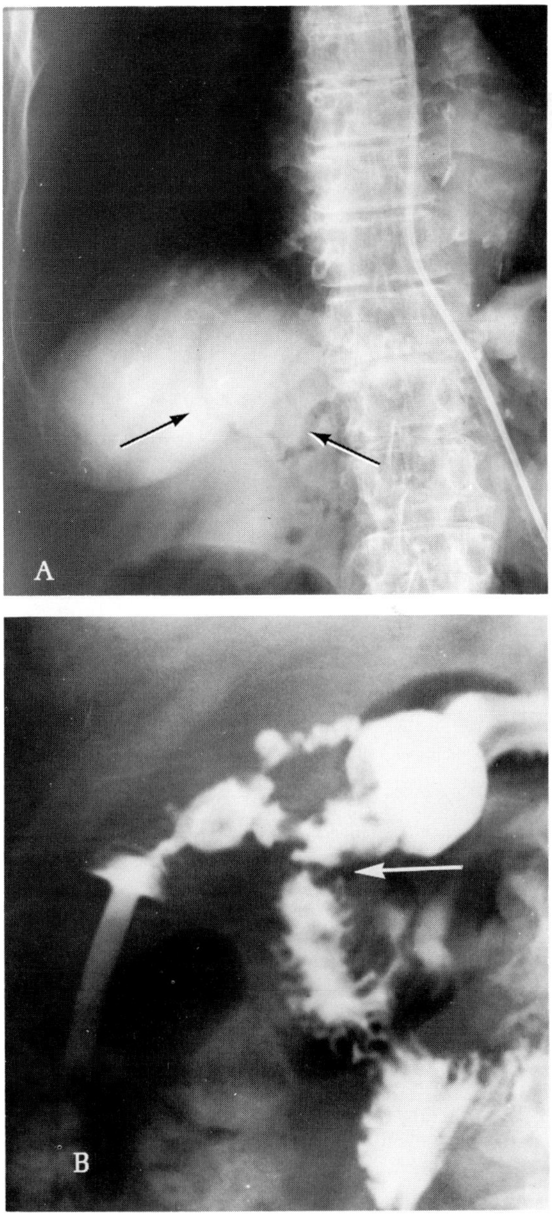

continued

continued

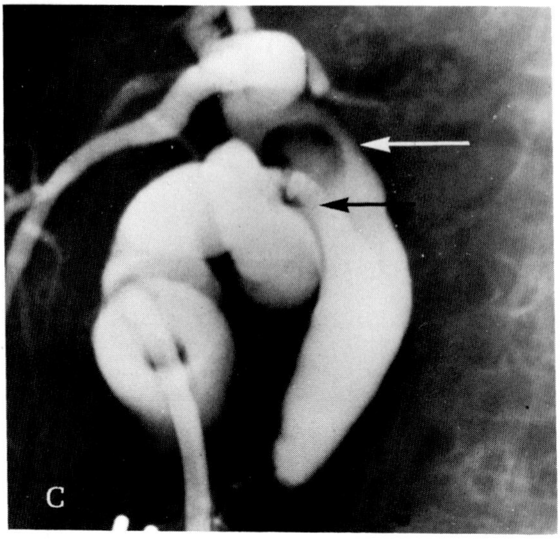

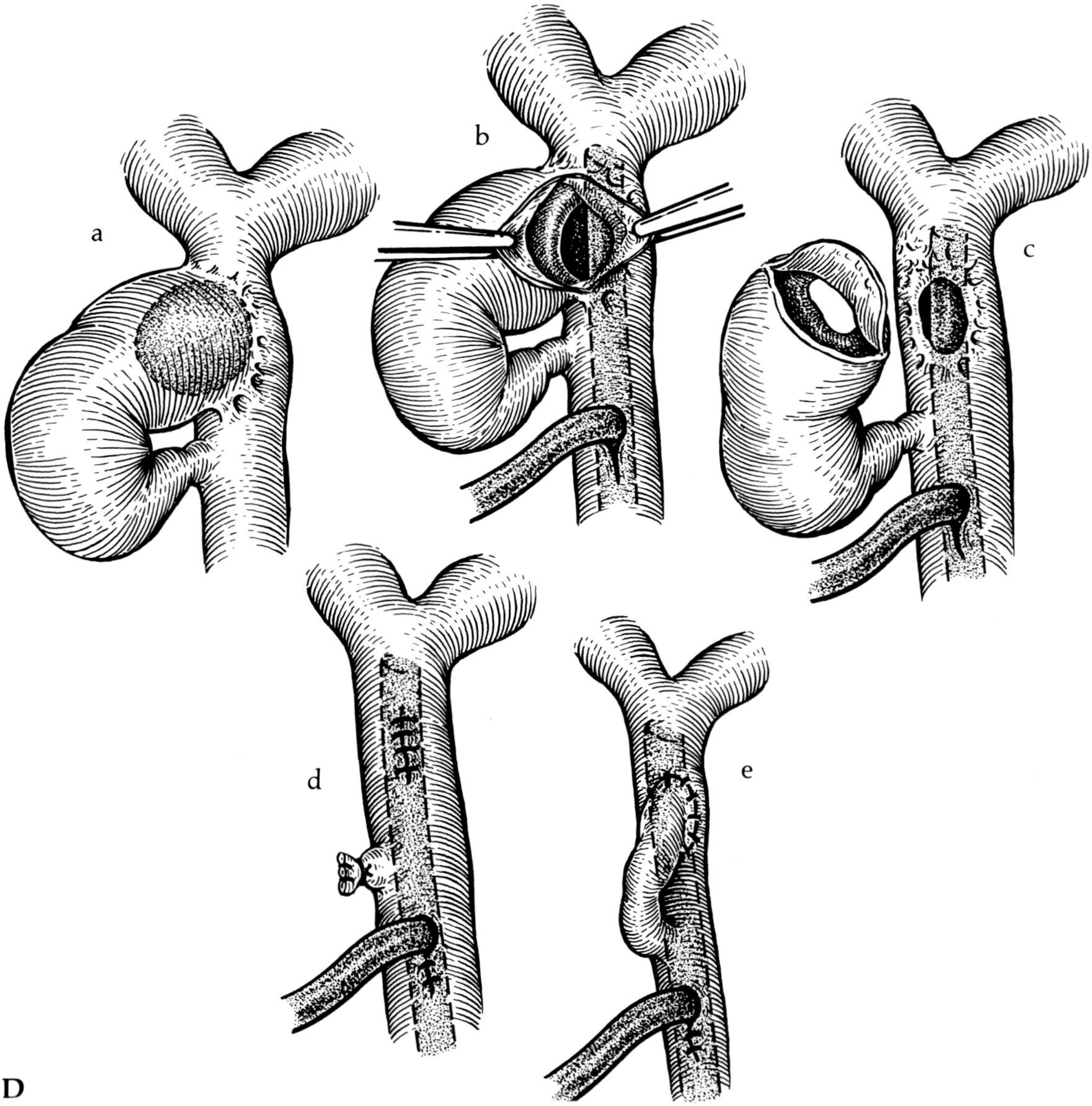

D

15 Biliary Dyskinesia

The concept of dyskinesia has been invoked to account for typical biliary symptoms on a functional basis in the absence of overt pathologic findings. The prefix **dys** means diseased, faulty, difficult, or impaired; **kinesis** is the Greek root for movement or motion. The term **biliary dyskinesia** is intended to indicate faulty choledochal motility (usually in the Vaterian segment) and impaired transit of bile from the liver to the duodenal lumen.

A DEFINITION OF TERMS

Oddi (451), in 1887, suggested that spasm of the sphincter could cause jaundice and colic. Meltzer (422), in 1917, and Berg (53), in 1922, suggested that functional disturbances might cause symptomatic biliary stasis. Westphal (626) in 1923, postulated autonomic nervous system imbalances that result in hypo- and hyperkinetic dyskinesias.

The most prominent contemporary exponent of functional biliary disorders is Mallet-Guy (397). His monograph on PCS includes his collected experience with the diagnosis and management of dyskinesias. The entity is by no means as clearly defined to others as to this investigator.

There is the danger of invoking an etiology and pathogenesis for an entity that is ill defined. For in particular terms, the problem is in the management of a harried, young to middle-aged parturient woman with typical biliary pain and dyspepsia, encountered after cholecystectomy. Liver function tests are normal, an intravenous cholangiogram is normal, and the findings on biliary drainage are normal (598).

The transit of bile to the sphincter depends upon the secretory pressure (30 cm H_2O) of the liver, which is sufficient to overcome the resistance of the normal (13 ± 7 cm H_2O) Odditic sphincter mechanism. The source of dyskinesia is presumed to reside in a malfunctioning choledochal sphincter, which is the sole peristaltic component of the ductal conduit. The character and function of the two muscular components of the sphincter are readily demonstrable on the cine cholangiographic studies referred to in the section on the choledochal sphincter in Chapter 2. The thick circular muscle simulates the pyloric sphincter of the stomach. Indeed the area has been referred to as a **pylorolus.**

It is assumed that colic results from distention or stretching of the sensory receptors in the duct wall. The intensity of the inciting factor is lowered in the presence of an inflammatory process. The studies of McGowan *et al.* (412, 413) have demonstrated in man that the distention is inversely proportional to the degree of the inflammatory reaction. Indeed this form of quasi-choledochal palpation is another index of the intensity of the reaction in the wall of the duct. The precipitousness with which the stimulus occurs is an important consideration, for the more insidious the stimulus, the less intense the response.

There has been one striking instance of dysfunction at the Vaterian segment. A 40-year-old woman was having an intravenous cholangiogram to investigate colic. During that examination she experienced her typical episode of pain. A film at that time showed that the duct had dilated. At the conclusion of the examination, the duct returned to its smaller caliber. She responded to hepatic plexus vagectomy by remaining symptom-free for 4 years (Fig. 15-1).

Manier *et al.* (399) reported on a patient who experienced pain during an intravenous cholangiogram. The film showed dilatation of the duct. Subsequent exploration of this duct revealed that it was normal, but they postulated a motor dysfunction in the sphincter of Oddi, and even though the duct was not dilated, did a choledochoduodenostomy.

FIG. 15-1. Dyskinetic obstructive choledochopathy. **A.** This intravenous cholangiogram was performed in a female with typical biliary colic **(arrows).** During the examination she experienced pain. **B.** A film obtained a few minutes later reveals that the entire extrahepatic system had dilated **(arrows).**

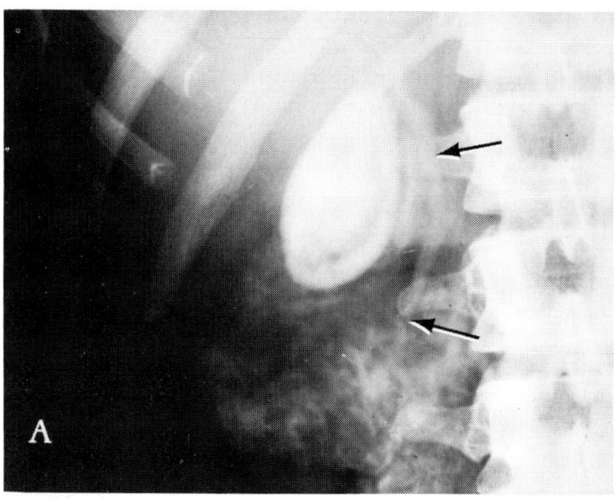

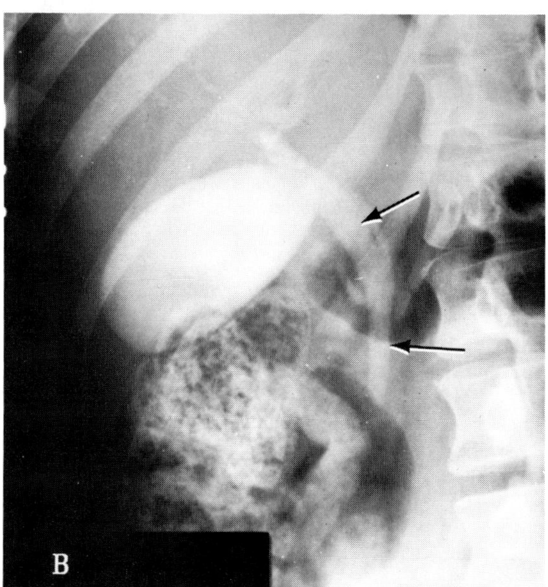

The patient was asymptomatic for 4 months thereafter. The interesting fact is that during the examination, the common bile duct enlarged to twice its original size during the height of pain and then receded as the pain subsided. This series of events of dilatation of the duct during an episode of biliary colic has also been documented by Sullivan *et al.* (580); in that instance dilatation was caused by calculous impaction during the diagnostic procedure.

The demonstration of duct dilatation during an episode of pain and its decrease in size with the subsidence of the pain suggests that some motor mechanism in the distal end of the duct was responsible for the event. (269, 327, 642).

Simplistically, it would appear that man relies for good gallbladder function on a well-functioning sphincter, for in that way, hepatic bile can remain in the gallbladder for concentration. Under certain conditions, functional disorders (dyskinesias) and anatomic changes (CDJS) in this area can produce postcholecystectomy complaints. This is a physiological paradox, for once the gallbladder has been removed, the functional significance of the choledochal sphincter is completely abrogated. It remains as a vestigial structure, no longer required to control preferential gallbladder filling rather than direct intraduodenal transit.

ROLE OF THE AUTONOMIC NERVOUS SYSTEM

If one accepts the concept of dyskinesia, then a fundamental neurogenic imbalance is implied. Experimental studies in the dog, as well as clinical experiences in man, indicate that the sympathetic and parasympathetic divisions of the autonomic nervous system do not have equal and contrary functions in relation to the choledochal sphincter (149, 626).

Vagal section in man reduces the passage pressure resistance at the normal choledochoduodenal junction by 30–42%. There have been no exceptions to this.

Lagerlof (343) treated 15 PCS patients with choledochal denervation. All these patients experienced pain relief, but this effect lasted no more than a few weeks to a few months.

The strong probability is that these denervations were not complete. From the anatomic description, only one nerve was divided, which means that the hepatic plexus, if this is what was severed, was incompletely divided hence no reduction to outflow resistance could take place. The operation of severing the nerve that Latarjet described as the *nerf-pancreaticocholedochien* is not the same as the division of the hepatic plexus. That type of choledochal denervation is not comparable to the hepatic plexus vagectomy. The relief of biliary pain with choledochal denervation has also been reported by Shafiroff and Hinton (553).

The vagus is the motor nerve to the biliary tract. It has its final outflow in the hepatic plexus, derived primarily from the left vagus nerve. The hepatic vasculature, on the contrary, is supplied by the sympathetic nerves. In the dog, at least, vagal section has no effect on the rate of bile production or on its viscosity.

Sympathetic block of T-4 to T-11 has no effect on the sphincter resistance passage pressure. It does induce a distinct increased tolerance to that variety of biliary pain that is induced by bile duct distention. The sympathetic system carries afferent pain fibers from this area; sympathectomy produces analgesia in the area without affecting the motor mechanism. Walters (606, 607) reports on pain produced by spasm of the common duct after sphincterotomy. At the height of an attack with intraductal pressure measuring 220–270 mm H_2O, immediate relief of the pain was accomplished by anesthetizing the left splanchnic nerve area. In two patients who developed postsphincterotomy pain, relief was obtained by alcoholic block of the splanchnic nerve (606, 607). This confirms our study of the sympathetic as the pain pathway.

The analysis of adrenergic receptors in the dog's biliary tract appears to have an analog in man. Passage pressures across the choledochoduodenal junction can be altered by specific adrenergic stimulating and blocking agents. Thus the fall in passage pressure that is invariably induced by vagotomy may also be induced with isoproterenol or phenylephrine (Neo-synephrine) in low doses. The effect can be reversed with propranolol, which is a specific beta-receptor blocking agent. Alpha blockage, however, did not always influence the passage pressure change induced by vagotomy. In the biliary system, the cholinergic system as well as the beta adrenergic mechanism is dominant (159).

It may be possible to identify dysfunctions in this area in terms of abnormal myoelectrical activity, by the latter's effect on the frequency of contractile activity at the sphincter. There may be an antogonism between the action of cholecystokinin and intrinsic muscle function, such as has been demonstrated in the irritable bowel syndrome (158).

There are also certain analogies to the abnormal lower esophageal sphincter as it contributes to the complex of disordered functions termed achalasia. These disorders have in common a satisfactory response to anticholinergic agents. It appears that the longitudinal muscle fibers are more cholinergically sensitive than are the circular fibers.

There is a cephalic phase to biliary excretion. In the trained laboratory dog, bile flow into the duodenum is initiated by the sight and smell of food. The phenomenon has been observed and filmed in the intact animal whose duodenum has been intubated with a Thomas cannula. The importance of this observation and whether it has a place comparable to the cephalic phase of gastric secretion in the genesis of duodenal ulcer is unknown.

Elman and McMaster (194) have shown that the anticipation of food raised the choledochal pressure in the dog. Puestow (484) demonstrated that the sight and smell of food caused bile flow before food reached the stomach. Doubilet and Colp (175) documented increased common duct pressure during excitement states.

Perhaps the legendary observation of the "bilious humor" has a basis in this mechanism. Certainly this would not be the first time that an ancient observation is shown to be a scientific fact. Perhaps the emotionally troubled female, who is so often the subject of the PCS, has some disorders of the neurosecretory mechanism as the basis for her complaints. At this time, this can only be a speculation.

Ritter (502) proposes that the finding of degenerated intramural ganglion cells in the common duct can be the anatomic basis for dyskinesias.

GASTROINTESTINAL ANALOGIES

Functional disturbances are readily recognized in regions of the bowel, where a direct endoscopic or roentgenographic approach is possible. Note, for example, the striking changes that can be observed in the human stomach under conditions of stress, as documented in Beaumont's Alexis St. Martin and Wolff and Wolff's Tom.

Subtle changes can be documented that would otherwise be completely undetected, as, for example, in the stomach with gastritis—changes that might be associated with dyspepsia before it bleeds, as well as with pyloric spasm before it becomes associated with peptic ulceration. In the same way the reactive hyperemia and superficial ulceration of stress situations can be observed in the rectosigmoid mucosa before a blatant colitis is in evidence. Manometric studies have now elucidated mechanisms in esophageal disease that are rooted in dyskinetic muscular incoordinations, diffuse esophageal spasm, scleroderma, and achalasia (450). Swallowing disorders have been demonstrated in patients with diabetic neuropathy. These have to do with the diminution in the amplitude of peristaltic contractions.

Every hollow part of the human gastrointestinal tract is influenced by the stress reactions of pain, hunger, fear, and rage, and by fight-or-flight situations. Why should one assume that the choledochus is not affected in a like manner (479, 506)?

The core of the problem is whether similarly functional changes occur in the postoperative biliary tree, and if so, how they are manifested symptomatically, and how they can be identified objectively (Fig. 15-2).

The cholecystokinin provocative test has been employed. The Jorpes compound, 1.5 cc/kg body weight, is given intravenously in 1 min. Results are positive if typical pain is induced in 10 min. Normal people do not respond with this kind of pain (352, 411).

In the MHMC experience, a provocative test with morphine alone has not proved rewarding. In the normal situation the intravenous cholangiogram will show a 0.2-cm increase in the lumen when morphine is given simultaneously with the iodipamide meglumine (Cholegrafin).

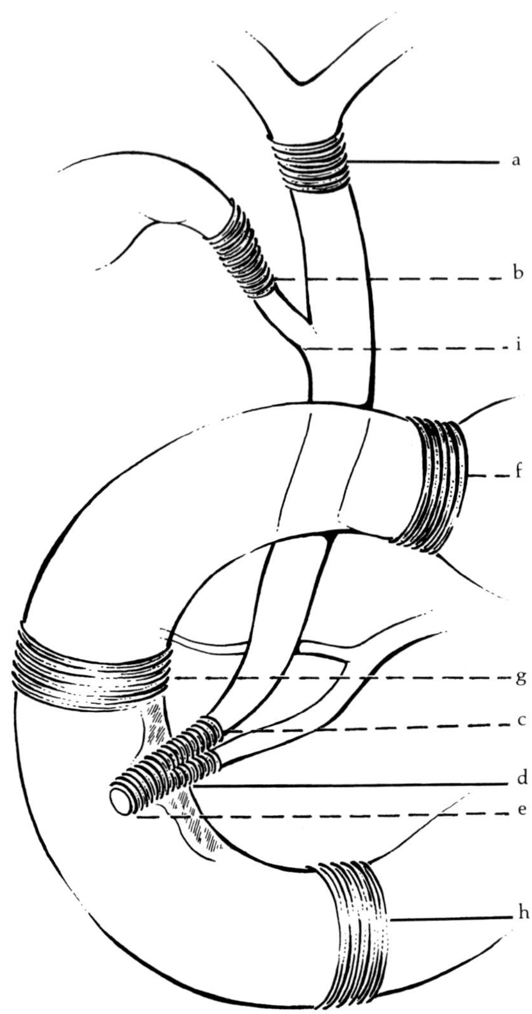

FIG. 15-2. Biliary duodenal sphincters. The sphincteric activity of the cystic duct (Lutkens) **(b)**, at the choledochoduodenal junction (Boyden) **(c)**, at the pancreatoductal-duodenal junction **(d)**, and at the pylorus **(f)** are well documented. The sphincter that Mirizzi describes at the hepatic duct junction **(a)** has not been recognized as a functional entity. The sphincter in the transverse portion of the duodenum (Ochsner) has been related to the pinchcock action at the site where the superior mesenteric artery comes off the aorta and passes over the duodenum **(h)**. The presumed sphincter (Kapandji, Villemin) at the supravaterian segment of the second portion of the duodenum **(g)** is not uniformly recognized. Functional disorders in the biliary tract have been described in relation to spastic, hypotonic, and achalasic states of these actual and presumed sphincter sites. Other sphincters illustrated are the sphincter of the ampulla **(e)** and the pyloric sphincter **(f)**. There is also a presumed valve (Puelch) at **(i)**.

DIAGNOSIS

The primary symptom must be one having the character, localization, and radiation that is ordinarily associated with biliary disease. Dyspepsia flatulence and fatty food intolerance are not specifically biliary symptoms. Price (482) reported that so-called fatty-food gallbladder dyspepsia was encountered in 28% of a group with normal gallbladders and in only 4% with diseased organs. These associations derive more from prejudice than fact.

Fatigue, headache pallor, irritability, constipation, migraine, and bloating are also unrelated to biliary disease. Anxiety may manifest pain, nausea, crying, or depression, as well as abdominal pain.

Childs (129) reported on patients who have undergone psychotherapy because no organic disease could be uncovered. At operation, some of these patients were found to have diseased gallbladders. The psychiatrist is sometimes able to suggest an organic disease, with or without a psychogenic overlay, by the nature and intensity of the symptoms. Neurotic people can also experience organic treatable disease. Rose (507) found that when patients with dyskinesia were studied psychiatrically, there was often a depressive illness, and biliary dyskinesia represented the somatic component of that disorder. When this is the mechanism, the depression is amenable to treatment with psychotherapeutic drugs.

None of these criteria for dyskinesia are specific, and the entire complex is so indefinite that I have reoperated upon only three patients with this presumptive diagnosis.

Depending upon one's viewpoint, this diagnosis is either missed too often or made too frequently. How can one define biliary dyskinesia in the presence of a normal cholangiogram, normal duodenal sediment and bacteriology, and normal liver function test? The role of periductal adhesions resulting from the initial gallbladder disease or the prior surgery is hard to evaluate. There are no data to support the concept of intermittent choledochal obstruction due to adhesions. This reported experience defies my ability accurately to screen out these cases. Possibly, others would group under dyskinesia the cases that I regard as choledochoduodenal junction stenosis. This albeit very limited MHMC experience has not proved satisfactory. I recognize that others may be more inclined to do sympathectomy that this experience has undertaken. The diagnosis of biliary dyskinesia remains vague and its treatment nonspecific.

Case Reports

Case 1. A 58-year-old male who had undergone cholecystectomy 8 years before suffered repeated colic. There was no evidence for infection clinically or by blood studies. On an intravenous cholangiogram the duct was 1.2 cm wide, with a normal emptying time. At operation there were dense adhesions about the duct, but the passage pressure and cholangiogram were normal. Lysis of periductal adhesions and choledochal exploration with T-tube drainage were performed. Results of postoperative cinemanometric studies were normal before removal of the T tube. The patient has been asymptomatic for 7 years. The mechanism is unclear and the therapy was nonspecific. The good result remains a puzzle.

Case 2. A 50-year-old female had undergone cholecystectomy 1 year before presenting with persistent colic that had begun 3 days after the first operation. The patient was obviously tortured by emotional problems. An intravenous cholangiogram was normal except for a 1.4-cm wide duct with a normal emptying time. At operation the duct was observed to be thickened but had a passage pressure of 16 cm H_2O. A choledochoduodenostomy was performed. The patient was well for 9 months, but the colics then recurred. She subsequently underwent a third operation at another institution, where the anastomosis was found to be patent and no other abnormalities were found. She was then referred to a psychiatrist.

Case 3. A 42-year old multiparous female complained of persistent recurrent colics following cholecystectomy 2 years earlier. The only abnormality was a dilated duct on intravenous cholangiography. At the second operation a choledochoduodenostomy was performed. Roentgen studies over the next 8 years have shown good functioning of the anastomosis. The patient still has colic, though it is less frequent and less intense. She has since had a pelvic operation by a gynecologist and another elsewhere for adhesions. The extent of this woman's neurotic background was not appreciated at the time the second biliary operation was advised. Obviously surgery has not solved her problem.

CONCLUSIONS

It is clear that my limited experience with dyskinesia has not been satisfactory. Perhaps the case selection was wrong and the criteria should have been even more carefully defined. Perhaps the surgery for this type of pain should be directed at interrupting the nerve supply rather than facilitating biliary drainage.

The problem is much more a lack of understanding the effect of emotional reactions on the biliary tract than it is one of overt misrepresentation on the patient's part. I am convinced that untreated biliary pain may produce emotional instability. I am equally certain that completely supratentorial problems may be expressed as biliary colic in which the abnormal roentgen and manometric deviations are deceptive anatomic chance incidents that are not the manifestation of intrinsic persistent biliary disease.

We know little of the precise relationship between the extrahepatic biliary system and the emotions. Only recently have the vagal factors in biliary dyskinesia and function been evaluated (493). We may be in the pre-Pavlovian era in this regard. Is it not possible that the emotion shown to initiate peptic ulcer may also selectively provoke biliary dysfunction? We recognize a predeforming stage of vagally mediated duodenal ulcer disease. Are we tardy in being able to document a similar type of prelithic biliary dyspepsia, first appearing as colic (with a normal cholecystogram), and later as the PCS?

16 Associated Disorders—Relevant and Irrelevant

Two varieties of associated or concomitant disorders have been, or can be, assumed to play a role in the initiation or maintenance of postoperative symptoms. One is represented by anatomic changes in the operated area; the second, by associated disease within the abdomen or by a systemic disorder. It is necessary to establish whether such associated disorders are the cause of the presumed PCS.

ABDOMINAL WALL

The most common complaints referable to the operative site are some variety of incisional pain and its equivalent discomfort and inability to lie on the right side, or a sense of bulge or mass. Some patients become aware of their normal costal arch flare only after operation. They conceive of it as an abnormal bulge. Comparison with the opposite side demonstrates the true situation (Fig. 16-1).

Heterotopic Bone Formation. Heterotopic bone formation has been reported in abdominal incisions and may cause pain. In the one case in which it was seen in the MHMC series, it occurred where the incision had extended far up into the costoxiphoid groove. It is possible that this resulted from an injury or avulsion of the costal periosteum. It is certainly an uncommon cause of incisional pain. In the review of this subject by Marteinsson (401), heterotopic bone formation was never reported in a transverse incision. The major problem is to distinguish the heterotopic bone formation from a neoplasm.

Scar. A scar may be so exquisitely sensitive that the patient covers it with cotton wadding to buffer it from contact with clothing. The hyperesthesia occurs in the postoperative course and usually disappears when the scar becomes completely fibrotic and is seen as a white line.

I have not been able to relate postoperative incisional discomfort to the width of the scar, keloidal reaction, or secondary wound healing.

Hernia. More significant is the demonstration of incisional weakness or hernia. If the incision extends high into the costoxiphoid groove, the weakness in this area can be considerable and cause a bulge that initially contains only the falciform ligament; later on the left lobe of the liver and omentum intrude. The hemispherical "derby hat" kind of hernia becomes quite obvious in 8–12 weeks; the predominant presenting complaint may be pain.

These hernias usually have large rings, the upper edge of which abuts on the costal margin. The direction of the original skin incision has important prognostic implications. Subcostal incisional hernias usually involve only the supracolic compartment, and small bowel is rarely present. Therefore, incarcerated small-bowel intestinal obstruction is uncommon. The vertical incisional hernia on the contrary, usually contains small intestine, and this hernia has the potential for small bowel incarceration.

Some patients do complain of pain in the costochondral groove, which disappears in a few months. I have regarded this as due to operative trauma to the costal cartilages.

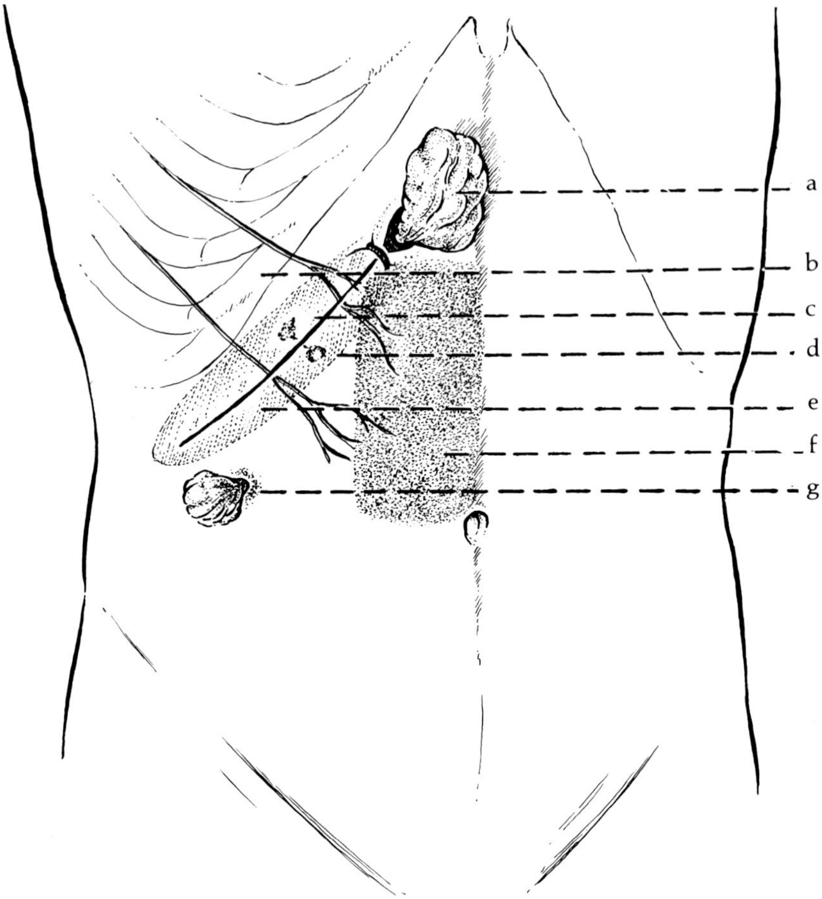

FIG. 16-1. Problems likely to be encountered in the abdominal wall of the postcholecystectomy patient are incisional hernia **(a)**, chondritis **(b)**, painful scar **(c)**, suture granuloma **(d)**, peritoneal adhesions **(e)**, area of anesthesia **(f)**, drain site hernia **(g)**.

Postoperative hernia through the drain site presents as an area of point tenderness; the hernia becomes obvious only on straining. It contains omentum or colon.

A third variety of postoperative hernia is often occult for a long time; it is of the superior Spigelian line type. It presents beneath the fascia just lateral to the linea semilunaris.

Wound Infection. In spite of antibiotics, operating room improvements, and one-time-use disposable equipment, the incidence of postcholecystectomy wound infection has not improved since the time of Kocher, who reported it to be 2.8%. In 1963, Larme (346) reported a 10% incidence of wound infections in those with positive bile cultures, versus a 1% incidence in those with negative cultures. The incidence of wound infection in those with infected bile at the time of choledochotomy has been reported by Engstrom *et al.* (195) as 27%.

SUTURE PROBLEMS

Some patients become aware of the fascial sutures and palpate these subcutaneous nodularities, which can be tender. In some, they produce pain beneath a tight undergarment. This has appeared as a problem with wire sutures, especially in a thin abdominal wall, in which subcutaneous closure either had not been done or its bulk is too sparse to be an effective cover. An especially tender and blebbed suture site frequently precedes the formation of a suture sinus.

Suture granulomas can present months

after an apparent primary healing. These sutures can be retrieved with a knitting needle. They are often multiple. It is occasionally necessary to reopen a large part of this incision and to remove all these sutures.

If localized subcutaneous pain persists, one must consider a foreign body as the cause. There were two such instances: One proved to be a small gallstone and the other, a short, rubber retention-suture boot.

INTERCOSTAL NEURALGIAS

The intercostal nerves segmentally innervate the muscles and skin of the abdominal wall. These nerves overlap so that the division of a single one rarely produces symptoms. However, if two or more of these nerves are divided, the patient can be left with a neurologic deficit (22).

The conventional vertical muscle-splitting or lateral muscle-retracting incision does not produce clinical neurologic residue. The subcostal incision—especially when carried laterally—can divide two intercostal nerves. The eighth and ninth are the ones involved and the patient is left with an area of hyperesthesia in the right supraumbilical area. It usually does not disappear. After an initial awareness and discomfort, the patient adjusts to it and often forgets it. In many ways it is analogous to the effect of the ilioinguinal nerve interruption in inguinal herniorrhaphy. I had the opportunity to evaluate 100 men in a geriatric facility for the latter problem. Seventeen of these had a diminished sensation to pinprick, but only five spontaneously mentioned it as a symptom.

I have not encountered unilateral abdominal bulge or muscle atrophy ascribable to nerve interruption, nor is skin hypesthesia accompanied by abdominal wall weakness.

THE POSTOPERATIVE GALLBLADDER BED

Periductal Neuroma. The common bile duct and cystic duct are interlaced by many nerve fibers. These are especially prominent about the cystic duct and must be divided to accomplish the straightening of the cystic duct. The division of these nerve fibers can result in a large periductal neuroma. Womack and Crider (640) postulated that this could be responsible for postoperative pain. There was a period during which there was a great interest in this finding as a cause of the PCS.

There are great variations in the anatomic prominence and complexity of the autonomic nervous system fibers. They appear as a complicated interlacing network in some subjects and are quite sparse in others. Adequate release and complete exposure of the cystic duct and anterior choledochal wall require that these tense white strands be lysed and stripped away. This nerve section is required to accomplish a a complete straightening out of the cystic duct. When they are thus stripped away, they need not be included in the cystic duct tie. The encompassing entrapment is thus possibly avoided (11).

The periductal neuroma is no longer regarded as a symptom-provoker. Neuromatous changes in the periductal area have been encountered in completely asymptomatic patients, and in one instance these bulbous enlargements of the nerve have been removed without clinical benefit. They can vary in size from 0.1 to 2 cm. Revisional surgery in this regard should not be primarily or solely directed at excision of the neuroma, nor should it be sought for.

Bodvall and Overgaard (72) found neuromas in 7% of patients with recurrent cholangitis and 15% of those with continuous severe distress. No patient in the latter group improved following neuroma removal.

Pyloroduodenal Adhesions. This portion of the bowel becomes directly adherent to the liver bed in all instances in which the omentum or hepatic flexure is not specifically interposed. The duodenum comes to blanket over the ductal structures and appears to be foreshortened. This is the normal position of the duodenum in PCS.

Inflammatory changes in this area can result in pseudo (traction) diverticula of the duodenum and in roentgen findings of antral gastritis. There has been no MHMC experience with such adhesions as the cause of PCS. The lysis of these adhesions and the interposition of the released hepatic flexure or of the omentum into this raw area has nevertheless been a routine part of my final peritoneal toilet.

Hepatoperitoneal Adhesions. These adhesions are of two varieties. In the first, the normally sharp edge of the right lobe of the liver adheres to the anterior parietes, obliterating access to the right anterior subphrenic space. The second consists of string and band adhesions between the anterior surface of the liver and the diaphragm. These are dense, diffuse, and more numerous than the violin-string adhesions that are assumed to be the result of gonococcal peritonitis as described in the Fitz-Hugh and Curtis syndrome.

Adhesions can represent something more than the usual postoperative reaction. They can be the residue of a postoperative right-upper-quadrant inflammatory process or the postoperative infectious sequela of the prior disease. This reaction is often encountered in secondary cases, but it is not of itself symptom-provoking.

Pericholedochal Adhesions and Lymphadenopathy. An indurative reaction in the hepatoduodenal ligament is the sequela of repeated bouts of biliary tract inflammation. The common bile duct can be embedded in this fibrous reaction. It is often associated with prominent pericholedochal and peripancreatic lymphadenopathy.

Such adenopathy is occasionally indicated on the cholangiogram by the beaded appearance of the contrast-filled duct. The nodes are soft, bean-shaped, and very friable. They fracture easily. Histologic examination reveals a nonspecific lymphadenitis.

The nodes are associated with disorders in the biliary–pancreatic system as well as with gastric or duodenal disease. They have no specific role in producing symptoms but are an indication of disease in the area.

GASTROINTESTINAL DISORDERS

Hiatus Hernia. A frequent finding in association with biliary tract disease is the hiatus hernia. The role of each in the production of symptoms can be impossible to define. One fact is of special importance: the sliding hiatus hernia is unlikely to produce significant symptoms in the absence of a complicating reflux esophagitis. The demonstration of gastroesophageal reflux alone need not be symptomatic. It is a good practice to esophagoscope patients with reflux. If esophagitis is demonstrated, the hiatus hernia should be repaired at the same time. If there is no esophagitis, it is best to disregard the hernia.

The indications for repairing this type of hernia in association with other abdominal dyspeptic disorders depends upon one's judgment of the finding solely as a radiologic demonstration or endoscopic finding, or as symptom-provoking. Fundal plication can be so readily executed that it should be done in the secondary operation along with the correction of the ductal disease. The results of the combined effort have been very satisfactory, even though it is hard to define what proportion of benefit can be ascribed to each component of the combined procedure.

Duodenal Ulcer. Duodenal ulcer and gallbladder disease coexist in 8–10% of patients. Ross and Pudvan (511) have found that 28% of gallbladder patients had peptic ulcer disease, and that 25% of peptic ulcer patients had a diseased gallbladder. In another study of 2161 surgical cases, 9% of those undergoing ulcer surgery had advanced gallbladder disease and 7% of those undergoing biliary surgery had a coexisting duodenal ulcer (511).

If duodenal ulcer is related to increased vagal activity, this same excessive vagotonia can produce increased contractility of the gallbladder musculature, operating against increased resistance in the cystic duct and choledochal sphincter. From the physiological viewpoint, this corticovagal axis influence on the cystic and choledochal sphincter area can be an explanation for the frequency of the association. Why isn't it even more frequent?

There is the uncommon problem of a duodenal ulcer perforating into the common bile duct. The source of trouble here is the posterior ulcer perforation. Treatment is preferably by vagotomy and gastroenterostomy, often with accompanying choledochoduodenostomy.

Some aspects of biliary and peptic ulcer dyspeptic symptomatology inseparably overlap. The latter is responsive to medical management in the majority of cases; the former, in only a minority. If the two diseases coexist, it is advisable to treat the biliary disease surgically and continue to have the uncomplicated ulcer treated medically, on the premise that one would not advise surgery on the patient if he had only the duodenal ulcer. In some instances refractory ulcer symptoms recede when the biliary problem is corrected.

A more aggressive prophylactic approach

is predicated on the proposition that since the area is exposed for bilary surgery, a procedure for the ulcer as well is a logical step. However, operative risk is increased, and the procedure for the ulcer may generate any one of the serious postgastrectomy syndromes: diarrhea, dumping, anemia, weight problems, and marginal ulcer. The indication for this major adjunctive surgical procedure on the stomach and duodenum should be very definite, not just because it is there. If the ulcer disease has been complicated by perforation, bleeding, obstruction, or intractibility to medical treatment, then it has its own rationale for corrective surgery.

The implications for alkali in the medical treatment have an experimental basis. The bile flow response to a fatty meal is interrupted by acid in the duodenum. Perhaps those with pyloroplasty and ineffectual vagotomy still produce enough acid to elicit this effect. The vagi must be intact to allow this acid effect on the sphincter. An important associated observation is that the normally alkaline bile that becomes infected with gram-negative organisms tends to become acid. Does this influence sphincter response?

Diverticula in the medial wall of the descending duodenum are roentgenographically encountered in 2% of routine gastrointestinal series. Occasionally the transmural portion of the common duct terminates in such diverticular outpouching. This cholangiographic observation has not been encountered as a serious consideration in evaluating the PCS.

Constipation. A correlation between the consistency and frequency of bowel movements and general well-being is part of folk lore, student jingle, and surgical skepticism. The relationship is hard to define in precise scientific terms; yet bile salts have traditionally been employed for their laxative action. In the MHMC clinical experience, the relationship of constipation to biliary disease is also inconstant.

Constipation in the male does not appear to have an increased frequency in association with gallbladder disease.

It has been demonstrated that the concentrating ability of the normal gallbladder can be influenced by constipation. (M-22) Regulated colonic evacuation can be associated with improved gallbladder opacification with orally administered contrast, when compared to visualization in the constipated state. Our own experimental attempts to correlate gallbladder function as seen on roentgenograms with partial distal colon obstruction in the rabbit were inconclusive.

Cholecystectomy should not be expected to improve the pattern of colonic evacuation. In my experience, the results of cholecystectomy are as fickle in this regard as they are with reference to flatulence and eructation.

In Anda's (16) series 66% of women and 36% of men subjected to cholecystectomy were constipated; about half of these were relieved by cholecystectomy. Fifteen of 28 patients who returned for postoperative study had constipation as the sole cause for the PCS. The observer comments that constipation "should be given a prominent place as a causative factor in the PCS"(16).

Diverticulosis. Saint's triad includes concomitant cholelithiasis, diverticulosis coli, and hiatus hernia. The first two anatomic associations, not necessarily diseases, increase in frequency with age. Thus, at age 50, at least 20% of people have gallstones and 30% have diverticulosis.

There can be a prophylactic aspect to the association in the sense that a symptomatically diseased gallbladder can be removed at the time of elective resection for diverticular disease. The converse is not indicated. However, functional disorders of the colon and of the biliary tract can have symptoms in common.

Pyloroduodenal Incompetence. The incompetence of the pyloric sphincter to the retrograde reflux of duodenal contents has been invoked in the genesis of the PCS. Numerous studies of this area have been done with by barium swallow and by transsphincteric intubation. Benevenato and Schein (46) evaluated this zone by the simple experiment of observing the frequency with which contrast material injected into a T tube positioned in the common bile duct would reflux into the stomach. One-third of 36 consecutive cholecystectomized patients demonstrated such sphincter incompetence. In no patient in this group was this reflux associated with gastric, duodenal, or residual choledochal disease.

The MHMC experience has not defined a relation between pyloric incompetence and flatulence or antral gastritis. It was concluded that such sphincter incompetence is a normal physiological variant (46).

Capper *et al.* (108) are of a different mind. They propose that duodenal reflux favors dysfunction of the oxyntic cells, causing gastric hyposecretion and flatulent dyspepsia. If the cardia is similarly incompetent, such duodenal reflux can cause esophagitis. In this viewpoint, dyspepsia is less likely to be associated with pylorospasm (as has been suggested) than with incompetence. These investigators found pyloric competence in only 2 of 18 patients with gallstones.

There is no evidence that cholecystectomy influences the competence of the pyloric sphincter. It is hard to ascribe the more than infrequent, but inconsistent, relief of flatulence that cholecystectomy sometimes affords to the assumed restoration of a competent pyloric outlet (136).

REMOTE SEPSIS

When a patient presents with sepsis or a fever of unknown origin, attention is ordinarily directed first to the urinary tract. The prior biliary surgery may have been remote in time and the scar so well healed in the skin lines of Langer as to escape casual inspection. Sometimes the patient does not recall the antecedent cholecystectomy. In the MHMC series we have encountered patients with cholangitis presenting 30 years after the initial surgery. There still should be a high index of suspicion that the biliary tract can be a source of late sepsis.

If the serum bilirubin is elevated, the problem is less of a conundrum. The only clue may be the elevated serum alkaline phosphatase. The preoperative diagnosis of residual disease can be clarified by intravenous cholangiography in the patient whose serum bilirubin is less than 3.5%. In the jaundiced patient, the situation is the ideal for endoscopic cannulation of the papilla of Vater, performed by an experienced endoscopist using the fiber duodenoscope. This avenue for cholangiography in the presence of jaundice is advantageous when the intrahepatic ducts are not dilated. The British Society of Digestive Endoscopy reports about 80% success rate for this type of cannulation. Percutaneous transhepatic cholangiography is a less complicated approach to the problem, in that it is easier to perform and has a slightly better diagnostic potential.

CARDIAC DISORDERS

The patient with heart disease can present differential diagnostic problems *vis-à-vis* the biliary tract. Congestive changes in the liver can mimic acute cholecystitis. Every large surgical service has had experience with this problem to the point that even the globular mass of presumed acute cholecystitis is palpated and later found to be the liver.

In the postcholecystectomy situation the commonest problem is establishing the differential contribution of the diseased common bile duct to the anginal pain of the diseased coronary artery. Biliary colic and angina have the same pain pathway. The symptoms overlap, and the colic of the common duct stone can aggravate or precipitate an established anginal syndrome (10).

There are conflicting data about the mechanisms involved, but these observations seem to be pertinent: common duct distention can produce anginal pain and electrocardiographic changes in the patient with coronary artery disease, and the association is often symptomatically improved by correcting the biliary disease (91).

Experimental data in the dog conflict with the observation in man that distention of the biliary tract does not produce changes in aortic or coronary blood flow. Others report contrary experiences (152).

The clinical role is even more difficult to individualize, and the term "biliary linked angina" has been employed. Friedman (205) stated that there is a "weak association with shared etiologic factors and the possible aggravation of cardiac symptoms by a diseased gallbladder." The facts are confusing.

In the MHMC experience, there have been six striking examples of symptomatic relief of angina in patients undergoing secondary operations for common duct stones and gallbladder remnant disease. Elective secondary biliary operation in the patient with coronary artery disease has been undertaken when residual anatomic biliary disease has been demonstrated and was differentially considered as being the probable source of symptoms. The improvement in cardiac symptoms is a gratifying unpredictable dividend that cannot always be achieved. In six instances in which common duct disease and coronary artery disease coexisted, the surgical correction of the biliary problem was undertaken first. Through happenstance in each of these instances, the cardiac problem was alleviated. Common duct stones have been encountered in "coronary deaths" and it has been hypothesized that they can trigger an arrhythmia.

The differential diagnosis can be difficult if based solely on clinical symptoms, intravenous cholangiogram, and enzyme blood studies. In several such problems, coronary angiography has been utilized as the final definite way of demonstrating the presence of coronary artery disease as the sole or concomitant cause of symptoms.

ALLERGY

Allergies of the respiratory tract and skin have no specific identification with biliary tract disorders. I have not recognized allergic biliary colic as a specific entity (21).

Jennings *et al.* (304) stated that postcholecystectomy colic can be mimicked by food allergy, especially to egg albumin. The bile of the allergic person was cultured, then centrifuged, the supernatant was discarded, and a vaccine suspension made from the killed organism. They cite cases of good response to benadryl and an elimination diet. Among 92 patients with PCS the investigators encountered a definite allergy in 45%; in addition, 21% reacted to a vaccine having its antigen in the bile organisms. It was postulated that postcholecystectomy colic may have its source in continued sensitivity to residual bacterial infection (304).

THE BILIARY NEUROTIC

Biliary calculi and their complications do not respect independent emotional problems. When a patient presents with persistent postcholecystectomy complaints of a subjective nature, it can be difficult to compartmentalize the abdominal disorder within an anxiety reaction. When repeated and adequate studies of the liver, bowel, and extrahepatic biliary tree are normal, there is a tendency to ascribe the symptoms of typical biliary pain to unknown causes, rather than offering a psychiatric diagnosis. Surgeons, by experience, have hesitated attaching that label to a postoperative symptom.

The right upper quadrant can be the somatic reference point for primary emotional problems in the same way that there is a cardiac neurosis, a neurocirculatory asthenia, or the psychiatric association with hyperthyroidism, asthma, duodenal ulcer, and ulcerative colitis. One must be alert to this problem and refrain from advising reoperation, no matter how typical the symptoms, in the absence of at least a significantly dilated common bile duct or cholesterol crystals in the duodenal tube drainage (66). I am aware of the failure of several such operations that had been undertaken as the "only way of being absolutely sure" (44).

Possibly some patients suffer an injustice when we ascribe a supratentorial origin to what is, in fact, our inability to define the psychophysiologic parameters of biliary dysfunction. Particularly pertinent is the frequent problem of symptoms that antedate the capacity to demonstrate roentgenographic changes.

Nash (440) noted choledochal sphincter "spasm" in a patient who overheard a conversation about his residual stone. Nash considered that hyperirritability of the area can be related to emotional factors.

On the other hand, there is the patient who for 3 or 4 years bitterly complains of colic but has normal roentgen studies. Later she turns up with the significantly dilated common duct of CDJS or a now clearly definable stone.

Our present unsophisticated study methods probably underdiagnose the problem. Lithogenic bile as a provocation of symptoms awaits precise definition regarding its role in clinical practice. Dreiling's study (178) of the functional component of PCS revealed that 82% of patients had either a major psychosis (schizophrenia) or a psychoneurosis—anxiety, depression, conversion hysteria, or cancerophobia. This is a common experience. However, it may be speculated that subtle pancreatic disorders can produce behavior disturbances, as in pancreatic cancer, which are frequently preceded or accompanied by a severe depression.

CIRRHOSIS

The problem in the patient with alcoholic cirrhosis is specific. The incidence of cholelithiasis in cirrhosis is increased as compared to that in the noncirrhotic population. The figures reported by Nicholas *et al.* (413) are 30.8% versus 16%. Gallstones are more common in the cirrhotic group at all ages. There is apparently an accelerated gallstone formation early in the course of cirrhosis. However, jaundice due to extrahepatic obstruction by these stones is uncommon.

These calculi are primarily pigment stones and their pathogenesis is chronic hemolysis secondary to hypersplenism. Cholesterol gallstone formation is not increased in cirrhosis. Although there is a decreased bile-acid pool in cirrhosis, tending toward lithogenic bile, impaired liver function produces an equivalent reduction in cholesterol synthesis. Thus the solubility of cholesterol in the bile is maintained. For the most part, gallstones in the cirrhotic patient are not provocative, and if asymptomatic, the stones should not be removed.

Common duct exploration in the established cirrhotic patient should be undertaker only on the absolute demonstration of significantly sized intracholedochal calculi. It has been suggested that the small friable stones usually pass spontaneously. A real hazard exists of excessive venous bleeding associated with portal hypertension.

OTHER ENTITIES

Other entities, on which there have been isolated or rare reports are mentioned for the sake of completeness: 1) Granulomas of the gallbladder bed are attributed to a talc reaction, inadequate resorption of cellulose gauze, and retained foreign bodies. 2) In disease of the hepatic artery, the extrahepatic vessels are implicated as a cause of cystic duct–cystic artery fistula and aneurysm of the hepatic artery—the latter reported to be a cause of postoperative jaundice (17). Unruptured aneurysm of the hepatic artery can be associated with a bruit. When it ruptures into the bile duct it produces the typical picture of hematobilia—pain, jaundice, gastrointestinal bleeding. 3) Sclerosing cholangitis has never been encountered in the entire MHMC experience with over 6000 biliary cases except in association with ulcerative colitis, Riedel's struma, or idiopathic retroperitoneal fibrosis. No case of calculus-related sclerosing cholangitis has been diagnosed (544).

17 Medical Considerations

The nonsurgical treatment of persistent postoperative biliary tract disease falls into three categories. Treatment is 1) solely symptomatic, 2) in anticipation of a further corrective procedure, or 3) still to be evaluated. In the first category are included the control of pain and the management of a wide variety of dyspepsias. In the second, infection is managed in the hope that the treatment can be definitive but is essentially preparation for an anatomic correction. The third category includes efforts to dissolve the stones by chenodeoxycholic acid. Osler's experience is generally still pertinent: "The medical treatment of gallstones is a chapter in our book of therapeutics the leaves of which are best turned very rapidly." Much of the medical treatment must be realistically viewed as procrastination within the triangle of either spontaneous remission or an unavoidable surgical indication (492).

SCOPE OF THE PROBLEM

Because surgery can be definitively corrective of anatomic abnormalities in an area in which medication has no true influence, the attendant physician must balance risk against probable operative result. Certainly it is hard to improve on the complaint status of the asymptomatic individual. Some tolerate defects that, in others, initiate serious PCS. For the bad-risk patient, (obesity, cerebral, cardiopulmonary, or multiple system disease) one can defer treatment until symptoms appear. About 50% of persons with documented calculus-related defects who are truly asymptomatic may be expected to remain so for an average of 2–5 years. There is less latitude in the diabetic or in the infectious or obstructive state.

A collateral problem is the effect of symptoms on the patient's general condition: Recurrent colic can debilitate, as well as trigger cardiac arrhythmias or angina (143). Passage, through the common duct, of calculi that had been asymptomatic can eventuate in a catastrophic pancreatitis. Judgment is difficult, and the prognosis for a specific patient is virtually impossible (572).

Acute catarrhal cholangitis will often respond to antibiotics. The period of remission is undeterminable. The suppurative variety of cholangitis, which is truly an intracholedochal abscess, makes the patient disoriented, as part of septic shock. For this variety of infection, the surgical risk has to be assumed (126).

Obstructive jaundice without infection can be tolerated for the time taken to improve the general condition. Definitive diagnosis is paramount in this situation. The fact that there has been prior biliary surgery does not always mean—although a suspicion should exist—that there is a persistent problem anatomically related to the earlier procedure. In the elderly bad-risk patient, there is one approach to jaundice-associated carcinoma of the pancreas and quite another to the impacted common duct stone.

There is no substitute for an aggressive diagnostic approach, provided there is an intent to do something upon the information that will be gained. If there is an adamant "no-matter-what, do-nothing" attitude, then ERCP or cholangiography need not be considered.

The variety of functional complaints that precede, and often follow, the first intervention are varied (358). They have been regarded as linked to biliary disease, but there is, in fact, no physiological basis for this association. The symptoms include headache, nausea, eructation, flatulence, constipation, coated tongue, fatty food intolerance, and episodic distention with bloating (635). The approach to these collateral or dyspeptic symptoms has to be predicated on the exclusion of organic lesions. The postoperative patient with headaches is not immune to a brain tumor or cerebrovascular disease, and the newly constipated patient may have a new, or until now unrecognized, colon tumor.

FUNCTIONAL ASPECTS

The management of functional disorders includes a regimen for weight reduction with a diet that is adjusted to the patient's tolerance. Diet is an ancient adjunct to management of disorders linked to biliary disease, yet it is largely empirical. Ingelfinger (292) has commented on the fact that one is puzzled about how to regulate the fat in the diet: Use it to stimulate function or restrict it for rest? The only constant thing about the diet is that it should be bland. The patient requires trial-and-error elimination of foods that are disturbing. There is the strong probability that diet in relation to biliary disease is as innocent a provocative factor as it is in the genesis of the exacerbations of duodenal ulcer disease. This time-honored association in folklore does not have a clear physiological basis (398).

Low-fat diets have been in the medical armentarium for a long time. Empirically they seem to work. In the ordinary case, the avoidance of fat and the use of a diet aimed at building hepatic glycogen reserve in the liver has been based on the assumption that there is "chronic hepatitis" associated with biliary tract disease. There is no support for this; there is no hepatitis associated with the common occidental variety of biliary lithiais (181, 196, 478). Nevertheles, the diet has to be worked out on a trial-and-error basis, for what works for one individual does not necessarily work for the other. Mallet-Guy (392) found that 23.8% of 820 patients required alimentary restrictions to prevent mild attacks of pain and digestive problems.

States of hyperchlorhydria or achlorhydria should be corrected with a knowledge of the gastric pH (148). Endocrinopathies should be sought for, especially a larval type of myxedema or hyperparathyroidism, which are associated not only with biliary tract disease, but with its associated constipation.

Constipation is the commonest associated complaint. It is difficult, ordinarily, for the patient to evoke sympathy from the profession, which view it as a fact of life. Moreover, the patient's concept of what constipation is may differ from the professional attitudes. A person who has fewer than three bowel movements a week can be regarded as constipated. Patients would prefer at least one easy movement daily. Constipation can be the most troublesome and difficult to manage of all the associated functional disorders. One rules out associated organic disorders, such as diabetes, neuropathies, amyloidosis, and the endocrinopathies, as well as local factors in the anorectal canal such as fissures, fistulas, and hemorrhoids.

There is a good correlation between colon stasis and biliary dysfunction that is based on the demonstration that the correction of colonic stasis can restore a nonfunctioning gallbladder to roentgenographic normality and on Ivy's observation (295) that colonic distention increases resistance at the choledochal sphincter.

Insofar as treatment is concerned, it may be difficult to influence psychiatric factors having their origin in childhood obedience or defiance of parents; in abdominal wall flaccidity, associated with lack of exercise and specific assumed toilet-facility needs; and in the chronic use of constipating drugs. However, sometimes the patient's bowel complaint has to be evaluated objectively by the use of radiopaque transit markers. Traditionally, a purely functional symptom is managed by reassurances regarding the benignancy of the problem. I have found this consoling to myself, but of little help to the troubled.

One may resort to a high-residue diet, the periodic use of enemas, magnesium sulfate before breakfast, and with patience the complaint can be alleviated but not cured. I have not encountered fecal impactions in association with dyspepsia related to biliary disorders, and in no case has an anorectal myotomy been required (285).

An evaluation of this problem in a Norwegian hospital (190) notes that almost half the patients who return for postoperative symptoms cite constipation as their sole complaint, even though more than half the 133 patients had been significantly relieved by cholecystectomy. Two-thirds of the patients were women. This complaint is not confined to one side of the Atlantic.

Certain attitudes toward the nonsurgical treatment of biliary stone disease and its presumably correlative functional disturbances have their basis in endocrine considerations. These are based not only on the higher incidence in women but on the fact, demonstrated by Nilsson and Slatten (445), that there is impaired emptying of the normal gallbladder during the progesterone phase of the menstrual cycle. This unrecognized physiological variant allows for the diagnosis of biliary dysfunction, unless the examination is repeated in the estrogen phase. The association has been referred to as the hepatoendocrine syndrome or cholecysto-ovarian "sympathy." During the progesterone phase, CCK-stimulated emptying is also impaired (217).

Anabolic steroids are said to alleviate symptoms. Adlercreutz (7) reported that 34 of 45 women were rendered symptom-free with progesterone—in one case after four laparotomies had failed. Men were improved with methyl estrenolase or allyl estratrienol.

NONSPECIFIC MEASURES

General hygienic measures will often improve the dyspeptic complaint: no smoking, minimal alcohol intake, mild sedation, and carminatives. Regularity of meals, the avoidance of overeating and rapid eating, and the proper rest all contribute to the general well-being. Some of the older clinicians placed a great deal of value upon fasting 1 day a week, except for 8 glasses of warm-water lemonade and a bromide–chloral-hydrate mixture.

The psychiatric aspects of biliary symptoms, in terms of Pavlovian concepts, have not received the emphasis established for ulcerative colitis or duodenal ulcer. However, the stress situations that produce colonic congestion and diarrhea in some people and gastric hypersecretion and ulceration in others have been shown also to evoke transitory choledochal hypertension. Therefore, the adjustment of emotional problems, insofar as this is possible, can assist in the relief of functional disorders in the biliary tract (362).

The spa treatment of biliary tract and associated disorders goes back to Roman times. There are well established resort areas with radioactive waters in Karlsbad, Montacatini, Vichy, and Marienbad as well as Saratoga Springs. The results of spa treatment can be attributed not only to laxative action of the salts and the stimulating effects of hydrotherapy, but also to the change of routine and the vacation aspects of this experience (73, 321).

"Little attacks just like before, but not as bad" are not uncommon. They tend to appear within the first several weeks after the initial surgery and often become increasingly severe. If they have no anatomic basis, they disappear in 2–5 years. They present a diagnostic problem when the intravenous cholangiogram is normal, indicating the absence of a grossly demonstrable defect.

It is wise to examine biliary sediment in these cases as in the diagnostic Lyon-Meltzer test. This is a rapid way to demonstrate that the patient may be passing small calculi or sludge. In such instances choleretics may be of help, and the biliary flush regimen, outlined here, can be curative.

1. Three tablets of dehydrocholic acid and belladonna after each meal and at bedtime

2. Magnesium citrate (6 oz) each morning before breakfast

3. Pure cream or olive oil (3 tbs) before noon and evening meals

4. One nitroglycerin tablet (0.02 gr) under the tongue before the evening meal

This regimen is employed for 3 consecutive days.

The pain of functional colic should not be treated by repeated doses of narcotics. Bilateral or left-sided sympathetic block with 1% procaine from T-6 or T-8 to L-1 has been effective. In several cases, it seemed to break a cycle so that the pain is less frequent and of lesser intensity. In the MHMC series there has been no experience with surgical sympathectomy of the type recommended by Mallet-Guy (397) although I have recognized that the sympathetic system is the afferent pathway for biliary pain.

I have not been impressed by the use of atropine derivatives as a choledochal sphincter relaxant. This is one of the considerations that led to the use of adjunctive hepatic plexus vagectomy with cholecystectomy. It is reassuring following cholecystectomy to know that the choledochal sphincter has been maximally relaxed by the denervation. When this is not done, the doses of atropine must be large and repetitive (210).

However, there has been considerable experience in Europe with methyl-4 umbelliferone as a noncholagogic choleretic that is said to have a specific, selective spasmolytic action on the sphincter of Oddi. The agent has been marketed in Europe extensively under the name of Cantabiline. The European reports are encouraging. I have had no experience with the drug.

We are now entering a new era in the management of the anatomic aspects of the PCS. New endoscopic techniques facilitate stone extraction and sphincterotomy performed in the awake patient via the duodenoscope. The approach represents an extension of ERCP from a purely diagnostic to a therapeutic modality. This highly specialized technique is less physiologically straining upon the patient than is a formal laparotomy. At this time, the general applicability and the possible early hazards and late results have to be more universally formalized and evaluated. However, the early reports are encouraging. Endoscopic surgery of the biliary tract may come to be the same kind of specialty within surgery that angiography is in radiology (130, 319, 329, 647, 648).

CHENODEOXYCHOLIC ACID

The basic problem in patients with cholesterol gallstones is that they have a decreased bile-acid pool and increased cholesterol synthesis and secretion so that their bile is incapable of maintaining the cholesterol in solution. Chenodeoxycholic (CDC) acid apparently acts to reverse this by increasing the bile acid pool and by decreasing the amount of cholesterol synthesized and secreted by the liver. CDC acid induces, therefore, a desaturated bile and rapidly dissolves the cholesterol in the bile that is present; in time it also dissolves the cholesterol stones that have formed in the gallbladder. The ordinary period of treatment required for this is 6–36 months. The limiting factor is the transfer of solidified cholesterol from the gallstone itself into the bile.

The final word on the effect of CDC acid on gallstone disease awaits the results of a double-blind study by the National Institutes of Health (275, 293, 340, 540, 541). However, the following facts have emerged:

1. Radiolucent stones less than 1.5 cm in diameter will disappear or decrease in size on doses of 15 mg/kg/day.
2. Calcified stones are not affected.
3. Solitary stones greater than 1.5 cm in diameter respond poorly (about 25% in the Mayo Clinic study).
4. The response is effected in 6–24 months.
5. Stones recur when the medication is stopped, but respond to reinstitution of therapy.
6. Liver biopsies show no diagnostic abnormalities.

The major criterion for the selection of patients for the CDC acid treatment is the radiologic demonstration of lucent stones. However, the work of Trotman *et al.* (592) points up the difficulty of this. In their series of 92 lucent stones, 13 were pigment stones. There were 18 opaque stones, but 6 of the latter were cholesterol. Thus the criterion of stone lucency allows for the inclusion of a sufficient number of subjects with lucent pigment stones, a factor that may account for some of the treatment failures. Moreover, exclusion of the patients with opaque stones (one-third of which were cholesterol) from CDC acid treatment may be unfair.

The role of CDC acid in the treatment of recurrent common bile duct stones in patients who have previously had a cholecystectomy is unclear. Hoffman and Thistle (275) report a small clinical trial indicating that some patients did not respond.

A pharmacologic approach to the solution of cholesterol stones holds great promise. The age-old desideratum of a drug that will selectively dissolve the stones without having any adverse effect seems to be on the threshold. Seventy-five percent of gallstones are mixed with cholesterol, accounting for about 70% of their weight. They tend to be medium-sized or small, multiple, and round or faceted. Ten percent of gallstones are pigment stones, consisting either of bilirubin, pigment or calcium bilirubinate. Pigment stones are most often dark-colored, hard, irregularly shaped, and found as multiple stones rather than solitary ones. The CDC acid is effective for the cholesterol stones but not for the pigment stones. As to the primary stones formed in the common bile duct as a result of stasis, it is not believed at this time that CDC acid will affect them.

In summary, the medical approach to nonorganic biliary disease is symptomatic, working within the periods of what appear to be natural remissions. The approach is most efficient when the entire personality is considered along with the physical problems.

IV

Secondary Biliary Tract Operations

18 Operative Techniques

Secondary biliary tract operations have their own specific problems. Their technical aspects are influenced by the effects of prior interventions as well as by the distortive sequelae of the residual biliary pathology (117, 324, 344).

Among the effects of earlier treatment are the changes produced by adhesions, synechiae, residual infection, foreign-body reactions, and hernias. These pathologic findings rarely occur singly. Thus there are combinations of gallbladder remnants and secondary common-duct stones, primary common-duct stones and choledochoduodenal junctional stenosis, biliary fistulas and cholangitis, ventral hernia and residual subhepatic infection.

Secondary procedures require a collaborative diagnostic evaluation to outline the entire problem. Certain instruments are of special value (Fig. 18-1).

This surgery cannot be satisfactorily accomplished with a struggling patient, or with heaving and hiccoughing that prevents the exposure from being maintained. Complete relaxation of the abdominal wall is a *sine qua non*.

The desideratum is to have direct access to the right upper quadrant in an area of anticipated changes, avoiding other organs as much as possible. It is best to stay completely in the subhepatic area without getting out of the supracolic compartment. The aim is to do what is required with minimal manipulation of the bowel except for the duodenum and hepatic flexure.

The pattern of adhesions is completely predictable, regardless of the number of previous interventions. Each of the areas of adherence corresponds to the anatomists' observations that there are the areas of normal anatomic impression of the colon and duodenum onto the dorsocaudal surface of the liver. The large gastric impression to which the stomach can be adherent is ordinarily well to the left and outside the area that is the intimate surgical field. Portions of the omentum adhere to the abdominal parieties and to the inferior margin of the liver. The plane of adherence is usually filamentous and relatively avascular. The hepatic flexure of the colon will be adherent to the gallbladder fossa in a broad band.

The most striking change involves the first portion of the duodenum, which appears considerably foreshortened and blankets over the choledochus to become adherent at the base of the gallbladder fossa, in toward the porta hepatis. Until this portion of the duodenum is completely lysed and mobilized inferiorly, the choledochus cannot be exposed.

The previous incision comes into consideration if it is infected, contains a sinus tract, or is the site of a hernia. It is sometimes wise to disregard a long-standing hernia and to plan the operative approach around it. This approach is safe when the hernia is known to contain only liver or omentum, but it is impossible to be sure. As a general policy, it is wise to plan a revisional procedure so that it is possible to repair the hernia during the final stages of the operation.

The most important incisional consideration, especially with revisional procedures, is that the exposure be appropriate. "This time it must be done right" is the idea. Without a perfect incision it cannot be accomplished. Two uncertainties can erroneously influence the choice of the incision. If a scar is well

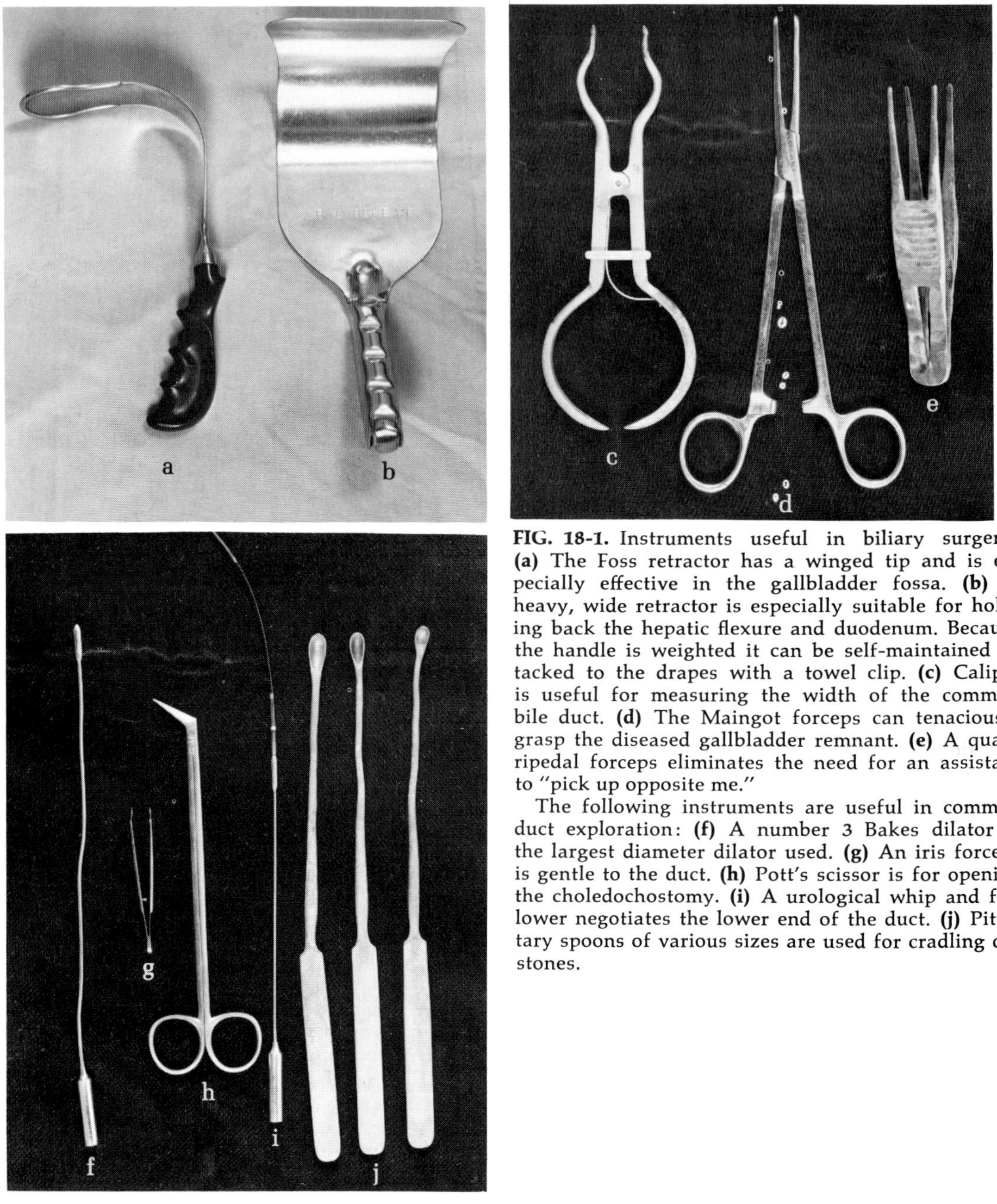

FIG. 18-1. Instruments useful in biliary surgery: **(a)** The Foss retractor has a winged tip and is especially effective in the gallbladder fossa. **(b)** A heavy, wide retractor is especially suitable for holding back the hepatic flexure and duodenum. Because the handle is weighted it can be self-maintained or tacked to the drapes with a towel clip. **(c)** Caliper is useful for measuring the width of the common bile duct. **(d)** The Maingot forceps can tenaciously grasp the diseased gallbladder remnant. **(e)** A quadripedal forceps eliminates the need for an assistant to "pick up opposite me."

The following instruments are useful in common duct exploration: **(f)** A number 3 Bakes dilator is the largest diameter dilator used. **(g)** An iris forceps is gentle to the duct. **(h)** Pott's scissor is for opening the choledochostomy. **(i)** A urological whip and follower negotiates the lower end of the duct. **(j)** Pituitary spoons of various sizes are used for cradling out stones.

healed, a second, parallel or crossing incision will not eventuate in necrosis of the intermediate skin flap. It is also safe to go through an old well-healed scar and then to open the fascial muscular component at a higher or lower level and to extend it in a medial or lateral direction.

INCISIONAL APPROACH

Skin Incision

The choice of incision depends partly upon the habitus of the costal arch and on the desire to avoid a tic-tac-toe scarification of the abdominal wall. One need not utilize a previously poorly placed scar just because it is there. The site of incision has to provide good exposure of the area to permit circumscribing sinus tracts, and, when at all possible, to permit repair of a coexistent incisional hernia (Fig. 18-2).

The older textbooks list and illustrate a wide selection of choices, many of which have become eponymic. In general, a wide costal flare allows for a transverse or oblique incision placed 2–3 cm below the costal arch. It can be extended across the linea alba into the left rectus, which can be retracted or sectioned. A better form of medial extensions can be achieved by vertical extension in the midline superiorly high into the costoxiphoid groove. This is akin to the original Kehr incision (322).

A great advantage of this approach is that it confines the surgery to the supracolic compartment and obviates the need to manipulate the small bowel. This subcostal incision can also be extended laterally beyond the semilunaris into the oblique muscles. The external oblique is sharply sectioned and the internal oblique split in the direction of its fibers.

With a narrow costal margin, there is no suitable alternative to a vertical incision. An absolute midline incision through the linea alba is an effective way of circumventing the wound complications of a previous incision.

FIG. 18-2. Incisional choices. **A.** A subcostal incision is preferred if the costal flare is wide. It may be extended up into the costoxiphoid angle or laterally across the oblique muscles. The stippled area becomes hypesthetic if intercostal nerves are divided. **B.** An exact midline incision is the best general utility approach. It is often extended into the costoxiphoid groove. Only in the extraordinary situation is the cross-lateral extension required.

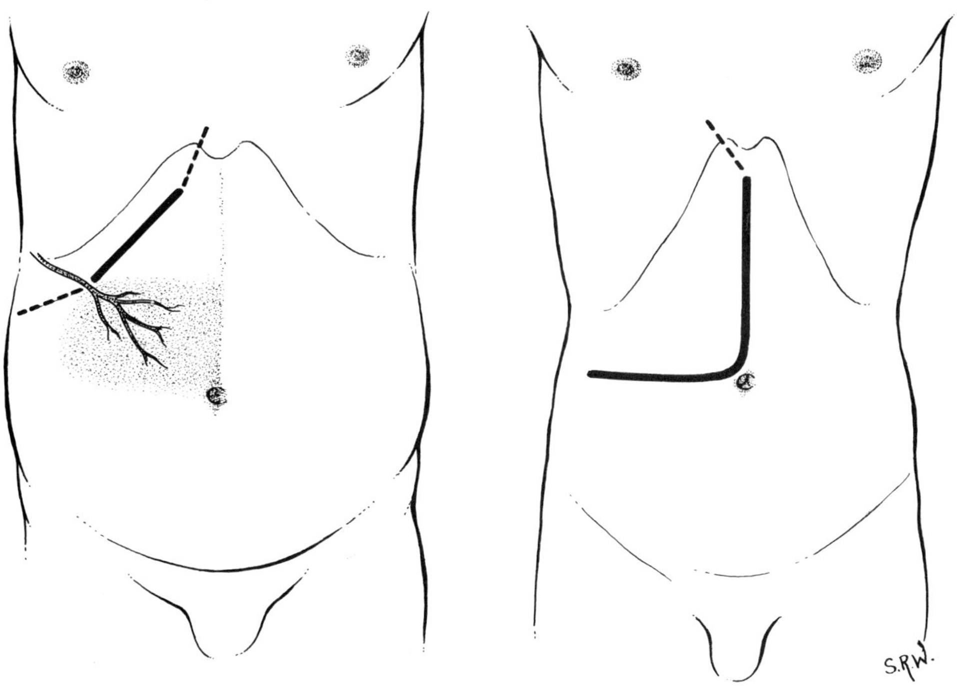

A B

That incision goes down to and through the middle of the umbilicus. In the obese patient, it can be extended 4–6 cm below the umbilicus. The skin incision should be longer than that in the other layers. One can retract its upper and lower angles to get another inch at each pole.

If the right upper quadrant skin presents difficult problems, satisfactory exposure of the area can be obtained by a left paramedian incision. I have never found it necessary to do revisional biliary surgery through a thoracoabdominal approach, although this has been recommended by others. The aponeurotic-muscular component need not be sectioned at the skin incision level. One can retract up or down for 1.5–2 in. There is sometimes that same advantage to sectioning the deeper layers over the coastal arch and the peritoneum at the skin incision level—a sort of staircase configuration.

It can be useful to cut the lower two costal cartilages in the midclavicular line. This is done subperiosteally with care not to enter the pleural space. A well-placed curved periosteal elevator of the duckbill type can be positioned posteriorly as a guard while the cartilage is being divided. This fracture allows for a hinge type mobility of the upper end of the incision.

If the incision is to be placed at the hernial site, that area should be approached elliptically with a sidewise or vertical extension on each side. At the time of entrance the dissection should go clear back to the peritoneal-fascial edges that will be suitable for later reapproximation.

Entering the Peritoneum

The skin incision should be opened full length down to the fascia. The well-healed old scar can be excised or incised; there is no difference. The exposed nonabsorbed sutures should be removed. The rectus muscle should be divided in the area where it is well defined, not where it is attenuated or scarred from the prior intervention.

The clue to an easy entrance into the peritoneum is to effect it in the area where there are least likely to be significant adhesions. Otherwise there can be inept entrances into the liver or bowel. For the vertical midline incision this requires going in at the extreme upper or lower end, hence the longer skin incision. For the horizontal incision it means getting in far laterally, by separating the oblique muscle. Hemostasis should be meticulous.

If the peritoneum is not thin and translucent, it is best to effect a keyhole entrance at the extremity of the incision. The area is then spread open with a curved hemostat to be certain that it is properly positioned. The index finger then goes through that opening and evaluates the extent of underlying adherence to the remainder of the scar.

A convenient method is first to open the full length of the transverse skin and subcutaneous area. The end of the incision is then retracted and elevated, creating a free space away from the underlying viscera, and the incision deepened through a 1-in. area that is the fasciomuscular envelope. Bleeders are ligated as encountered. The area is then reached where the fasciomuscular envelope of the abdominal wall reflects onto the lateral gutter at the upper pole of the right kidney. The colon is right there; so I prefer to nick the translucent peritoneum and then to perforate and widen the aperture bluntly with the finger or the back of the scalpel.

The edge of each side of the peritoneum is then grasped with a Kelly or Mikulicz clamp and everted. The second and third fingers of the left hand are inserted onto the posterior surface of the peritoneum and the adhesions are bluntly separated. The muscle and fascia are elevated from within and are sectioned in one plane. The full length of the incison is thus opened. Unless this precaution is observed, it is possible inadvertently to open the bowel or to make an incision into the hepatic parenchyma.

I have seen the sequelae of such accidents as small-bowel and colonic fistulas. Such accidents can be a disheartening note at the outset of a revisional procedure. The complication is best avoided. If the bowel has been opened, it is not enough to close the opening. It is also necessary to lyse the adherent loop so that there is no tension on the line of closure.

After the two fingers in the intraperitoneal area have freed all adhesions in the line of entrance to the abdominal wall, and while the edges of the peritoneum are thus exposed, it is advisable to prepare on the way in for the closure on the way out. This requires clearing the peritoneum on each side. The lysis is accomplished to include both angles for an area at least 2 cm in all directions. The upper end of the incison can be adherent to the liver. One must avoid incising this organ in the liberation and must also avoid going too far superiorly because there is an advantage to preserving the existing adhesive obliteration of the subdiaphragmatic space. If these precautions are taken at the beginning of the procedure, adequate definition for the peritoneum will have been accomplished so that the closure is prepared for.

Exposure of the Common Bile Duct

Except for specific indications, it is not necessary to expose other areas of the peritoneal cavity, and it is not necessary, ordinarily, to lyse small-bowel adhesions. This advice, of course does not pertain when an infracolic exploration is required to evaluate that area. The anatomic basis for the exposure was anticipated by the older anatomists, who described the areas of impression on the liver. The clue to exposure for secondary biliary procedures is the freeing of the liver from these sites of adhesion and their retraction into a position that maintains the common bile duct, gallbladder bed, duodenum, and pancreas in the operative field. It is axiomatic that the neophyte will regard the choledochus as being farther to the left and more posterior than it is in fact (Fig. 18-3).

The omentum has usually been separated during the freeing of the undersurface of the peritoneum. However, it can still be adherent to the edge of the liver. The hepatic flexure is invariably adherent to the undersurface of the liver. The constant relation to the gallbladder is a fact that has also been noted by the radiologists. It is best to start to free the hepatic flexure by mobilizing the upper end of the right colon, as in doing an ileocolectomy. This entire area is liberated sufficiently

FIG. 18-3. Patterns of adhesions usually found when the abdomen is opened a second time. **A.** The omentum is adherent to the undersurface of the peritoneum and to the liver edge. **B.** The hepatic flexure is attached to the liver edge by broad or bowstring adhesions and is often socked into the former hepatic-gallbladder fossa. (From Schein CJ, Stern WZ, Jacobson HG: The Common Bile Duct. Operative Cholangiography, Biliary Endoscopy and Choledocholithotomy, 1966. Courtesy of Charles C Thomas, Publisher, Springfield, Illinois)

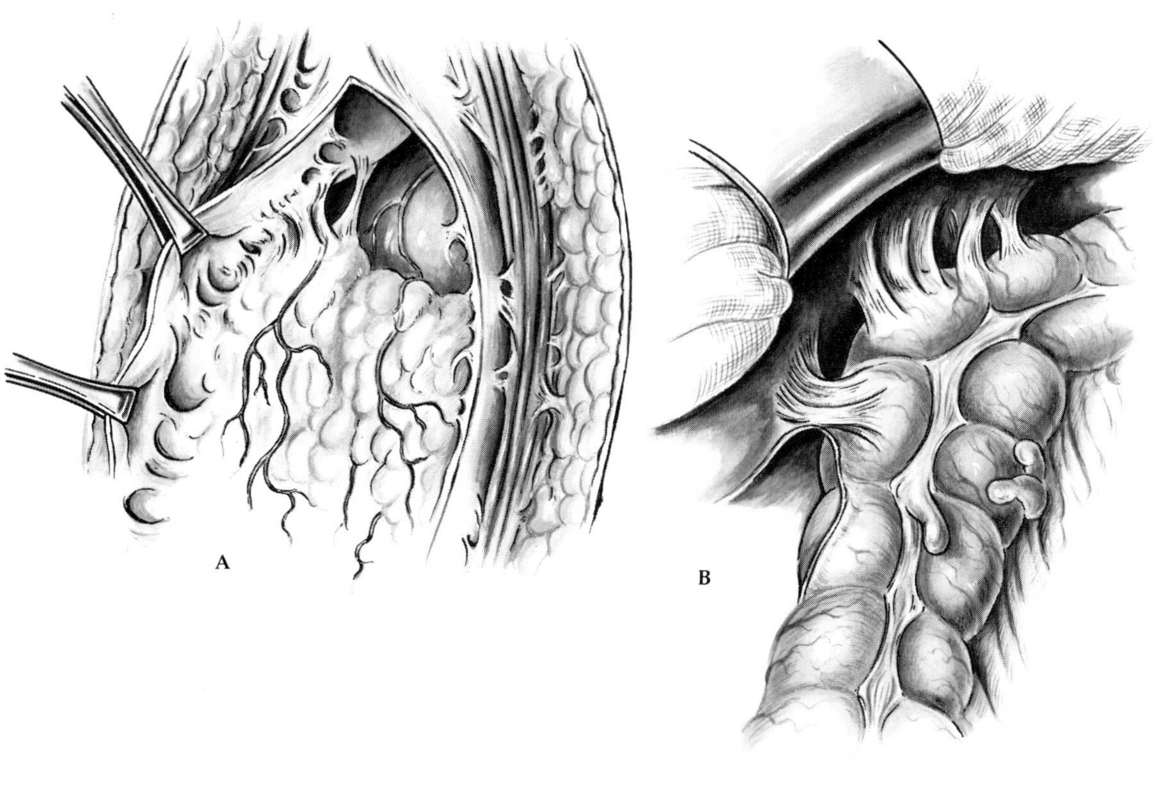

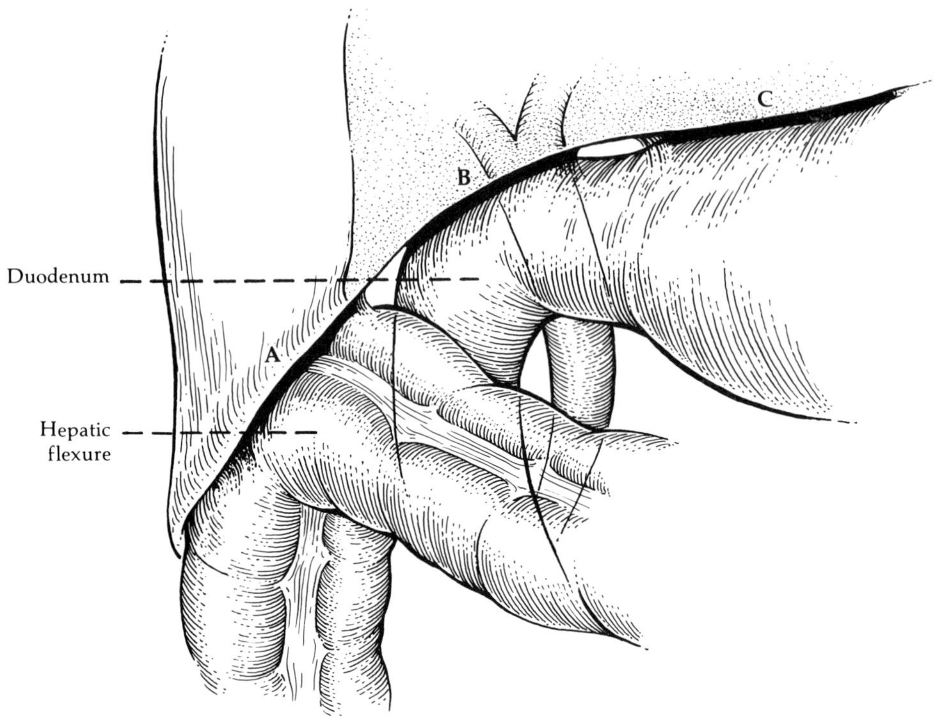

FIG. 18-4. Pattern of adhesions. The hepatic flexure and omentum must be separated from the gallbladder bed and liver edge at point **A.** The duodenum blankets over the entire supraduodenal choledochus and must be freed from area **B.** The lesser curvature of the stomach is adherent to the liver in the area of its gastric impression. **C.** This latter site does not always have to be mobilized.

to expose the underlying second portion of the duodenum. In this way the hepatic flexure can be accurately lysed from the liver. It is retracted inferiorly and to the left (Fig. 18-4).

The ascending duodenum cannot be visualized until this has been accomplished; its postbulbar segment is usually densely adherent to the liver, blanketing over the common bile duct. It must be lysed from the liver to identify the ventral aspect of the duct. This lysis can be difficult, and the serosa and muscle may be split in accomplishing it.

The entire duodenum must be mobilized to facilitate manipulation of the entire "C" area. The lesser curvature of the duodenum is dissected away from the area of hepatic adherence. The concept in exposure is that the adherent duodenum will roll back readily if the detachment is initiated in the normal zone. Rarely is it easier to start the approach from the pylorus, going to the right.

The duodenal mobilization frees the area for anastomotic procedures, and permits palpation of the pancreatic head, ampulla, and infraduodenal bile duct. The paraduodenal peritoneal incision is diaphanous. It is incised with due regard to the underlying vena cava. This is an avascular zone. The capillary ooze that can come with this mobilization is readily controlled by pressure with a laparotomy pad. The stomach does not have to be liberated from the liver, although the pylorus can be followed as a lead to the adherent distorted duodenum.

With the duodenum now retracted, the full length of the supraduodenal segment of the bile duct and of the gallbladder fossa is exposed (117). This position is maintained by three retractors. The hepatic flexure and the small bowel must be kept out of the field. A large towel serves this purpose better than the conventional laparotomy pad. The liver tilt from below provides accessibility to the hilus. This is well done with the Foss or broad Harrington type retractor. The upper pole of the kidney is clearly seen, and a laparotomy pad in the hepatic renal fossa serves to catch the effluvia of bile duct exploration.

Maneuvers in this area are facilitated by good retraction that does not necessitate constant repositioning. This is especially true with regard to the southern end of the operative field. I have modified the Deaver retractor by increasing its width to 6 in., with some slightly increased convexity. The handle is weighted so that it can be maintained in position or hooked onto a drape. This makes another hand available. The width of that single wide retractor is sufficient to restrain both the hepatic flexure and the duodenum.

In this position the common bile duct is tense and appears somewhat flattened. Relaxation of the retractor allows it to balloon out, rendering it accessible to aspiration by a number 19 needle with a 2-ml syringe.

Evaluation of the Extrahepatic Bile Ducts

This pertains to gross morphologic evaluation. The cholangiographic features have already been detailed. Duct width is the most important factor. The only pertinent value is that determined on the hepatic side of the cystic duct so that a parallel cystic duct is not included in the mensuration. Accurate determination by number—not by eye alone—requires a simple caliper, ruler, or comparison alignment with a Bakes dilator. Duct width of 1.4 cm or greater is an absolute indication of obstructive choledochopathy. A narrow duct (less than 0.8 cm) suggests either a more proximal disorder or a nonobstructive situation. Such narrow ducts are less likely to have stones. A diseased duct is indurated (ascertained by indentation) and lacks the normal sheen and translucency. The freely pulsating, readily visible small arteries that are part of the epicholedochal plexus are less prominent. Transillumination is impaired.

Intrahepatic bile lakes can be seen as well as palpated. These confirm the diagnosis of an advanced obstructive disorder. Hepatic nodularity and excessive bleeding are strongly suggestive of cirrhosis; with such findings one should be prepared to revise the preoperative diagnosis.

It is a wise and safe rule always to aspirate the presumed duct before incising it. I know of aggressive, inadvertent incisions into the portal vein and hepatic artery. Aspiration can be safely accomplished with a number 19 needle on a 2-ml syringe. It is not far-fetched to caution against going too deeply, in which case one perforates the posterior wall of the duct. If the portal vein is thus entered, simple digital pressure will control it. The aspirated bile is used for culture and sensitivity studies.

The pericholedochal lymph nodes, by their number and consistency, offer an indication of the present or antecedent inflammatory reaction.

CHOLEDOCHOLITHOTOMY

The cardinal principle of intraoperative stone extraction is to manipulate the stone out through the choledochostomy ostium rather than to extract in a dental sense. It is truly impossible to know the remote effects of inept instrumentation unless there are gross manifestations of perforation or traumatic pancreatitis. Smith *et al.* (568) have indicated how postoperative complications in the form of pancreatitis, intraabdominal abscess, and intestinal obstruction have their source in faulty handling of instruments. Such a cause and effect are often not appreciated in considering complications following choledocholithotomy. It remains impossible to correlate less-than-catastrophic symptoms with surgical manipulations. Perhaps there are none.

Surgical maneuvers in this area should be so delicate and purposefully directed as to avoid damage to the epithelial lining of the duct. Choledochoscopic observations have indicated how easily this epithelium becomes edematous and hemorrhagic with intraductal manipulations.

It is not possible to explore the duct properly unless it is well mobilized. Although one can visualize only the supraduodenal segment, it is possible to get a sense of the intraduodenal portion by palpation, from behind the pancreas, of an indwelling catheter. This requires mobilization of the second part of the duodenum, eponymically referred to as Kocher's maneuver (Fig. 18-5). Kocher originally described this technique as adjunctive to gastroduodenostomy. That type of mobilization is required for virtually all intraductal manipulations, and is mandatory for anastomotic operations (379).

The peritoneum along the lateral wall of

the descending duodenum is incised for 2–3 cm. The duodenum is then rolled off the vena cava toward the superior mesenteric vein. The head of the pancreas is thus completely mobilized.

Opening the Duct

There is always a small bile leak at the site of needle puncture for aspiration to identify the duct (Fig. 18–6). This opening is first enlarged with the point of a number 11 saber-shaped scalpel blade and then spread to a 10- to 12-mm aperture by spreading a clamp blade within its lumen. The edges are then held open by in–out looped, tagged sutures that evert the edges. This method has the advantage of avoiding the troublesome bleeding that can come from sharply dividing one of the epicholedochal vessels or of penetrating the posterior wall of the duct.

Triangulation of the opening is accomplished by two full-thickness lateral traction sutures and a vein retractor placed anteriorly. These sutures should be tagged with light weight clamps to avoid their tearing through. Now one can get a good, direct inside look for several centimeters in each direction. This direct visualization through the surgical ostium is a valuable type of naked-eye choledochoscopy that is often neglected.

A sucker should be positioned over a laparotomy pad in the subhepatic fossa, so that the latter will catch stone fragments and the former will keep the field free of fluid. The stoma may tear open further during the intraductal manipulations. In the dilated duct, I have often taken a 1.5-mm full-thickness biopsy of the duct at the site of one of the sutures for the purpose of documenting the extent and chronicity of the diffuse extrahepatic ductal inflammatory reaction (529).

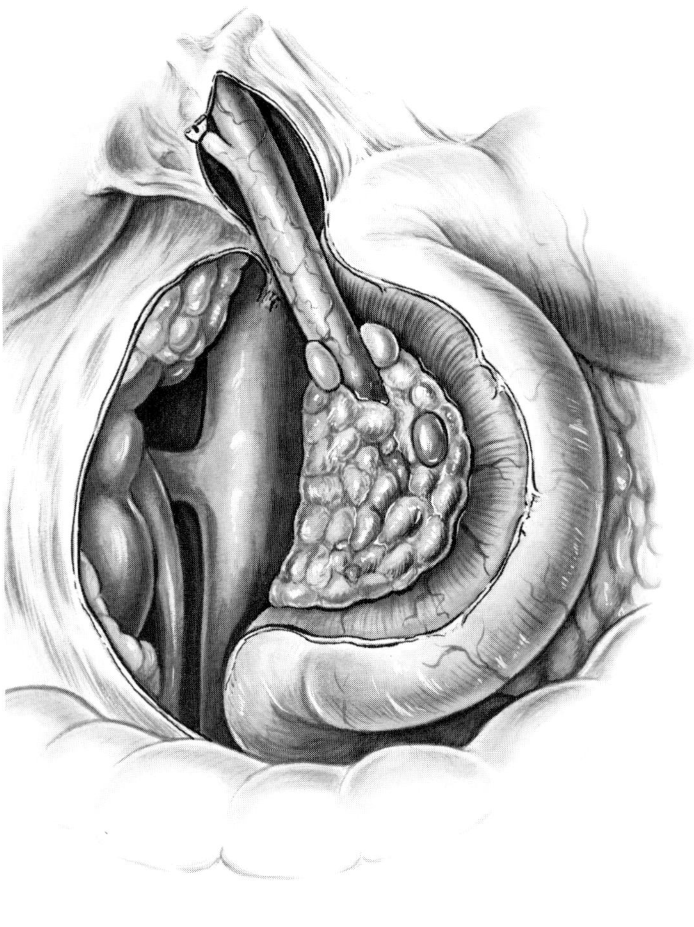

FIG. 18-5. Exposure by Kocher mobilization, showing extent to which the lateral duodenum must be mobilized. The entire pancreatic head and retroduodenol choledochus must be exposed and available. (From Schein CJ, Stern WZ, and Jacobson HG: The Common Bile Duct. Operative Cholangiography, Biliary Endoscopy and Choledocholithotomy, 1966. Courtesy of Charles C Thomas, Publisher, Springfield, Illinois)

FIG. 18-6. Choledochostomy. **A.** Common bile duct is identified by aspiration in an avascular area. **B.** The site of the needle aspiration is then speared open with a bayonet type blade. **C.** That opening is then spread with a clamp in both planes of the choledochus to permit adequate exposure. **D.** This type of opening of the common duct is preferred to incising it with a scissor.

E. The exposure of the common bile duct that is required for adequate inspection, diagnosis, and intraoperative maneuvers is complete. **F.** There is a problem of the choice of choledochotomy incision when there is a long parallel type of cystic duct. In this instance the cystic duct has been opened, not the common bile duct. This faulty incision is appreciated when a probe is inserted retrograde. (From Schein CJ, Stern WZ, Jacobson HG: The Common Bile Duct. Operative Cholangiography, Biliary Endoscopy and Choledocholithotomy, 1966. Courtesy of Charles C Thomas, Publisher, Springfield, Illinois)

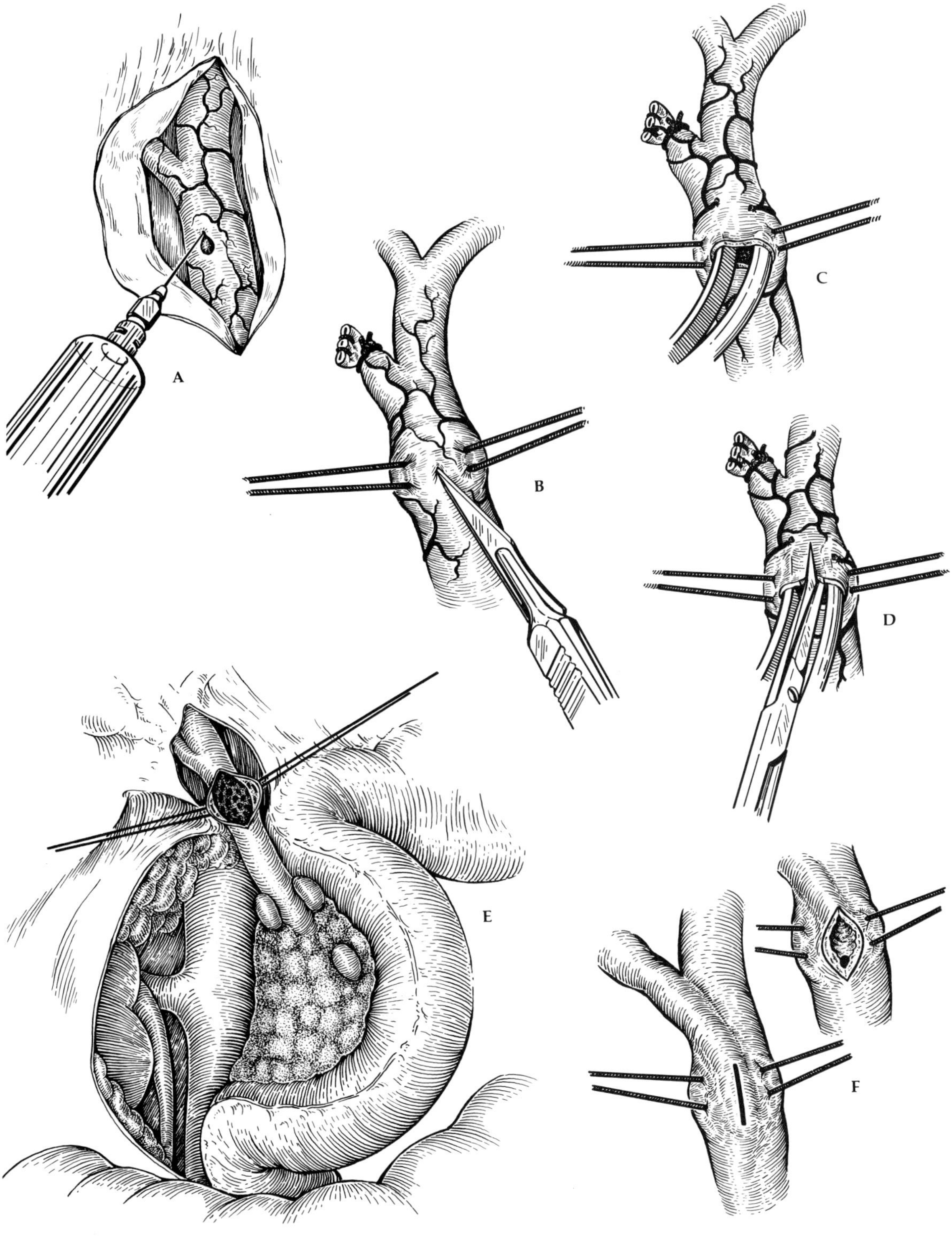

FIG. 18-7. Choledocholithotomy. **A and B.** Stones are ejected from the duct by milking from below and from above. Intraductal manipulation should be done only after this method of extrusion. **C.** Intraductal manipulations are done with a moistened pituitary spoon. **D.** The spoon serves as a scoop to cradle stones out. Palpated stones are delivered into the jaws of the forceps rather than attempting to search blindly by opening and closing the forceps jaws. (From Schein CJ, Stern WZ, Jacobson HG: The Common Bile Duct. Operative Cholangiography, Biliary Endoscopy and Choledocholithotomy, 1966. Courtesy of Charles C Thomas, Publisher, Springfield, Illinois)

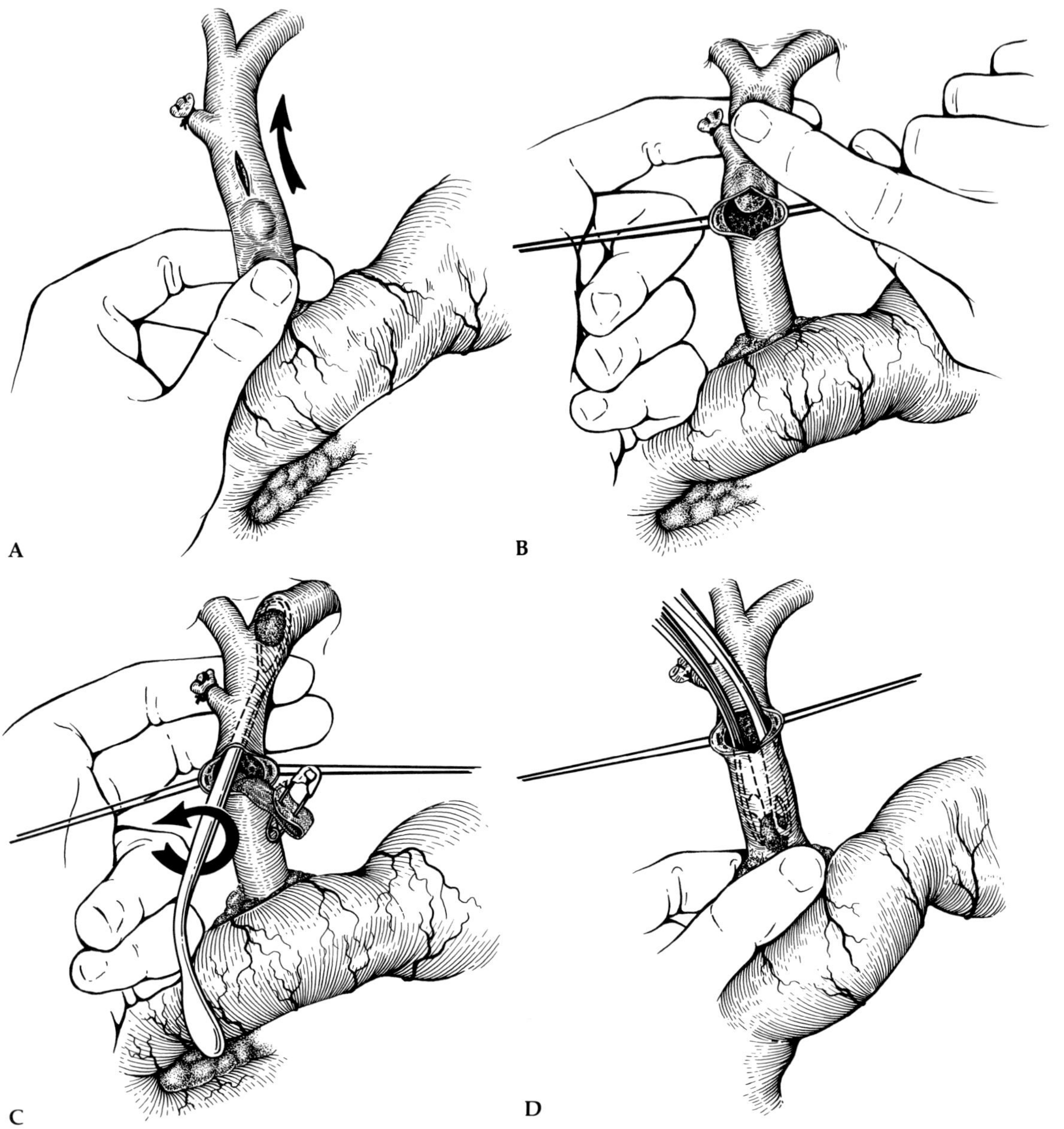

EXTRUSION OF CALCULI

Calculi and stone debris often spontaneously extrude as soon as the duct is opened. With the surgical ostium held ajar, the anterior duct wall is gently milked from the hilus toward the opening. This is done several times with the forefingers or with the belly of an appropriately curved clamp. The same procedure is carried out on the distal duct, milking from behind in the common duct groove of the pancreas toward the center. This procedure of milking from without clears the duct of most free-floating calculus material (Fig. 18–7).

Duct exploration, especially in the difficult problem, is best done with the operator on the patient's left. One has the advantage of holding the duodenum and the head of the pancreas (*i.e.*, the entire retro- and infraduodenal portions of the duct) between the thumb and the second and third fingers. This position allows for more sensitive palpation during the intraductal manipulation. It works particularly well for the impacted distal stone, which can be fixed by the left hand while the stone-crushing forceps are delivered by the right. The lumen of the duct is now explored intraluminally with moist, graduated, malleable pituitary spoons. These are inserted centrally and withdrawn circumferentially so that each quadrant of the duct is systematically swept. Obviously, the hollow of the spoon is cleaned after each fruitful sweep. At the conclusion of these two procedures one should come away believing that ducts are sanitized, but the exploration is not completed until the ducts have been washed out (248).

The duct is irrigated with warm saline through a moist number 12–14 rubber catheter. The injection is likely to be most rewarding with intermittent forceful bursts. The catheter should be inserted to its full depth before the irrigation is started; otherwise the stones are forced ahead into smaller radicles on the proximal side or are sometimes only rotated about on the distal side. Good evacuation requires that the saline push will so distend the duct proximally as to wash out the stones on the "off the backboard" outflow. At the distal end, observe whether the duodenum becomes distended by the fluid passing through the Vaterian segment. This procedure is carried out in both directions and is discontinued when the flush is repeatedly clear.

Hepatic Duct Stones

There are several types of hepatic duct stones. There are uncommon ones that are associated with intrinsic liver disease, and abnormalities of intrahepatic ducts, such as are seen in the Far East or in Caroli's disease. These are quite distinct from the usual variety of choledocholithiasis in which some stones get into the hepatic duct (212). It is with the latter that this text is concerned.

In the vast majority of instances hepatic duct stones are introduced into the peripheral bile duct by intraoperative manipulation (266). When hepatic duct stones are found in the bile ducts, they have frequently been driven in by a maneuver that fails to empty the duct before it is irrigated. The order of priority of bile duct exploration has been violated. 2) When these stones are present, and there is a chance of leaving them behind, it is well to provide for their postoperative passage through a wide choledochoduodenostomy (520). It has been my policy to do this procedure in every instance in which the bile duct is dilated to 1.2 cm or more and contains hepatic duct stones. I will accept a slightly narrower duct for choledochoduodenostomy in the presence of hepatic duct stones than I would in the case without hepatic duct stones.

The solitary hepatic duct stone in one of the major radicles can be difficult to retrieve because of the pericalculus reaction. It can be retained because that area has not been properly explored. This is especially true with reference to the left hepatic duct. This is a common site for retained calculi, if the conventional exploration is not monitored. Shore and Berci (558) would have missed hepatic duct stones in 18 of 31 cases. In 10%, the detected calculi could not be removed. If a hepatotomy fails to solve the problem of hepatic duct stone removal, then one must make provision for extrusion by choledochoduodenostomy or some type of sphincter relaxation.

One or several stones high up in the liver are often retained *in situ*. The subsegmental area that is blocked by such a stone (or stones) can atrophy without harm. The problem occurs when these stones pass into the common duct and produce obstruction. It is advisable, therefore, to anticipate provision for their evacuation into the intestine.

Longmire and Tompkins (371) indicate that an obstruction of a segmental hepatic duct not associated with infection will allow that portion of the liver to atrophy without clinical symptoms. The obstruction becomes a problem only when infection is present. If infection is introduced by the surgeon, it is possible to convert a dormant situation into an intrahepatic abscess that can then only be managed by drainage or resection. It is not necessary to remove every intrahepatic duct stone, especially in the bad-risk patient. Many patients can tolerate these stones for many years without either cholangitis or liver abscess (389).

Sometimes the position of a stone is made evident only by choledochoscopy or cholangiography. It can be dislodged by shaking the liver and then grasping it with the intraductal forceps. The stone is frequently fragmented, and the individual fragments are then washed out. Others have described passing the tip of a Fogarty catheter beyond the stone, and then forcing it out with the distended balloon (184). Sometimes a stone can be retrieved only under direct operative choledochoscopic control.

The Stone in the Distal Duct

True impaction of a calculus in the distal segment is an unusual circumstance. In such instances the patient is usually jaundiced. When there is no hyperbilirubinemia, it is likely that the stone was forced into this position by ductal maneuvers. There are three methods of attacking this problem: forceps extraction with probable fragmentation; an attempt at catheter balloon expulsion; or duodenotomy with sphincterotomy. The last is the original McBurney procedure, in which the sphincter sectioning can be viewed as an episiotomy. These three procedures can be tried sequentially. There is a danger of overdistending the balloon and producing a large hematoma, which bleeds into the duct.

I know of instances in which it has been impossible to get the stone by any of these maneuvers. In such circumstances one has to be diagnostically cautious about combined diseases. In one circumstance, there was an associated cancer of the distal bile duct. The cancer became apparent when fragments of tissue were removed with minor stone chips. Frozen section confirmed the diagnosis. The truly impacted stone is probably not as common in fact as the frequency of its diagnosis would suggest.

The Dormia stone dislodger, used so successfully for postoperative stone retrieval, has an applicability in this problem. The instrument is delivered past the stone, and then opened and rotated on the pullout. There has been but a single experience when it was difficult to get the instrument back through the sphincter.

In general, these stones are better cradled out with a pituitary spoon than grasped with a forceps. The conventional grasping forceps is of limited use in the problem of an impacted suprasphincteric stone. For the impacted stone, the alternatives beyond the instrumentation suggested are 1) crushing and washout, 2) trying to retrieve under choledochoscopic vision, 3) doing a transduodenal open sphincterotomy (episotomy type) and delivering it, or 4) leaving it in and bypassing with a choledochoduodenostomy.

When a stone or stones cannot be removed —and this is rare—a bypass procedure is indicated. For the distal stone, a choledochoduodenostomy completely solves the problem. It serves as well to eliminate the stasis at the choledochoduodenal junction, which may be a factor in the genesis of calculi. It will serve as an outlet if stones move spontaneously. However, fixed stones may cause backup stasis, cholangitis, intrahepatic abscess, or focal cirrhosis. It should be emphasized that these are rare problems in current surgical practice. They were more commonly encountered in the past, in long-neglected cases.

In a general way the instruments available for intraductal procedures are far more effective for sweeping and cradling out stones than for grasping them. The leverage angle does not permit the grasping end of the forceps to open for more than 1 cm. Such stones are invariably fragmented during the grasping. The use of urologic instruments in the bile duct is not always effective or safe. For the small, soft stone there are several alternative instruments. For the larger, faceted, hard stone there is no one instrument that is effective in all instances (135).

Postlithotomy Evaluation

As a final step, the patency of the Vaterian segment is confirmed by inserting a silk, woven, flexible urethral catheter from the surgical ostium into the duodenum. It is sufficient to feel or see the catheter in the duodenal lumen. In the routine case, when calibration of the lumen of the choledochal sphincteric segment is unimportant, I prefer this catheter to the use of the Bakes dilator (33, 276). It is less likely to produce a false passage or a submucosal hematoma.

When the Bakes dilator is used, it is best to limit it to the number 3 or 4. One does not and cannot dilate the choledochal sphincter. The instrument is a probe, used only to establish patency. The difficulty resides in the fact that a probe may push the ampulla ahead without having actually traversed the normal opening (Fig. 18–8). However, certain observations help: The saline stream distends the duodenum; a filiform catheter is palpated in the lumen; the "silver" of the Bakes dilator is clearly visualized; or a malecot or red rubber catheter stretched on a mandrin is delivered into the duodenal lumen via the choledochostomy. The local reaction to manipulations makes subsequent manometric and debimetric findings impossible to interpret.

FIG. 18-8. Ampullary patency. When the large Bakes dilator is used to demonstrate patency of the ampulla, it may bypass a stone, or produce a mucosal abrasion. The patency of the ampulla is demonstrated when one can "see the silver" of the dilator pouting against the anterior duodenal wall. The evaluation of patency is much better done with a whip and follower. (From Schein CJ, Stern WZ, Jacobson HG: The Common Bile Duct. Operative Cholangiography, Biliary Endoscopy and Choledocholithotomy, 1966. Courtesy of Charles C Thomas, Publisher, Springfield, Illinois)

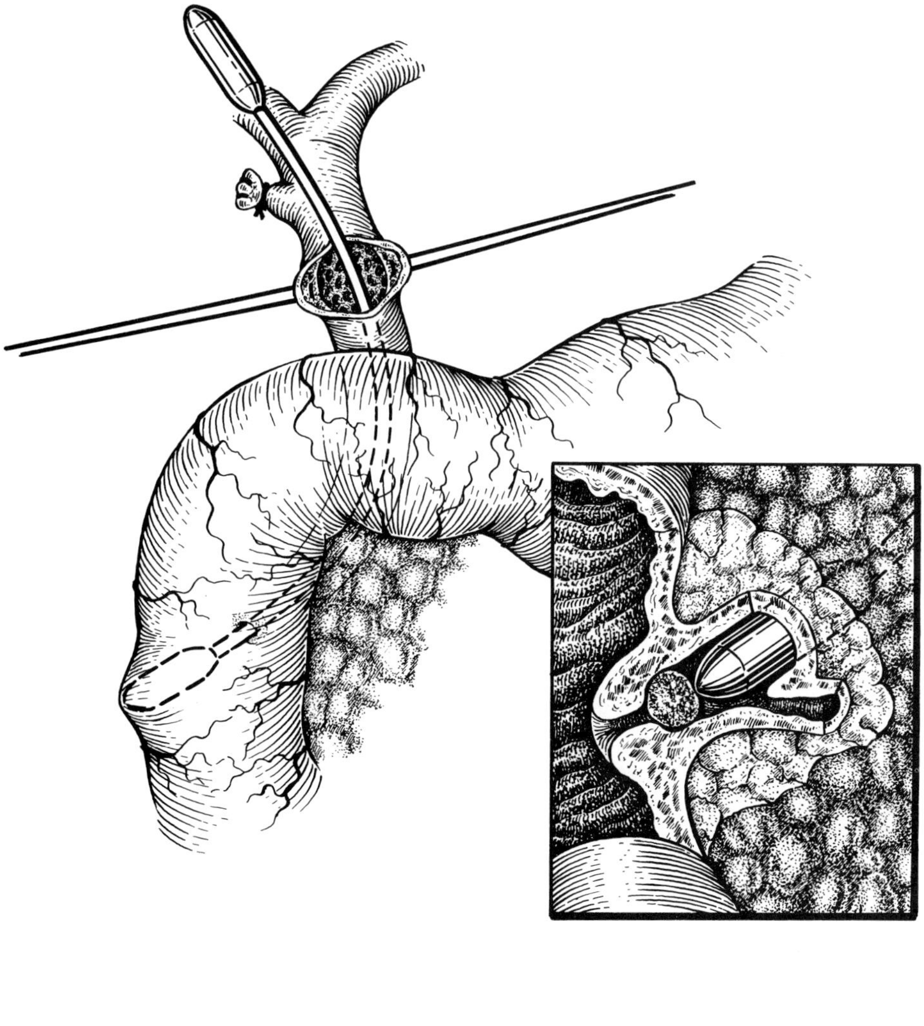

It is at this point that choledochoscopy has its greatest value. Visualization of a cleared ductal system is reliable asurance that no stones have been left behind. Endoscopy can reveal the special problem of the small radicle hepatic duct stone or the bypassed suprasphincteric incarcerated calculus (especially if the latter is embedded in a calculus decubitus or diverticulum).

MANAGEMENT OF RETAINED STONES DEMONSTRATED BY POSTOPERATIVE CHOLANGIOGRAPHY

If the stone is smaller than 7 mm, there is a good chance that it will pass either spontaneously or be well tolerated. The reported experiences are detailed in Chapter 9. In the absence of symptoms, one clamps off the T tube and has the patient go about his affairs. At least half of such stones will pass in 6 weeks. Reevaluation cholangiograms can be repeated at 3- to 6-week intervals.

If the stone does not pass because it is caught about the upper limb of the T tube, it is wisest to wait for a good tract to form (4–6 weeks), then remove the T tube, allowing the stone to be spontaneously extruded or to pass into the distal duct. A straight catheter is then re-inserted into the fistula tract, both for subsequent reevaluation and as a route for extraction. Sometimes merely passing the catheter through the ampulla for 24 hours allows stones to pass after it is withdrawn (97, 104) (Fig. 18-9).

If the distal duct is normal cholangiographically and manometrically, spontaneous passage of the stones can be expected (52). With one or two such small stones I have sometimes advised that the tube be removed, in anticipation that the subsequent course will be benign. This approach, under these specific circumstances (small stone and normal x-ray and dynamics), has been completely satisfactory. Theoretically, it would be well to reevaluate such patients by later intravenous cholangiography. My view is that this is not necessary in the asymptomatic patient.

The "wait" or "disregard tolerance" approach is not applicable to the symptomatic patient, to the larger stones or to altered dynamics. There is then the choice of 1) perfusion techniques or 2) basket retrieval via the T-tube fistula, or 3) reoperation.

FIG. 18-9. Stone passage facilitation. **A.** This patient has a retained stone in the distal portion of the common bile duct **(arrow).** The T tube was removed and a straight catheter was passed through the Vaterian segment. A second study 48 hours later failed to reveal the stone. It is assumed that passage of the catheter facilitated the passage of the stone into the duodenum. **B.** T-tube cholangiogram demonstrates a retained stone in the proximal bile duct just distal to the carina. The stone is 4 mm in diameter. Silver clips **(arrow)** are at the site of a hepatic plexus vagectomy that had been carried out as an adjunct to cholecystectomy, in the presence of a minimally dilated duct. A repeat cholangiogram 5 days later showed that this stone had passed. One may assume that the hepatic plexus vagetomy facilitated the rapid passage of this stone, but it is probable that a stone of this size would ordinarily pass.

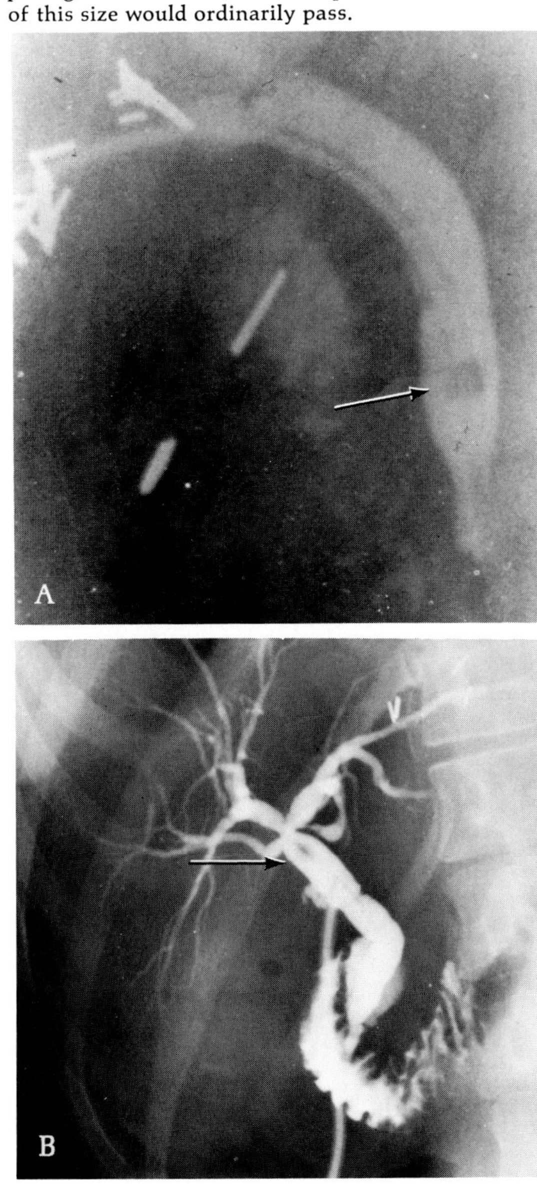

Perfusion

An old method of perfusion that was largely unsuccessful in the past was a technique initiated by Walker (526) in 1892. He dissolved a cystic duct stone via a cholecystostomy fistula by the topical application of ether and glycerine. Pribram (481) popularized the use of intracholedochal ether; some of these patients were said to have fallen asleep. Cole and Harridge (138) reported disappearance of stones with the daily oral administration of 3–4 gr of bile salts. In a way, perfusion techniques were a prefunctory approach prior to suggesting that because they had failed, the next resort had to be surgical. Sometimes the method worked not because of the solvent action of the medium but because of spontaneous passage or mechanical flushing. The agents used were ether, alcohol, or chloroform (because they could extract cholesterol), or bile salts (for their suface tension effect and role in altering cholesterol solubility in bile). Some satisfaction with the method persists based on the use of different perfusates.

The techniques have been variously modified with the use of local and systemic drugs that are supposed on the one hand to relax the sphincter and on the other to increase the flow of bile. Sasson has summarized the experience with the solvents (526).

Washout flush techniques alone have been successful. Catt (116) reports that flushing the T tube with 100 ml of saline containing 40 ml of lidocaine on three successive days cleared residual calculi in six of ten patients.

There has to be the consideration that stones can be simulated by mucus, blood clots, or sludge, in which instance the effect of perfusion alone is readily comprehended.

Tubes have also been modified for this purpose: A urethral catheter has been passed through the T tube so that the drip was directly on the stones. MacDonald (380) used a two-way T tube for continuous perfusion. Those who advocate the procedure emphasize that it requires persistence and patience.

The MHMC experience is limited to the use of heparin and in two instances, to sodium cholate perfusion that had to be terminated because of unfavorable side reactions.

Gardner *et al.* (215) have reported on the satisfactory use of intraductal heparin. The technique involves the use of 25,000 units of heparin in 250 ml of saline every 8 hours as a constant T-tube drip. They ascribe the efficacy of the method in 31 of 43 patients to the marked increase in zeta potential of particles suspended in heparinized bile. With this approach the stones are believed to dissolve or be so fragmented as to pass spontaneously. The published cholangiograms (215) are indeed impressive, with dissolution accomplished in 5 days. The MHMC experience with this technique was not successful in any of the six instances in which it was attempted.

Perfusion with bile acids is based on improving the ratio of bile salts and phospholipid to cholesterol and on the *in-vitro* demonstration that the cholesterol matrix in the stones can be dissolved in micellar bile salt solution. The crumbled fragments would then pass. A bile salt solution of sodium cholate (100 mm) in saline is buffered to a pH of 7.5. Prefiltration is performed by passage through a 0.45-μ millipore filter. Then the solution is continuously perfused through the T tube by a gravity drip at 30 ml/hr, at a pressure of 15–20 cm. The greater the concentration of bile salt solution the greater the chance for dissolution of human gallstones. If the stone has a ring of calcium around it or is mainly of pigment, then it is unlikely to dissolve because the concentration of bile salts around the stone is not sufficiently high. All these patients suffer diarrhea, which is managed with cholestyramine, 4 g every 2 hours during the day. When this method is effective, the results are evident in 10–14 days. Lansford *et al.* (345) were successful with five of six patients, and Way *et al.* (615) with 12 of 22.

Other successful intraductal perfusion or instillation methods have used 5 ml of 2% lidocaine preceding simple 500-cc saline perfusion and followed by 10 cc of olive oil.

The present status of perfusion depends a good deal upon persistent confidence that it will work. It requires strict adherence to the criteria established by those who have been successful. On the basis of my experience, I prefer to avoid this approach except as a temporary expedience in the very-poor-risk patient. My position is that the stone will either pass spontaneously with flushing alone or it can be extracted. The satisfactory experience of others with perfusion contradicts this viewpoint. I concede that in special cases perfusion has a place. My negative attitude is based on the failures and complications that I have observed.

Basketing Controlled by X-ray Visualization

The approach to the retained stone has been totally altered by the method of closed extraction. This technique requires only that a T tube be *in situ*, preferably at least a number 16 tube. Smaller tracts are more difficult to manage, but Mazzariello (405) has emphasized that most of these can be serially dilated over several days or weeks to permit this access route. It is best if the tract exists laterally, as it is more difficult to maneuver through the midline.

The method should not be applied until there is a well-formed fibrous tract. Ordinarily this takes 3–6 weeks. In the interval, one can try the perfusion-dissolution techniques.

Basketing is done without anesthesia in the x-ray department equipped with image intensification (361, 384, 550). The patients are ambulatory. Some are given prophylactic antibiotics. The methods used are, for the most part, those worked out by Burhenne (99, 100) in San Francisco and Mazzariello (406) in Buenos Aires.

The T tube is withdrawn, and a catheter is directed through the fistulous tract so that its tip is near the stone or the closest of several stones. The closed Dormia stone basket is introduced, and the catheter is withdrawn. The closed Dormia catheter bypasses the single stone and is expanded to grasp it on the pullout.

If the stone is crushed on removal, as it may be, the duct is then washed out. Within the duct, the skilled person manipulates the stones like a series of marbles and manages to engage and retrieve them (Fig. 18-10). Mazzariello also has a specially designed forceps that is inserted directly into the tract to

FIG. 18-10. The technique of basketing for the removal of calculi during x-ray visualization. **A.** After the T-tube fistula has matured, the tube is removed and a catheter is introduced in its place and steered toward the stone. The Dormia catheter is inserted into the steerable catheter. **B.** The sleeve is partially retracted, and the closed Dormia catheter is then positioned at the stone. **C.** The Dormia loop is opened and snares the stone, which is then removed, trailing the sleeve segment of the catheter. The stone is either removed completely or is fragmented and then washed out. Several passes are made to retrieve all the stones.

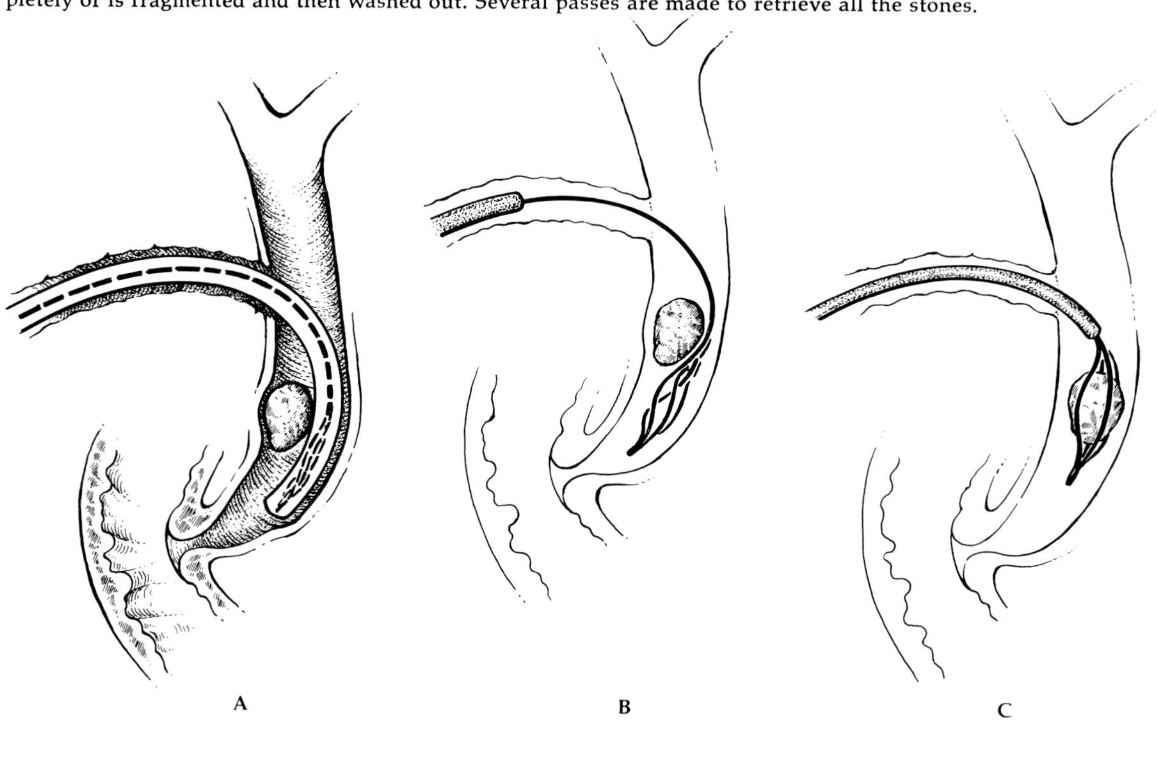

remove the stone. A 1973 survey of 50 institutions (101) revealed that this roentgenographic technique is done by radiologists. There has been a 5% morbidity and no fatality in 612 reported extractions. Only 9% of the 612 patients required reoperation (101).

It is apparent, then, that no patient should have a secondary choledocholithotomy without a prior attempt at stone removal by basketing. Exceptions are the septic patients, those with CDJS, or those with retained gallbladder remnants who require bypass or excisional adjunctives to stone removal.

Endoscopic choledocholithotomy is an approach to the retained or re-formed stone in the patient who does not have an indwelling T tube. The duodenoscope that is used for ERCP has been modified so that the Vaterian segment can be dilated to facilitate either the subsequent passage of stones or their endoscopic basket manipulation. This is adjunctive to endoscopic electrosurgical sphincterotomy or papillotomy (141, 517).

CHOLEDOCHODUODENOSTOMY

Choledochoduodenostomy is the most effective time-tested form of bypass for the management of calculus-related disorders of the distal common bile duct. The procedure was advocated by Riedel (500) in 1888 and first successfully popularized by Sprengel (489). Sasse (525) stimulated further interest with his report on use of the procedure for a variety of indications in ten successful cases. There are reports on the benignity and efficiency of the procedure by many investigators with larger series (107, 165, 262, 382, 394, 524, 539). Rathcke's monograph (489) summarized the published experience to 1956. One may be unconvinced by any one report, but repeated confirmation from so many sources puts the technique's value in perspective.

This anastomosis obviates obstructive disorders of the distal duct by providing a proximal detour. Indications for the procedure have varied from one surgical epoch to the next. The early enthusiasms were related to using the technique to avoid an external biliary fistula with its accompanying fluid losses (417). A pragmatic attitude was that choledochoduodenostomy offered a most satisfactory prophylactic approach to the retained stone problem.

Some of the earlier enthusiasm was then tempered when the advances in image-intensification operative cholangiography considerably reduced the incidence of the retained stone. Choledochoscopy offers another way of policing the duct to avoid the retained stone, and the experience reported with that modality has supported its acceptance. One of the largest published satisfactory experiences with choledochoduodenostomy is Rathcke's monograph (489). In a recent letter, however, Rathcke states that because of the advances with choledochoscopy, he has now limited its indication. In a general way, as judged by already cited publications, the endoscopic advances have now restrained some of the former European enthusiasts for bypass. On the other hand an increasing number of American publications deal with the satisfactory results of choledochoduodenostomy.

Theoretical Considerations

It has been assumed that choledochoduodenostomy introduced two potential problems: 1) cholangitis arising from anastomatic stricture, and 2) possible detrimental effects from the accumulation of debris in the blind end of the choledochus distal to the anastomosis. The threats of cholangitis have proved to be unwarranted if the anastomosis is properly performed—with a stoma that is at least 2.5 cm wide. This can be accomplished in every situation in which the procedure is indicated.

The theory was that cholangitis could result because a nonvalved anastomosis will allow regurgitation of intestinal contents into the bile ducts thereby introducing bacteria and food particles that would initiate an inflammatory process. This potential has not been realized either experimentally or in actual practice. Hess (263) found four reasons for dissatisfaction with choledochoduodenostomy: narrowing of the anastomosis; obstruction by retained stones and foreign bodies; overlooked pancreatitis, because of stenosing papillitis; and intolerance to the biliary duodenal reflux. He suggests that, in general, one can count on the fact that these anastomoses shrink about one-third of their original width. I have seen none of these problems.

Experimental anastomosis of the bile duct to the colon is possible without infectious complications, provided that the anastomosis is wide enough to allow for unimpeded in- and outflow. The pressure and directional flow of hepatic bile favors this self-cleaning mechanism. In fact, the reported cases of cholangitis have been the consequence of an inadequate anastomatic ostium. When there is no stricture and no obstruction to bile flow, there is no cholangitis despite the reflux of intestinal contents into the ducts (Fig. 18-11).

In the MHMC experience with the first 100 cases of choledochoduodenostomy embracing a 15-year follow-up there has been no instance of cholangitis (537). Similar reports have been collected by Madden (382) and Degensheim (164). Problems that have been reported, were the result of technical imperfections.

FIG. 18-11. Anastomosis of choledochus **(arrow a)** to an accessory hepatic duct. Oral barium study of a patient who had had biliary enteric bypass performed 4 years before reveals air bubbles in the biliary tree. There is a patent anastomosis between the duodenum and a long accessory right hepatic duct. This is not a choledochoduodenal anastomosis. However, the stoma to the accessory duct **(arrow b)** is wide enough to provide good outflow. No cholangitis is present.

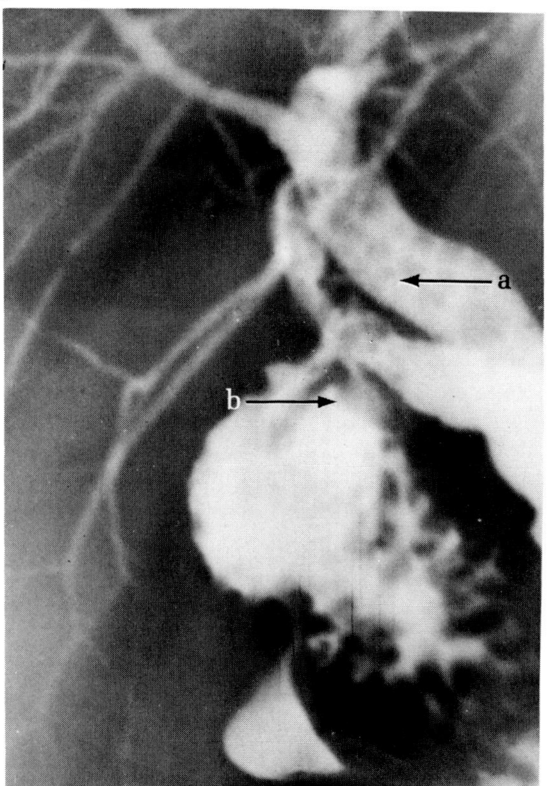

The barium swallow offers a good way of remotely evaluating this anastomosis. Optimally the barium should not only opacify the anastomosis and the biliary radicles; it should also be completely voided within 12 hours. Such an anastomosis is functioning well. The presence of air in the biliary tree, evidenced on the flat abdominal film as a pneumocholangiogram, is not *per se* evidence of an adequate anastomosis, for it can appear in the presence of significant stricture. Sorby and Ham (569) present an interesting method of evaluating the stoma after choledochoduodenostomy. A guide wire, of the type used in arterial catheterization and superselective arteriography, is passed via the nose through the stomach into the duodenum and then guided through the anastomosis. After this is accomplished, diatrizoate sodium is injected, and films are made of the entire ductal system.

Endoscopic manipulation of the stoma of the anastomosis has not been required in any case in this MHMC series, although this would appear to be a good way not only of visualizing it, but of mechanically irrigating it, should this be necessary (249). The possibility of intra-anastomatic manipulation makes possible the endoscopic management of the faulty anastomosis. It is difficult to evaluate the role of the bypassed blind remnant. I have not recognized a problem with this area even in association with choledochoduodenal junction stenosis. Nor have I encountered retrograde obstructive scarring in stone-related inflammatory disorders.

After decompression of jaundiced patients, there is occasionally a secondary rise in the serum bilirubin on the second or third day, but thereafter it declines consistently at a rate that reaches its half value by about 10 days. This average fall of serum bilirubin can be used to forecast when the jaundice should clear if the operative relief of the biliary obstruction has been satisfactory (516).

Indications

A dilated duct is the *sine quo non* for this procedure. It should not be performed with ducts less than 1.2 cm in diameter and preferably only in those at least 1.4 cm. A duct narrower than 1.2 cm is an absolute contraindication (308). The circumstances in which this bypass has been effective in association with a dilated duct are:

1. Retained or recurrent calculi in the choledochus or hepatic ducts
2. Cholangitis
3. Choledochoduodenal junctional stenosis
4. Presence of primary choledochal calculi or stasis bile
5. Tubular stricture of the transpancreatic portion of the choledochus, where there is associated choledochal hypertension (320)
6. Combinations of these
7. After unsuccessful sphincterotomy or sphincteroplasty

Bypass is contraindicated if there is 1) hemorrhagic pancreatitis, 2) significant duodenal ulcer disease, 3) a quasi-dilated duct with a small lumen and very thick wall.

Operative Technique

1. The common duct is opened to a measured length of 2.5 cm. Since the vertical incision has already been made to explore the duct and to determine the indication for the procedure, this simply involves lengthening the incision. No matter how wide the duct, the vertical incision is preferred (Fig. 18-12).
2. Seromuscular horizontal mattress sutures of an absorbable type are used to approximate the posterior wall of the duodenum to the adventitia of the bile duct. The sutures serve only to approximate the two structures. They are best guttered as far posteriorly as possible.
3. The duodenal incision is placed as far away from the pylorus as can be conveniently accommodated. It should be transverse in the long axis and measure 2.5 cm in length. Small submucosal bleeders are cauterized. Although this is a side-to-side anastomosis, the opening should be anteroposterior.
4. The midpoint of each opening of the duct incision is tagged with a catgut suture. It is then pulled to one side to achieve the maximum spread from each lateral suture to the center. Interrupted through-and-through catgut sutures now approximate the posterior walls by the method of bisection (Fig. 18-13).
5. A triangulation "slap onlay" of the anterior duodenal wall allows for the wide stoma. The midpoint of the anterior duodenal wall is sutured to the midpoint of the anterior duct wall, forming one side of an isosceles triangle from the anterior wall anastomosis site. The anterior wall is approximated with through-and-through catgut sutures. No secondary anterior layer is required (Fig. 18-14).
6. The omentum is tied in over the anastomosis by the outer lateral sutures.

No drain is positioned near the anastomosis and no stent is required.

There are the obvious advantages to this procedure: it detours bile away from all the problems distal to the stoma; it allows for the spontaneous extrusion of retained calculi; the status of the anastomosis is easily evaluated by barium swallow or endoscopy; its technical execution avoids the problem of iatrogenic pancreatitis; and it allows a large stasis duct to drain via an adequate stoma.

Results

The published experience supports the attitude that a properly performed choledochoduodenostromy, undertaken for justified reasons, will serve as an effective bypass. It is the best solution to stone disorders occurring in association with a dilated duct. In the PCS problems, the illustrated cases indicate the variations in indication for sphincteroplasty, choledochojejunostomy, and choledochoduodenostomy. Certainly the latter is the simplest in terms of technical performance and the least hazardous in terms of postoperative mortality and morbidity (421).

The MHMC experience established the following facts: The procedure can be safely and widely applied to all ducts that are at least 1.4 cm wide. It can be done in the presence of extensive cholangitis at either the primary or revisional operation. In a personal experience, the only death in 50 consecutive patients was due to liver failure and occurred 6 weeks after the operation. There have been no leaks and no intraperitoneal complications. An initial wound infection rate of 12% has been reduced by the use of pre- or intraoperative antibiotics in all patients undergoing the procedure (503, 585). The technical safety of the procedure is analogous to that of gastroenterostomy for obstructed duodenal ulcer disease. No patient so treated has required an additional biliary tract operation.

In the elderly, very sick patient it can be performed more rapidly, if time is the factor, than the procedure required for monitoring the conventional common duct exploration. The median age of patients in this series was 70 years. I have come to believe that with the dilated duct in either the primary or secondary situation, the question should not be, "Why do this procedure?" but "Why not do it?" (258, 421, 458, 578, 579).

Fezig and Tonelli (197) indicate that in any single study the incidence of complications with choledochoduodenostomy is smaller than that with procedures on the papilla. Their approach is papillostomy for the initial operation and bypass in secondary procedures. My point of view is that if it works in the secondary procedures, why should it not be done in the primary?

Madden's review (382) of the collective literature reported an incidence of cholangitis of 0.4% in 1225 operations. In each of these cases the cholangitis was related to stomal stricture, which must be viewed as a technical problem. The long history and follow-up

FIG. 18-12. The alternative incisions for choledochoduodenostomy. **A.** This combination is the one most often employed. **D.** The **arrow** indicates the course of bile as it passes through the surgically created stoma.

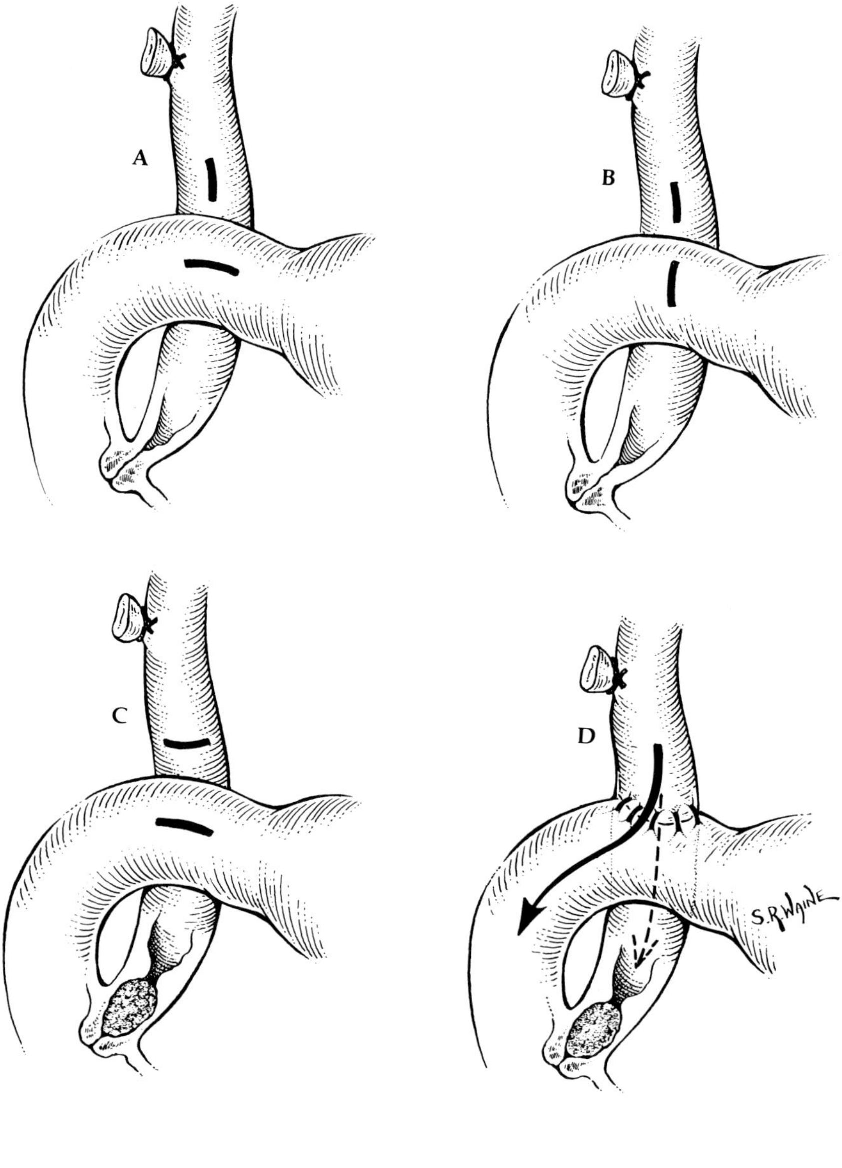

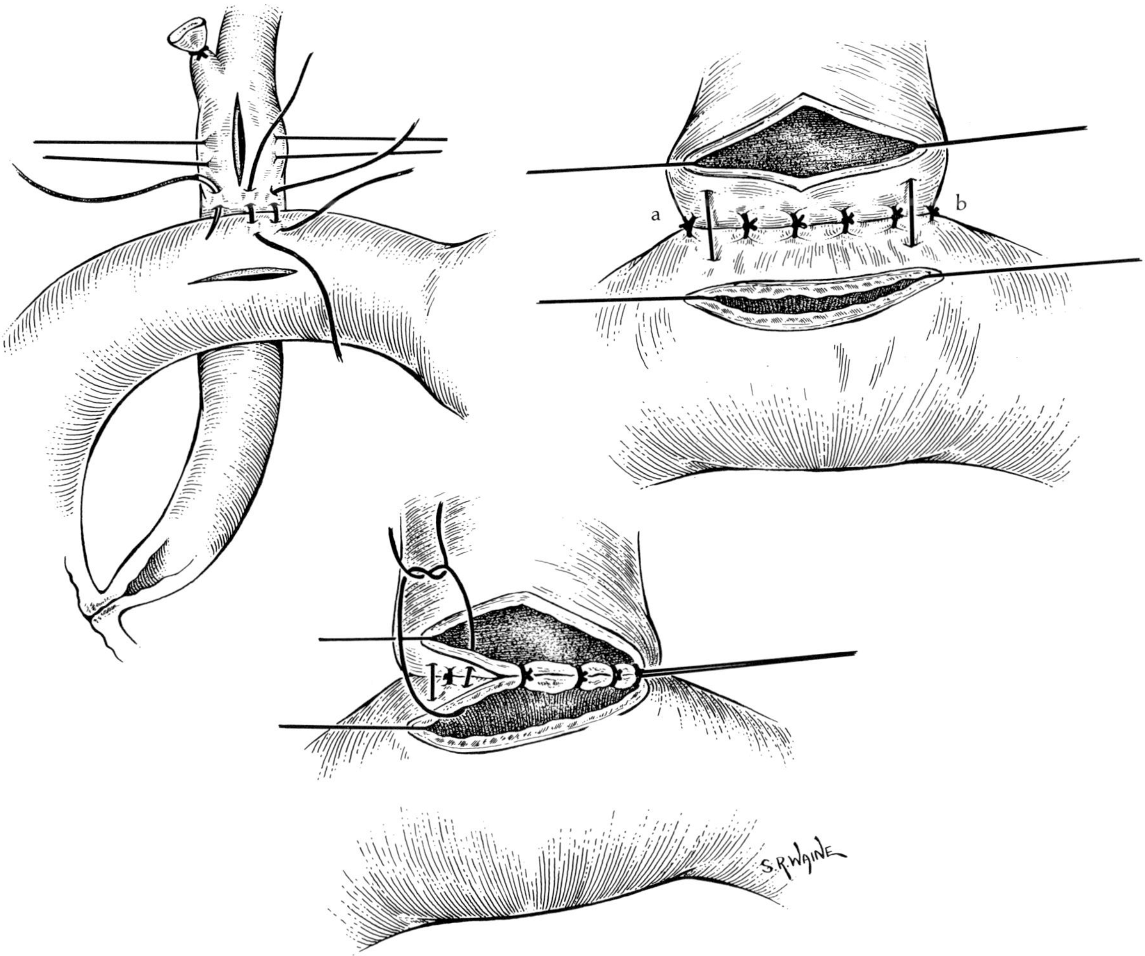

FIG. 18-13. Choledochoduodenostomy anastomatic technique. The incision in the common bile duct is made much longer than is shown in this figure. A two-layer anastomosis is depicted, but usually a single-layer anastomosis is adequate. The most important consideration is the size of the duct stoma. It should be at least 2.5 cm in width. Interrupted absorbable sutures are used throughout. Silk sutures are avoided in either wall since these can find their way into the duct lumen and be the subsequent nidus for a new concretion. The posterior suture line **(a–b)** is intended solely to approximate the two structures. It does not bite into the choledochal wall. The anterior wall is completed with a series of interrupted inverting catgut (00) sutures.

indicate there are no ill effects from incontinent drainage of bile into the duodenum and from possible reflux of duodenal contents into the bile duct. The anathema of the blind segment between choledochoduodenal anastomosis and the ampulla of Vater has not been a source of difficulty in any of the reported cases.

One of the first five patients upon whom I performed choledochoduodenostomy returned 6 months after the operation with a cancer of the ampullary area. It was probably missed at the time of the first procedure because of the associated calculi. I have since been alerted to the observation that 15–20% of Vaterian segment cancers have choledochal stones. I now routinely palpate the papilla through the duodenostomy incision prior to completing the anastomosis.

HEPATIC PLEXUS VAGECTOMY

The place for contraselective parasympathetic (hepatic vagal plexus) section in biliary disorders has not been clearly established, even

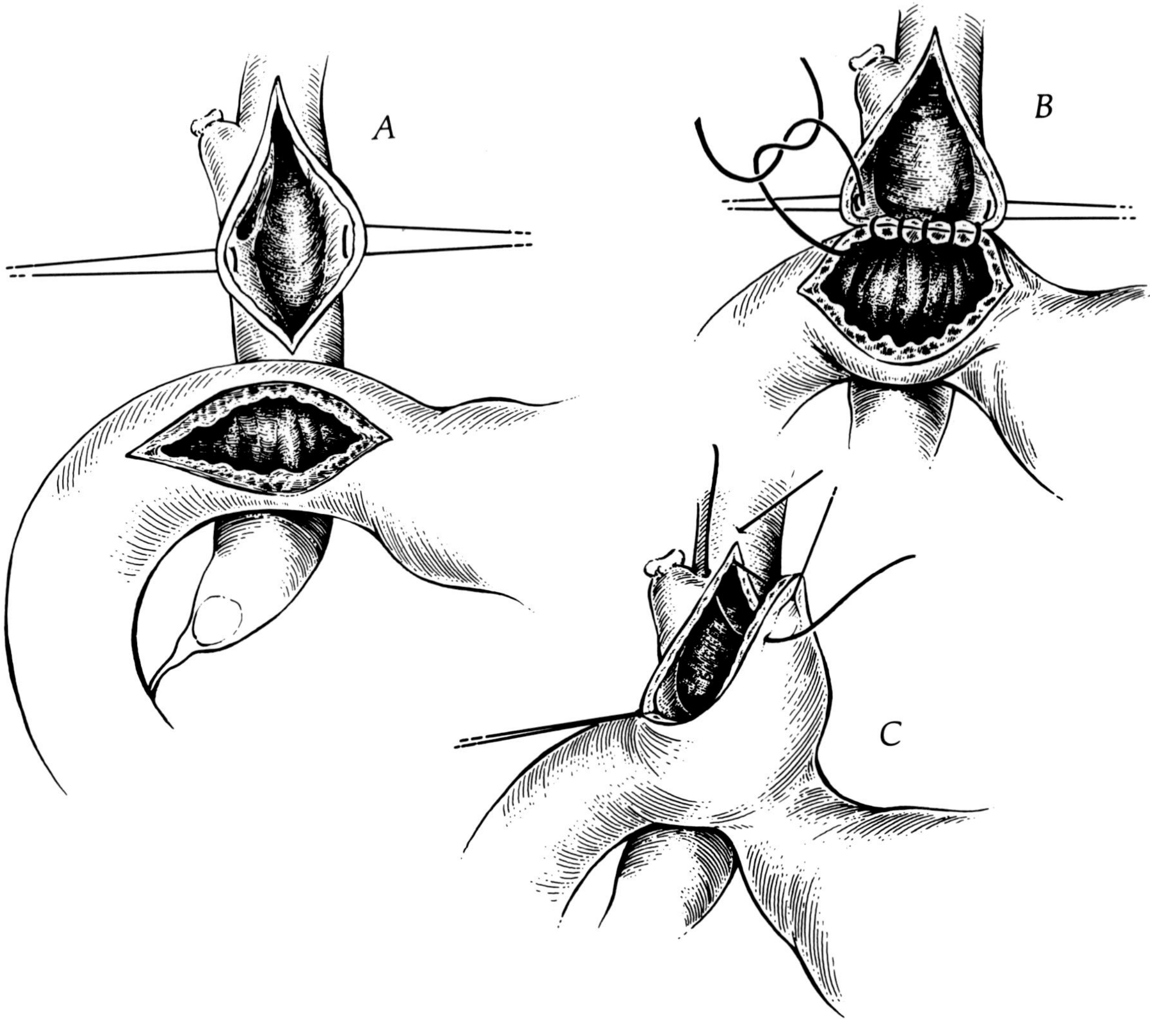

FIG. 18-14. Choledochoduodenostomy with onlay flap. **A.** The anterior wall of the 1.2- to 1.4-cm duct is opened longitudinally for 2.5 measured centimeters. **B.** A single posterior layer of interrupted catgut sutures is inserted. **C.** The middle of the anterior duodenal wall is sutured to the apex of the choledochostomy incision. In this way a triangular onlay flap is created.

though vagal section at the truncal, selective, or parietal cell level has become a standard operative procedure in the surgical management of various disorders related to peptic ulcer. Is it possible that we are in a "prevagal" phase of this adjunctive surgical procedure for a disorder in which vagolytic drugs have been a standard part of the medical armamentarium for decades?

Physiologic Basis

Vagal section has its physiologic basis in certain clinical and laboratory observations:

1. There is a cephalic phase in biliary excretion that has a central localization and is vagally mediated. The folklore identification of bilious personality may be no more farfetched than it is in regard to the ulcer type. The influence of stress factors on common duct dynamics in the form of Cannon's pain, rage, hunger, and fear has been demonstrated by several investigators.

2. The tone of the choledochal sphincter is maintained by an intrinsic muscular mechanism as well as by a vagal factor. This tonicity is responsible for the preferential flow of hepatic bile into the gallbladder rather than the duodenum. When the gallbladder has been removed, the function of this choledochal sphincter is abrogated. Selective hepatic plexus vagectomy obliterates the neurotonicity of the sphincter and decreases its resistance to bile flow. The normal pressure of 13 ± 7 cm H_2O is reduced by an average of 32.1% during the operation, and by 42.3% in the remote evaluation. Vagal section does not result in regurgitation, and the competence of the ampullary segment is maintained by the obliquity of the intramural portion of the bile duct (533).

Experience with vagal section in the stone disease has been reported by Hess (262), Iliescu (290), Mallet-Guy (394), and Schein (533). The results have been favorable, or—perhaps more accurately expressed—not unfavorable, since it is impossible to evaluate this specific contribution to the total correction of the biliary outlet.

Indication

I have chosen this procedure for those cholecystectomized patients who present with a duct that is not suitable for choledochoduodenostomy (*i.e.*, a duct whose lumen is less than 1.4 cm), in all ducts exhibiting choledochal hypertension, and in all cases of choledocholithiasis. In the overall spectrum of indications for sphincter operations, I favor this form of neurogenic sphincterolysis, whereas others utilize sphincterotomy or sphincteroplasty.

The hepatic plexus vagal section has the distinct advantage of not requiring the opening of the duodenum, and avoids the not insignificant 1–5% fatal pancreatitis that follows the major series of reported sphincter operations. Furthermore, the efficacy of the nerve section can be immediately evaluated by demonstrating an immediate post-section fall in choledochal–duodenal passage pressure. There have been no complications from this procedure in the 22 patients who have been followed for 7 or more years.

The logic for the operation includes these facts:

1. The choledochal sphincter is no longer required in the cholecystectomized patient.

2. Various dysfunctions have implicated the role of the sphincter in the postcholecystectomy syndrome.

3. An atonic sphincter favors bile outflow and would avoid the stasis that generates primary duct stones.

4. An incompetent sphincter favors the spontaneous passage of retained calculi.

5. Sphincter "spasm" is eliminated as a cause of colic.

6. The patient is restored to his non-stone-producing, acholecystic, phylogenetic state.

7. The final outflow tract for vagus-mediated supratentorial stimuli is interrupted (*i.e.*, the result is analogous to what supraselective vagotomy is to the duodenal ulcer personality).

In addition, there have been no undesirable side effects.

Technique

The hepatic plexus courses in the upper end of the gastrohepatic omentum where the latter is a veil-like "sail" over the caudate lobe of the liver. Exposure of the area is obtained by retracting the greater curvature of the deflated stomach toward the left lower quadrant and rotating the liver upward to expose the caudate lobe. The latter is maintained in position by a hoe retractor of the Weinberger type or a very broad Deaver retractor. (Fig. 18–15).

There are three to five white strands coursing transversely in this rather transparent mesentery. These are the cords of the hepatic plexus. The transparent areas of the mesentery are perforated and spread transversely to isolate these cords from the fat and small blood vessels that are also present in this omentum. Each of these cords is clipped and sectioned. The intermittent segment is submitted for pathological examination. It is especially important to divide the highest nerve cord that is actually in direct contact with the visceral peritoneum of the diaphragm; if it is not sectioned the pressure will not fall (Fig. 18-16).

The clips are delivered by a long holder, which facilitates getting into the area from afar. Ties can be difficult to get in behind a high narrow costal arch. There are small vessels in the mesentery that are caught with these clips. The nerve of Latarjet and the descending branches of the left gastric artery are readily visible and easily avoided. They do not need to be especially cleaned since appropriate traction exposes them.

In the obese patient, a sterile light is positioned in the lesser sac to transilluminate the mesentery and facilitate identification of the cords.

Neurogenic sphincter lysis has been especially applicable in those situations in which the disease or previously resected duodenum makes an anastomotic or sphincteric procedure hazardous. The effect appears to be a purely motor one on the choledochal sphincter (Fig. 18-17). There have been no postoperative changes in liver-functon tests, pancreatic reflex, or gastrointestinal series. Some patients exhibit a remarkably increased pain tolerance to high-pressure, high-volume perfusion of the common duct.

FIG. 18-15. Method for exposing and sectioning the hepatic vagal plexus. The stomach is displaced to the left and inferiorly, putting the hepatoduodenal ligament on stretch. Through this ligament one can see the caudate lobe of the liver, and overlying it are the white strands that are the hepatic plexus. There is ample room to dissect out those cords so that a 1-in. segment can be removed for biopsy confirmation. (Schein CJ, Beneventano TC, Rosen RG, et al.: Surg Gynecol Obstet 128:241, 1969. By Permission of SURGERY, GYNECOLOGY & OBSTETRICS)

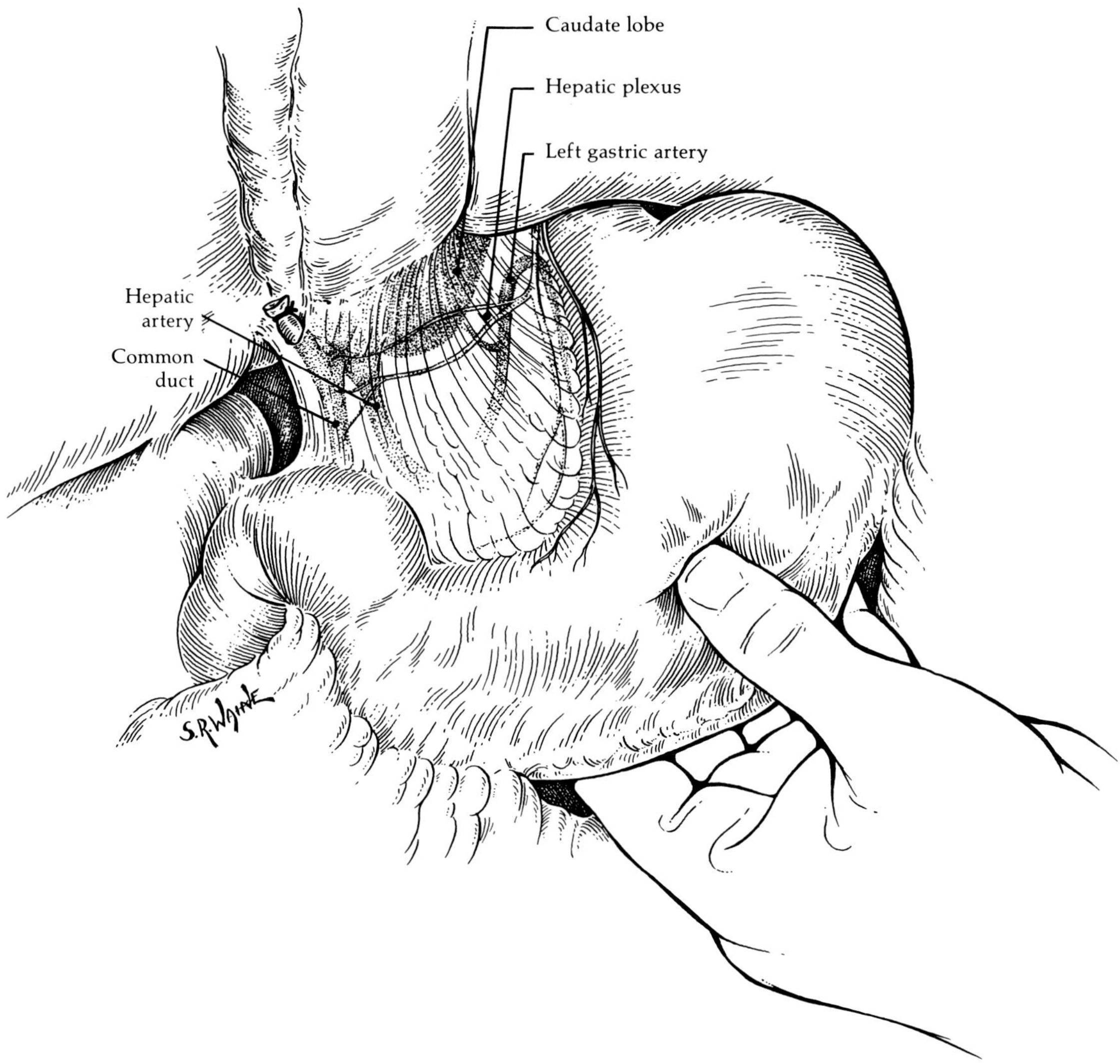

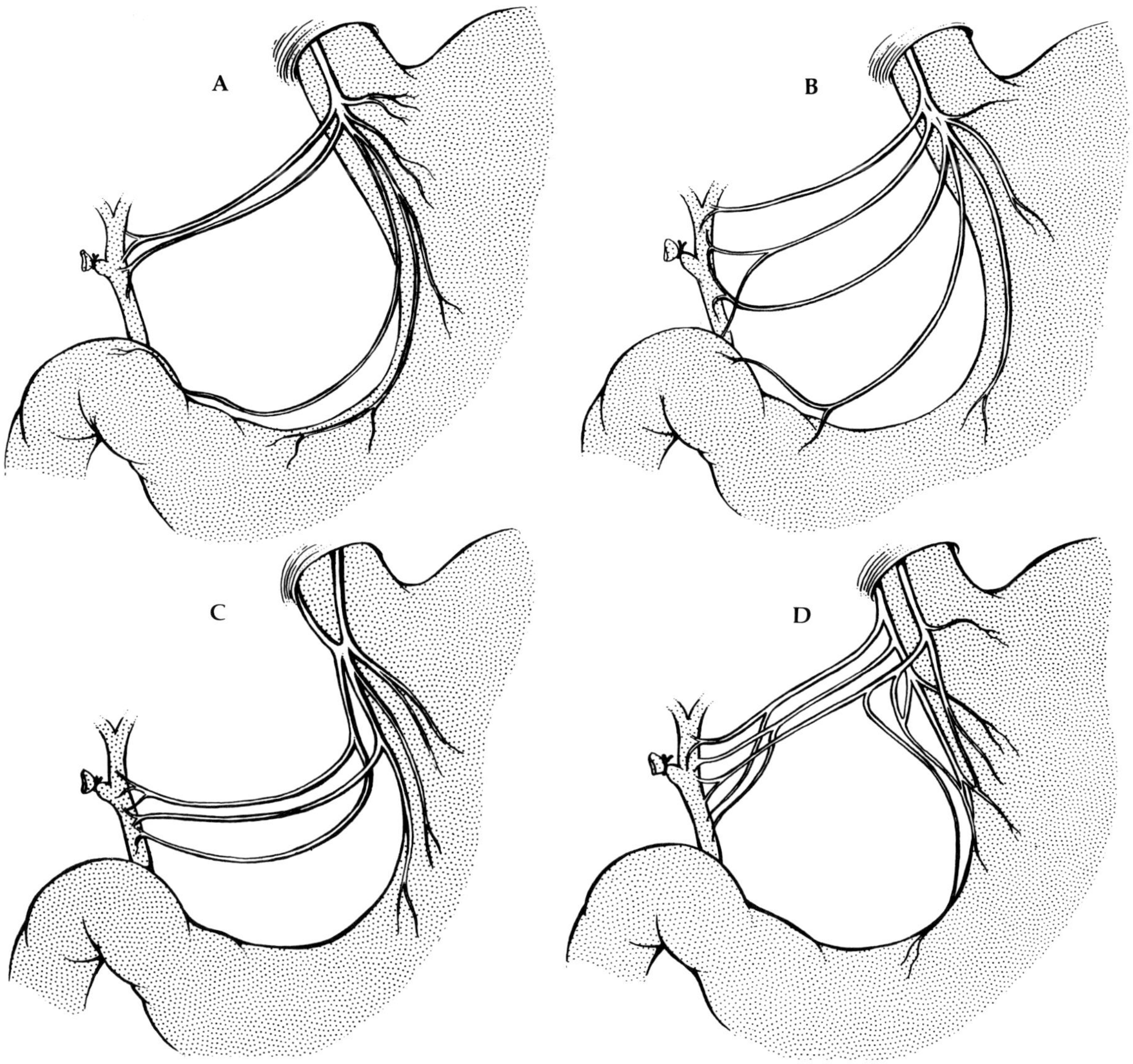

FIG. 18-16. Diagrammatic representation of the most frequently encountered neural distribution pattern of the hepatic plexus. It courses transversely in the "sail" that is the hepatoduodenal ligament, and the arrangement of the cords may vary as follows: **A.** There is a large fatty areolar area between the upper and lower cords. **B.** The cords are symmetrically arranged. **C.** The cords are in midsegment of the sail. **D.** The cords are juxtadiaphragmatic. Their number varies from three to as many as six cords. (Schein CJ, Beneventano TC, Rosen RG, et al.: Surg Gynecol Obstet 128:241, 1969. By Permission of SURGERY, GYNECOLOGY & OBSTETRICS)

EXCISION OF GALLBLADDER REMNANTS

The technical problem in gallbladder remnant disease depends upon how much of the organ had been resected. If the prior operation was a simple fundectomy or partial cholecystectomy, then the technical solution is basically that of cholecystectomy. A more difficult task is the management of the smaller, retained diseased ampulla or the true calculus-containing cystic duct remnant.

These problems share several anatomic features: 1) The remnant tends to be densely attached to the floor of the gallbladder fossa or to the side wall of the common duct. 2)

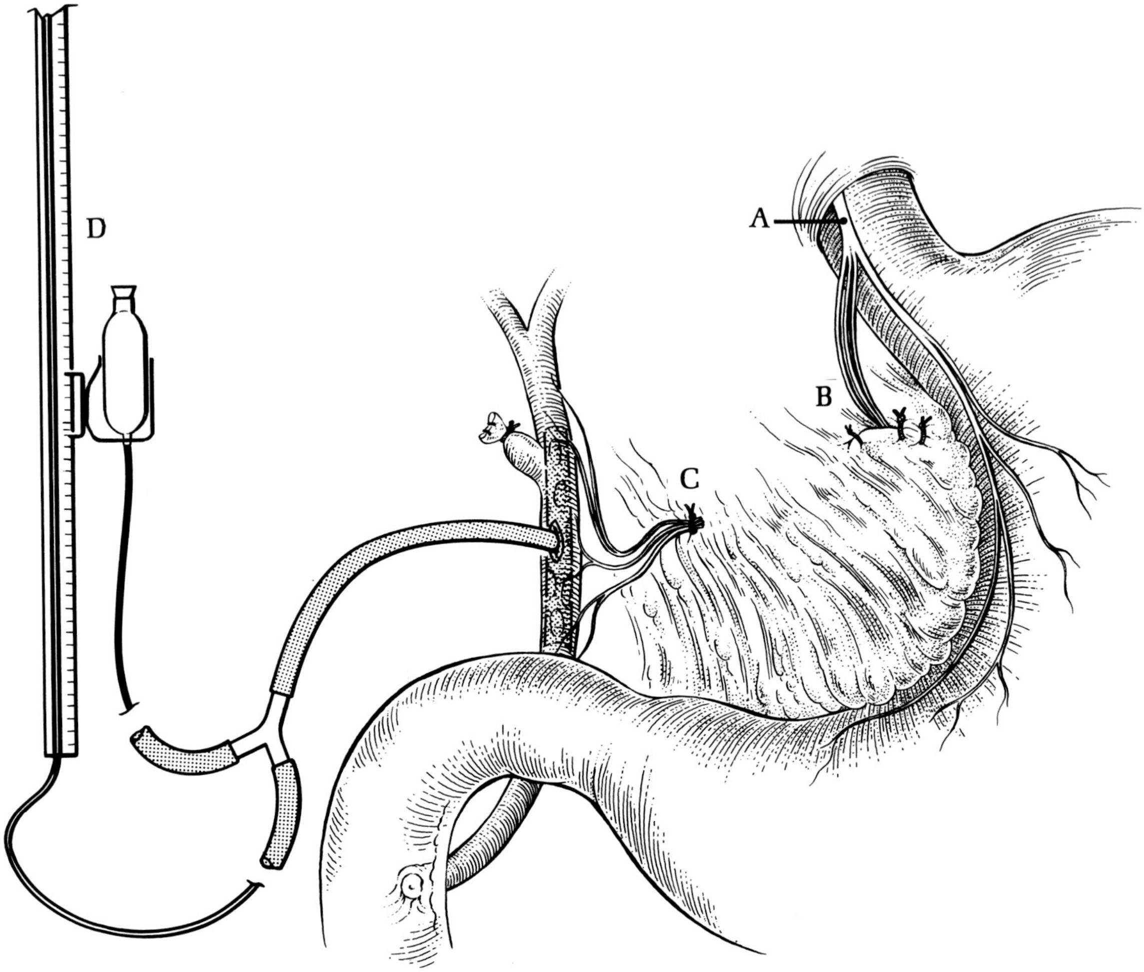

FIG. 18-17. Demonstrating the completeness of the hepatic plexus vagectomy. **D.** The passage pressure before and after the vagal section is documented with the Caroli manometer. Failure of the pressure to fall indicates that the nerve section has not been complete. **A.** Left vagal trunk from which the hepatic fibers usually originate. **B and C.** Severed ends of fibers, with intermediate segment removed for histologic confirmation. (Schein CJ, Beneventano TC, Rosen RG, et al.: Surg Gynecol Obstet 128:241, 1969. By Permission of SURGERY, GYNECOLOGY & OBSTETRICS)

The cystic artery is usually intact. 3) There is often a marked reaction about the remnant —especially in the duodenum and omentum; this sometimes masks a hitherto unsuspected fistula.

If the remnant is dome-shaped and contains a solitary round stone, there must be the suspicion that the cystic duct is partially or completely effaced and that there is, in fact, a cholecystocholedochal fistula. If this is not anticipated, the common duct can be injured before it is recognized (Fig. 18-18).

Although the operation may be no more demanding than a secondary cholecystectomy after a cholecystostomy, in some situations it can be formidable in terms of definition and mobilization. In this combination of circumstances, especially, nothing should be ligated until the gallbladder remnant is completely mobilized and the common bile duct and common hepatic duct are clearly defined. A rare occurrence is the confusion of the remnant with pancreatic head calcification or simulation of the remnant by an accessory hepatic duct containing stones.

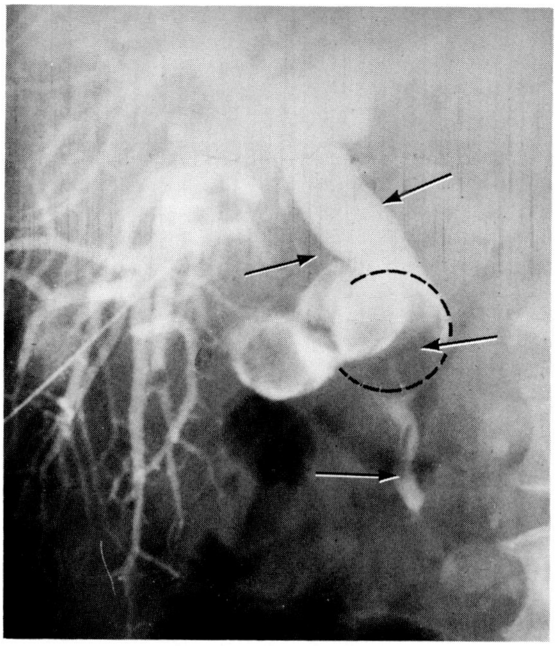

FIG. 18-18. Confluent stone. Transhepatic cholangiogram reveals a dilated common hepatic duct (between **arrows)** and a distal collapsed duct **(bottom arrow).** The gallbladder contains several large stones, one of which intrudes into the common bile duct and obstructs it **(dashed line** and **arrow).** The cystic duct has been effaced. If this anatomic situation is not appreciated, the common duct can be divided. The situation is best managed by open cholecystostomy, cholecystolithotomy, and partial cholecystectomy over a Pezzar catheter, leaving the distal 1 cm of the ampulla as a broad, relatively flat, choledochal diverticulum.

Several technical considerations are pertinent:

1. Free all adhesions to the remnant, working inferiorly first, then to the dome, and finally lyse the remnant away from the liver and ductal adhesions.

2. If a hepatic plane cannot be developed, it may be necessary to leave the posterior wall attached. That lining epithelium can be rendered inert by electrocoagulation.

3. If the cystic artery cannot be isolated in the dense obliterative fibrosis of the hepatoduodenal ligament, then the anterior and posterior divisions should each be underrun separately and tied with a fine vascular silk suture on the remnant wall, pushing away the proximal divided part of its invested thickened serosa.

4. If a remnant choledochal fistula is suspected, opening the remnant and removing the stone is usually sufficient. At that time one determines how much wall must be resected to maintain choledochal continuity. The stone-free, relatively shallow, broad-based diverticulum is compatible with normal flow and dynamics (144, 581).

5. The intravesical dissection method (Fig. 18-19) will sometimes define an area that is otherwise baked in with totally obscured landmarks. This technique requires that the dome of the remnant be opened and a finger or instrument be inserted into the lumen. Then, as in an indirect inguinal hernia sac, the structure is defined by dissection from without while providing guarded traction from within (535).

6. It has never been necessary, in the MHMC series, simply to remove the stones, insert a tube, and retreat, but it is conceivable, and preferable when the common duct cannot be definitively demonstrated.

Because remnant disease is often associated with common duct stones and ampullary disorders, a second part of the procedure requires the evaluation and correction of changes in those areas as well.

SPHINCTEROTOMY AND SPHINCTEROPLASTY

In 1899 McBurney (407) reported on transduodenal sphincterotomy as a means of delivering a large stone incarcerated in the ampulla. When McBurney read his report before the New York Surgical Society, he had already done this on at least six occasions. At this time the T tube was not yet in use and a choledochotomy was treated by either primary closure, with the insertion of a drain, or with the realization that "successful suture may be quite possible." He chose the duodenal route because it was much easier, in his opinion, at that time, to suture the anterior wall of the duodenum than to suture the incised wall of the common bile duct. He anticipated much of later thinking when he pointed out that it was the way to explore the common duct and that the orifice could be dilated, so that there would be less likelihood of overlooking thick bile or grumous

FIG. 18-19. Intravesical dissection. If the gallbladder remnant is firmly attached to the liver or to surrounding structures and the adhesions are dense, it is frequently advisable to open the fundus of the gallbladder and insert one's finger and manage it as a hernial sac, thereby decreasing the possibility of injury to surrounding structures. (Schein CJ, Hurwitt ES: Surg Gynecol Obstet 102:113, 1956. By Permission of SURGERY, GYNECOLOGY & OBSTETRICS)

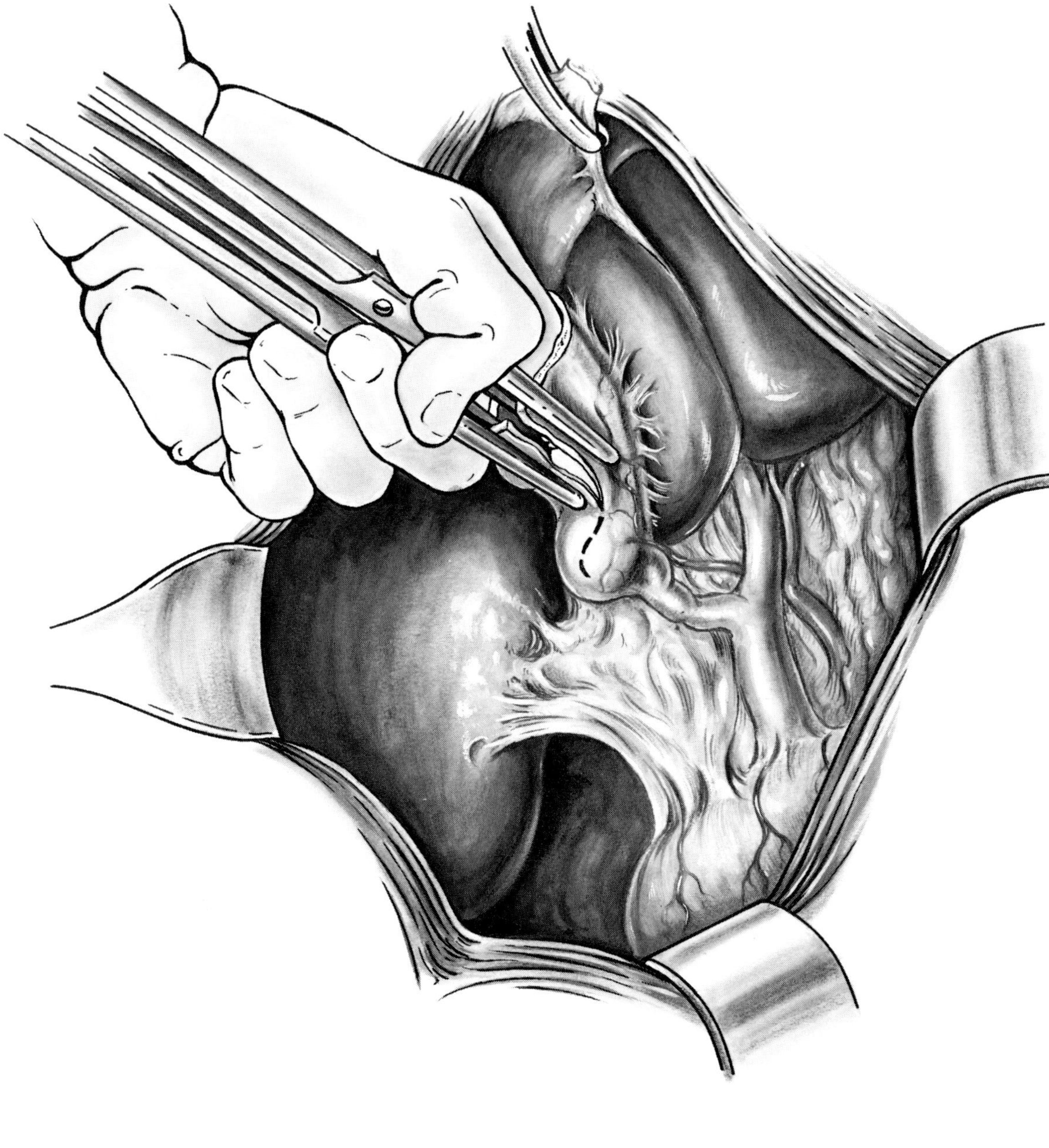

material. The concept is akin to that of an episiotomy for the delivery of the after-coming head. Kocher (331) reported on transduodenal sphincter section with anastomosis as an internal ampulloduodenostomy. These are the antecedents of the present direct attack on the choledochal outlet for biliary tract disease (400, 480, 499).

Concept

The indications for sphincterotomy and sphincteroplasty has been misinterpreted by those who have employed it to correct presumed common-channel regurgitation believed to cause pancreatitis due to alcoholism. The early promise of that operative procedure has not been fulfilled. It is important to be aware that the pancreatic disorder linked to biliary disease differs in etiology, pathology, and prognosis from that associated with alcoholism. Therefore, one should not draw inferences of any sort from former experiences as being applicable to the problem of the postcholecystectomy stone.

The concept of sphincterotomy is that an obstructive, distorting, etiologically significant element (fibrosis, muscular hypertrophy, ulceration, "spasm," "dyskinesia") is present in the intramural portion of the duodenal duct or the duodenal papilla. It is considered that these changes produce obstruction of the bile duct and/or the pancreatic duct.

The surgical attack is directed at completely opening this approximately 1-cm transmural area of the most distal portion of the common bile duct. This is not a meatotomy or papillotomy. It transects the entire transmural common duct sphincter. The nature of the operation is determined by how far in the duodenal wall the incision extends, and by whether the edges are left to heal or are sutured back in a mucosa-to-mucosa approximation. This approximation is intended to prevent adventitious scarring that may result in an obstructive cicatrix at the operative site (42).

Experimental and clinical data indicate that sphincterotomy-induced widening is at best only temporarily effective and that postoperative scarring can result in restoration of the original status and even in aggravation and increased resistance to the bile flow (186, 189, 354, 597, 616, 617, 618). A principal hazard of the sphincter-severing procedure is the complication of postoperative pancreatitis, which is reported in virtually every large series (37, 64, 69, 303, 373, 425, 460, 609).

The strict indication for sphincterotomy is the presence of a phimotic type of stricture at the duodenal papilla (which is very rare) or an incarcerated stone. The procedure is contraindicated in the presence of pancreatitis or a tubular stricture in the transpancreatic portion of the common duct or if retained hepatic duct stones are larger than 1 cm in size. However, some surgeons consider the indications for sphincterotomy as being so broad that they have applied the procedure as an adjunct to common duct exploration (74, 77, 154, 180, 242, 629). Kourias (337),

FIG. 18-20. Transduodenal stab sphincterotomy. A small incision in the anterior duodenal wall is a sufficient vent through which to deliver the sphincter. As the tapered catheter **(a)** is pulled out, the sphincter hugs it, prolapsing out of the duodenum into a good position for sectioning **(b).**

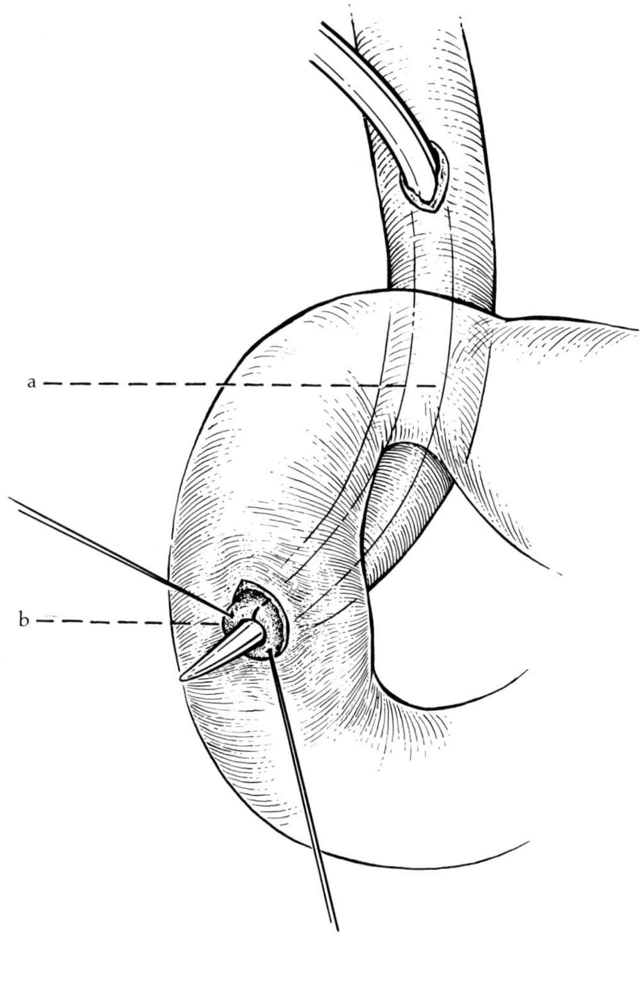

FIG. 18-21. Transduodenal sphincterotomy. **A.** The duodenum is opened widely. **B and C.** Each of the orifices is identified. The edges of the slit duct are sutured to the duodenal mucosa as a variety of ampulloduodenostomy.

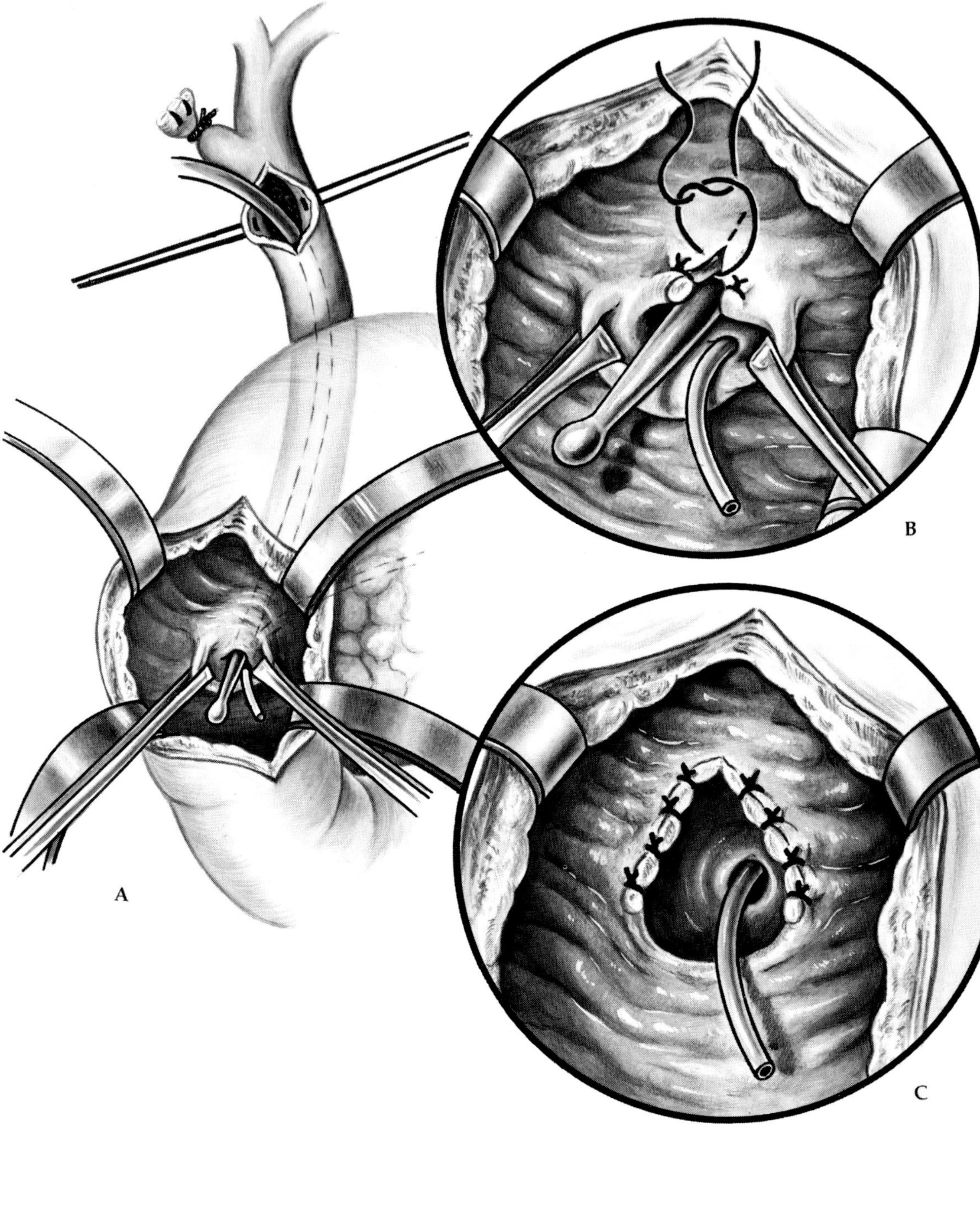

TABLE 18-1. SALIENT DIFFERENTIAL FEATURES OF SPHINCTEROTOMY AND CHOLEDOCHODUODENOSTOMY

	Sphincterotomy	Choledochoduodenostomy
Size of incision	Must be limited	At discretion of surgeon
Effect of operation	Limited to decompression of terminal common bile duct	Decompresses entire choledochus
Duration of effect	Transitory	Permanent bypass
Complications	Risk of postoperative pancreatitis	No significant technical complications
Postoperative evaluation	Difficult to evaluate remotely	Easily accomplished by barium swallow or endoscopy

Hess (259), and Arianoff (24, 26, 27) are enthusiastic about its role in the management of minor and major degrees of papillitis.

Jones's sphincteroplasty (310), in contrast to sphincterotomy, is intended to avoid later cicatrization by dividing all the muscle, removing a wedge of ampulla, and suturing the duct to duodenal mucosa. Reflux is less often seen after sphincterotomy (15%) than after sphincteroplasty (100%). There are a number of differences between sphincterotomy and choledochoduodenostomy (Table 18-1).

It has been my personal practice to limit sphincter procedures to the incarcerated stone problem. In the MHMC series that situation has been encountered only twice in 200 instances. Contrariwise, I have a broad indication for choledochoduodenostomy and have done it in almost every secondary common duct exploration in which the anatomic situation made it possible. Others take the same attitude toward sphincterotomy.

Fritsch (207) has combined sphincterotomy with choledochoduodenostomy when there is both papillary stenosis and choledochalectasia. He reported that postoperative flow rates are increased.

Whatever the method used to obtain a wide-open sphincter, one must be aware of the hazard of going completely through the full thickness of the duodenal wall, thereby creating a duodenal fistula and possibly compromising the pancreatic duct orifice. At the other extreme is the sphincter slit that may not be sufficient to actually widen the orifice. In this regard, one must steer between a surgical Scylla and Charybdis (242).

Technique

The procedure is best performed over a catheter, which is introduced via the choledochostomy exploratory incision. The choice of catheter is of some importance. If the orifice is difficult to traverse, a moist bougie followed by a sound is a good method.

The duodenum is submitted to kocherization. The tapered hard rubber follower engages the papilla. This is appreciated externally, and a small incision (0.5–0.7 cm) is made in the duodenal wall. The catheter is grasped and pulled through the duodenostomy (Fig. 18-20). This prolapses the Vaterian segment into and then out of the duodenal lumen (342). Sutures are placed to approximate the duct and duodenal mucosa at the right midlateral and left midlateral walls. A 1- to 1.2-cm incision is made anteriorly at 10–11 o'clock, and the apex is closed with a crown suture. The apex is that point where the pink mucosa of the duodenum meets the yellow of the bile duct. There is often a small vessel at that site. The catheter should now pass easily in a to-and-fro direction, so that the opening may be assumed to be 1 cm in circumference. The pancreatic duct orifice should be visualized. Unless there is good reason, it should not be manipulated (Fig. 18-21).

The catheter is withdrawn and a T tube inserted at the choledochostomy site. It is irrigated to check for ooze or leak. The duodenum stab incision is closed with several interrupted sero-muscular silk sutures. No transduodenal splint is used.

V

Case Studies

19 Case Studies in Postcholecystectomy Syndromes

The data are briefly presented in capsule fashion and include only the pertinent facts. Interesting irrelevancies are not included. The format is not meant to simulate a clinical pathological conference; it is rather that of the bedside case presentations of residents and attending staff that have proved to be a satisfactory teaching vehicle at this institution. These cases were encountered in office consultation, in the operating room, at the bedside, and in hospital corridor conversations.

The **history** encompasses the pertinent details presented by the patient and retrievable from prior studies. The **findings** consist of data obtained from physical examination, laboratory tests, and pertinent x-rays done in the investigation of postcholecystectomy situations. The **diagnosis** is the presumptive one for the patient to be operated upon and the conjectured one in the patient evaluated and treated by means other than secondary surgery. The diagnosis includes considerations of rationale for attitude toward management. The **operation** contains no technical details because those have been presented in the text; it gives only the findings and the procedural choice. The **results** are based on follow-up obtained by discussions with the patients and their attending physicians. The latter is the only recourse in patients seen only once. The **epicrisis** epitomizes the instructive features of that problem.

1. PANCREATIC DUCTAL LITHIASIS SIMULATING CYSTIC DUCT REMNANT LITHIASIS

History. A 40-year-old female has been suffering severe recurrent bouts of abdominal pain with several episodes of jaundice. Cholecystectomy 6 years ago did not relieve symptoms. Common duct exploration 3 years later failed to retrieve the common duct and cystic duct calculi that were regarded as identified on the operative cholangiogram. Severe abdominal pain persisted and the patient became addicted to meperidine (Demerol) and lost 30 lbs. A third abdominal operation was undertaken for adhesive intestinal obstruction. At that time the appendix was removed. Alcohol consumption has been excessive for 15 years.

Findings. The patient is acutely and chronically ill. Abdomen is flat with a sense of mass in the epigastrium. Hematocrit, 35. Serum and urinary amylase are normal. Review of the cholangiogram (Fig. 19-1) reveals that the common bile duct is normal. The stones presumed to be in a left-sided cystic duct remnant are, on lateral view, shown to be in the head of the pancreas.

Diagnosis. This is an instance of pancreatic duct lithiasis and chronic pancreatitis. The venous phase of a mesenteric angiogram demonstrated segmental occlusion of the portal vein. The symptoms of pain are significant enough to attempt surgical relief.

Operation. Splenectomy and subtotal pancreatectomy to the side of the superior mesenteric artery are carried out. The remaining (head) pancreatic duct is cleaned out and the end of the pancreas is invaginated into the stomach by a longitudinal slit in its posterior wall. The pancreatic duct is intubated with a polyethylene catheter that is exteriorized.

Result. Pathology report is pancreatic calculi and chronic pancreatitis. Patient has regained weight, requires no analgesics, and is back at work. She

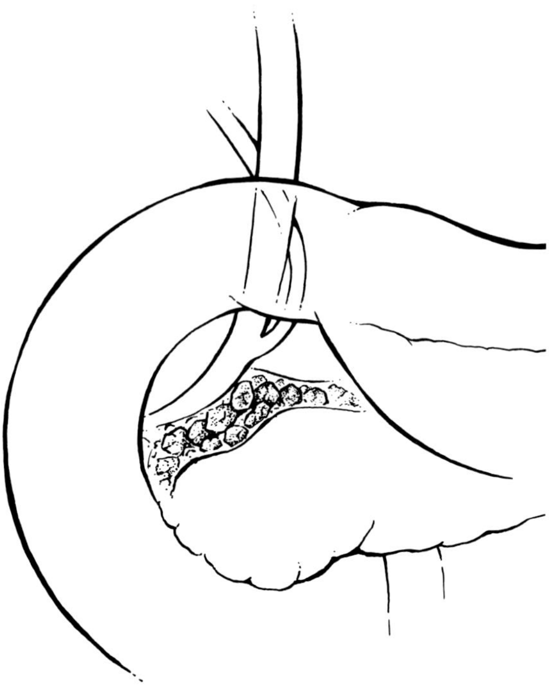

FIG. 19-1. Pancreatic duct lithiasis. Diagram of the cholangiogram in Figure 8-8. A clinical suspicion of a pancreatic lesion is suggested by the patient's alcoholism. A lateral view clarified the problem of localization.

abstains from alcohol and has no signs of pancreatic insufficiency on a normal diet.

Epicrisis. It is probable that the original gallstones were an incidental finding. Pancreatitis associated with alcoholism appears to have been the diagnosis from the beginning. Lateral and oblique views are required definitively to show that the stones were never in the cystic duct and that the indication for common duct exploration that was the second procedure was an error due to misinterpretation of the film. Pancreatic resection is probably the best method of managing the symptomatic disease at this stage in a young patient. The periportal fibrotic reaction contraindicated a Whipple or 99% type of resection, at least as the initial procedure.

2. ACCESSORY BILE DUCT LEAK

History. A 50-year-old female underwent uneventful cholecystectomy for cholelithiasis. Her postoperative course was complicated by subphrenic abscess and continued bile leak.

Findings. The incision is well healed. There is a bile leak through the Penrose drain stab site.

Diagnosis. Intravenous cholangiogram shows the common bile duct is normal. A sublobular segment of the right lobe of the liver is drained by an accessory duct that leaks into the subhepatic space and is the source of the persistent right-upper-quadrant infection (Fig. 12-3).

Operation. The accessory bile duct, 3 mm in diameter, is mobilized and intubated with a polyethylene tube. It is stabbed through a purse-string suture into the posterior wall of the stomach. The right upper quadrant is debrided, irrigated, and drained.

Result. Healed.

Epicrisis. This accessory bile duct was probably interpreted as a string adhesion, and the lumen in the strand was not recognized. This duct exited via the gallbladder or cystic duct, and when this pathway was severed, it continued to drain liver bile. Some of these accessory ducts close spontaneously in a few weeks, and are never recognized for what they are.

It is not possible, in this instance, to know whether the bile in the stomach after operation is related to pyloric sphincter incompetence or to the duct's continuity. This accessory duct could well stricture off, and that part of the liver would then drain via intrahepatic collaterals or become fibrotic. Clinically, it makes no difference so long as there is no infection and there is sufficient functioning hepatic parenchyma.

3. CHOLANGITIS WITH SPONTANEOUS PNEUMOCHOLANGIOGRAM

History. A 53-year-old female had an emergency gallbladder operation 6 years ago in another country. She knows no details except that she became suddenly ill and was operated upon. She was told: "You're lucky to be alive." She was well until 3 weeks ago when she experienced chills and fever and was treated for a urinary tract infection. She then became jaundiced with a serum bilirubin of 5.7 mg/100 ml. Chills and fever recurred.

Findings. There are tenderness and rigidity in right upper quadrant. Flat film of the abdomen reveals air in the common bile duct and hepatic duct; there are numerous calculi in the distal system; white blood cell count is 24,600, with 89% leukocytes (Fig. 19-2).

Diagnosis. The diagnosis of cholangitis is based on chills, fever, jaundice, and leukocytosis. Air in the biliary tree suggests a fistula (biliary enteric) or the rare incompetent ampulla, or the still rarer emphysematous cholangitis due to gas-forming bacteria. Urgent surgery is required.

Operation. A 3-cm portion of the ampulla of the gallbladder is retained. It contains cholesterol stones. Its dome has a wide-mouthed fistula to the duodenum. The cystic duct is 0.5 cm wide and patent. Common bile duct is 1.4 cm wide and contains a virtual cast of primary duct stones. The gallbladder remnant is removed and the duodenal side of the fistula is closed in one layer. The common bile duct is cleared of stones and a choledochoduodenostomy performed.

The stones are of the primary type, amorphous, and lacking calcium. Bile culture grows out *E. coli*.

Fig. 19-2. Gallbladder remnant, duodenal fistula. The retained gallbladder segment has fistulized to the lateral wall of the duodenum. The common bile duct also has stones (see Fig. 8-5).

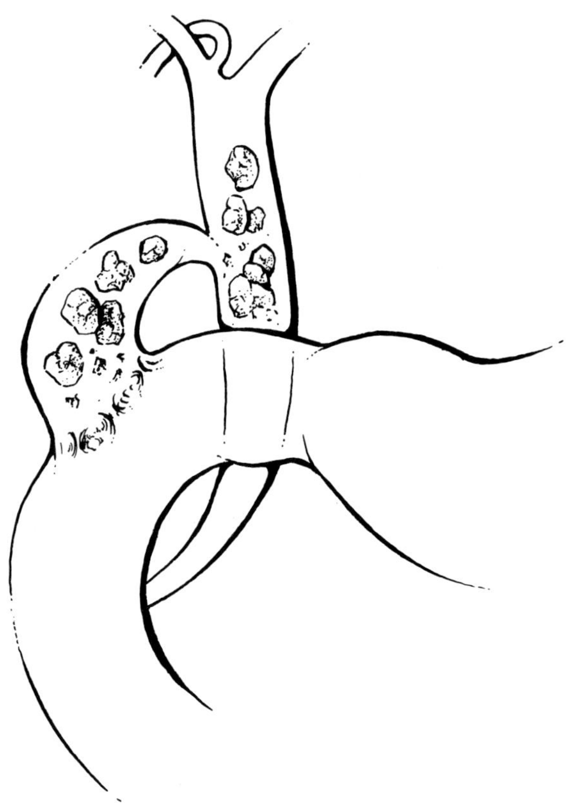

Result. There is a postoperative wound infection (*E. coli*). No further episodes of cholangitis occur. Barium swallow opacifies the intrahepatic ducts with virtually complete passage of the contrast on the 4-hour film.

Epicrisis. The initial cholecystectomy was incomplete. Hartmann's pouch may have been purposefully left behind because the first surgeon encountered difficulty in this area of impending or actual fistulization. This fistula may have been the sequel of acute perforative cholecystitis, for which a subtotal cholecystectomy had been performed.

The finding of primary stones in this greatly dilated duct indicates that there was significant choledochal stasis. The difference between the spontaneous pathologic fistula and the surgical choledochoduodenostomy is not only in the site, but, and more importantly, its functional width. Choledocholithotomy and T-tube drainage would have been a less satisfactory approach to duct stasis with primary stones.

4. CHOLANGITIS WITH IATROGENIC CHOLECYSTOJEJUNAL FISTULA

History. A 69-year-old jaundiced male underwent cholecystojejunostomy 2.5 years ago for a presumed cancer of the head of the pancreas. No biopsy was taken. The jaundice disappeared and his general condition improved. Starting 1 year ago he began to have chills, fever, and abdominal pain.

Findings. There were no palpable abnormalities and no roentgen evidence of metastatic disease.

Diagnosis. Patients with cancer of the pancreatic head rarely survive this long in this state of good health. It is highly likely that the initial diagnosis was erroneous. The cause of the present symptoms is probably cholangitis and cholecystitis due to anastomotic stricture.

Operation. There is no evidence of metastatic disease. The pancreas is indurated with loss of sharp margins. This is assumed to be chronic pancreatitis. The gallbladder contains purulent bile. The common bile duct is thickened and its lining granular; the lumen contains flaked pigment stones (see Fig. 13-1). The cholecystojejunostomy is dismantled, and the jejunal side of the fistula closed. A cholecystectomy and choledochoduodenostomy completes the surgery.

Result. Patient is well 4 years later.

Epicrisis. For long-term decompression, as required for benign disease, duct-to-bowel anastomosis is far superior to the technically easier gallbladder-to-bowel anastomosis. In general, when the diagnosis is uncertain, the former is to be preferred. If the clinical course does not fit the diagnosis, it is better to proceed with the premise that common complications of common diseases are more likely than uncommon presentations of an unproved diagnosis.

5. PERSISTENT EPIGASTRIC PAIN AND NORMAL WORK UP

History. A 44-year-old female, gravida 3, and a heavy smoker, reports onset of symptoms after second child. Cholecystectomy was performed 3 years ago. She had no jaundice or colic and the indication for initial operation was epigastric discomfort. She complains of being uncontrollably flatulent, having fatty food dyspepsia, and says the dietary factors "prevent me from living a normal life. My social life is circumscribed by my need to avoid embarrassment." The gallbladder disorder had been interpreted as "noncalculous chronic cholecystitis—mild." The pathology report described focal fibrosis. No cholangiogram was done.

Findings. The overweight patient is pleasant and garrulous and has no palpable abnormalities. Blood chemistries are normal. Gastrointestinal series shows hiatal insufficiency. Barium enema and intravenous cholangiogram are normal. Present symptom is that of epigastric discomfort and burning sensation.

Diagnosis. Neither the symptoms nor prior findings are consistent with anatomic biliary disease. No reoperative surgery is advised, but it is suggested that she stop smoking.

Result. Patient feels better when not smoking.

Epicrisis. The indication for the initial surgery is questionable. The epigastric discomfort could well be cigarette-related esophagitis. Flatulence is not a symptom of biliary disease. The diagnosis of noncalculous cholecystitis should be made cautiously and only in the presence of radiographic demonstration of a "fighting" gallbladder or after a provocative test or a positive duodenal drainage. The patient has no anatomic biliary disease.

6. ALLERGIC YOUNG WOMAN WITH RECURRENT EPIGASTRIC PAIN

History. A 23-year-old female, weighing 110 lbs, presents with a long history of multiple allergies manifested by urticaria and neurodermatitis; she has also had episodes of bronchospasm. There is a difficult family situation, and the patient has had intermittent psychiatric advice. A cholecystectomy was done 2 years ago because of "typical symptoms." No contrast studies were performed because of the allergies. She has the same symptoms: episodes of severe epigastric pain waking her up at night, bringing her to tears. "Everyone thinks it's all psychosomatic." The pain does not radiate. During one such episode, the bilirubin was recorded as 1.9 mg/100 ml. A flat film of the abdomen is unrevealing. Serum calcium, phosphorus, and urinary amylase had been normal on several examinations. Gastrointestinal series were normal on many occasions.

Findings. I saw her during one of these episodes and her pain was pitiful. There was a distinct point tenderness in the right upper quadrant without signs of peritoneal irritation. The radiologist preferred not doing an intravenous cholangiogram unless that was to be the last clinical resort. A Meltzer-Lyon drainage was performed, but no cholesterol crystals were found. Review of the previously excised gallbladder specimen revealed no true inflammatory reaction; the wall was infiltrated by numerous eosinophils. The diagnosis of allergic cholecystitis had been offered. An intravenous cholangiogram was performed, with anesthesia standby. The procedure went uneventfully. There was no untoward reaction. The study was normal. Percutaneous liver biopsy was normal.

Diagnosis. There was no indication for abdominal surgery in this patient. Treatment has to be directed to the allergy and emotional situation.

Epicrisis. The earlier "typical gallbladder" findings may have been the manifestation of an allergic pancreatitis. The first surgeon had the best opportunity to evaluate the total problem. Since the abdomen was opened unnecessarily, it is unfortunate that his operative note does not detail the examination of the pancreas and small bowel. He might have helped anticipate subsequent diagnostic problems by removing the appendix. Allergic cholecystitis has been described as an experimental and clinical entity (304). The diagnosis remains to be established. For the first surgeon it was another instance of being misled by "typical symptoms," for which there was no anatomic or chemical documentation. Until these are evident, the second surgeon should not be led into an exploration for "what has been missed."

7. SQUAMOUS-CELL CARCINOMA OF THE GALLBLADDER AS AN INCIDENTAL FINDING

History. A 72-year-old female has known of gallstones for 20 years. She has had repeated episodes of pain that she does not want to endure any more. Preop blood studies are all normal. A cholecystectomy for calculi is uneventful. There is no intraoperative cholangiogram. Casual examination of liver reveals no abnormalities. Histologic examination of gallbladder tissue reveals a squamous-cell carcinoma of the fundus, extending to but not through the muscular layer. There are several generations of the cholesterol stones. Is anything further advised?

Findings. No physical abnormalities are found 3 weeks after operation. Serum bilirubin and alkaline phosphatase are normal. Cystic duct lymph node is not in the operative specimen.

Diagnosis. The histologic diagnosis is definite. There is no known extension of the disease.

Operation. Reoperative surgery is not required to excavate the liver bed, to do a hepatic lobectomy, or to intubate the CBD prophylactically.

Result. Because there is no evidence of residual tumor, I did not advise cancer chemotherapy.

Epicrisis. Carcinoma of the gallbladder is a not-infrequent feature of the chronic calculous gallbladder in patients over age 70. At the time of surgery, the resected organ ought always to be opened and the mucosa inspected for this possibility. Having made the diagnosis at that time, I would undertake 1) careful evaluation of liver and regional lymph drainage area for evidence of extension as a further clue to prognosis and predictable course; 2) do a cystic duct cholangiogram—not only as a base line, but also as a way of monitoring the local invasiveness of the tumor. I might intubate the common duct. The spread of these tumors is such that they are difficult to manage surgically because they often metastasize to the peripancreatic and pericholedochal lymph nodes, show direct invasion of the liver substance and diffuse peritoneal spread. There is no effective surgical treatment at this time.

There is a difference in the behavior of gallbladder carcinomas that is related to histologic type. If the patient has a carcinoma *in situ* in the gallbladder, the experience of Bivens *et al.* (63) suggests that those patients followed from 4 to 6 years give no evidence of recurrence of the tumor. However, in the patient with microinvasive carcinoma of the gallbladder, there is often evidence of recurrence within a few months.

It has not been my policy to reoperate on patients with carcinoma of the gallbladder for the purpose of resecting the right lobe of the liver or of revision in the gallbladder fossa. I recognize that this is one point of view and that others may have a more aggressive attitude. A search of the literature fails to reveal convincing evidence that extended resection of the gallbladder, liver, and lymph nodes in the hepatoduodenal ligament is better than cholecystectomy. Squamous-cell cancers are less common than adenocarcinoma in this area and probably represent the metaplastic response to a prior chronic inflammatory reaction in the gallbladder.

This specific patient's situation appeared to be most favorable for cure. However, she returned in 10 months with evidence of pyloric outlet obstruction. At reoperation she was found to have diffuse peritoneal metasteses. Another example of the unpredictability of cancer in this organ.

8. PORCELAIN GALLBLADDER WITH LEFT HEPATIC DUCT TUMOR

History. A 75-year-old man underwent operation for symptoms of chronic cholecystitis. A flat film of the abdomen demonstrated a calcified gallbladder. A cystic-duct cholangiogram during operation was interpreted as normal. Nevertheless, a common-duct exploration was performed because of elevated alkaline phosphatase. The film was read as normal. The postoperative course uneventful. Repeat T-tube cholangiogram demonstrated a stricture in the left hepatic duct.

Findings. The only significant finding is in the cholangiogram: a stricture in the left hepatic duct with a fusiform dilation behind it (Fig. 19-3).

Diagnosis. The cholangiographic finding is specific. There is no lesion that produces this configuration except a primary bile-duct cancer. This lesion is easily missed by routine intraoperative probing. The area is rarely palpated as a routine. Choledochoscopy can be a collateral way of identifying the lesion, but the roentgen diagnosis is so specific that biopsy confirmation is not required.

FIG. 19-3. Porcelainized gallbladder. Diagrammatic representation of a characteristic cholangiographic finding **(arrow).** The fusiform dilatation of the left hepatic duct is proximal to a bile duct cancer stenosis (Fig. 5-7). This association is frequent enough to require concern when cholecystectomy is performed for a calcified gallbladder.

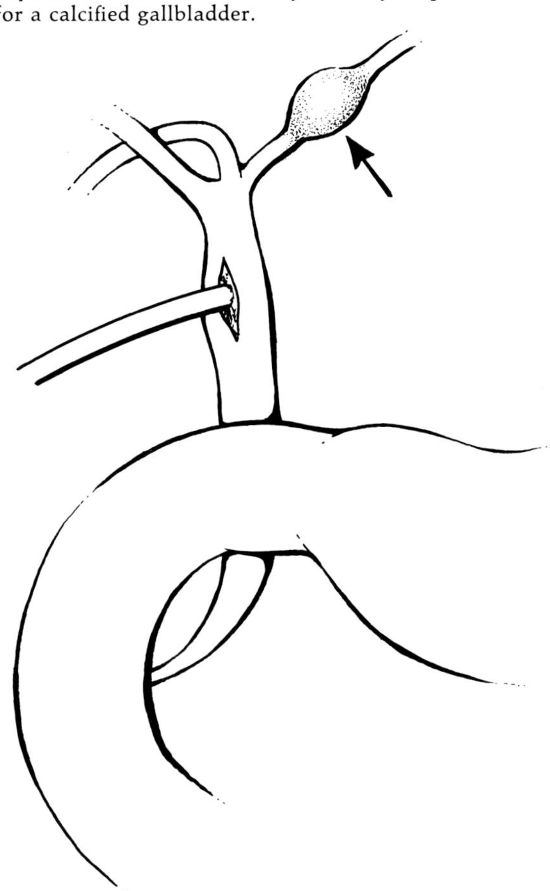

Operation. At reoperation, the tumor is found to extend beyond the duct into the hepatic parenchyma and around the vessels—more extensive than the cholangiogram indicated. A rubber tube is inserted through the tumor, one end going out through the liver onto the anterior abdominal wall and the other into the common bile duct.

Result. The patient is alive 2 years later. There have been several bouts of cholangitis, but there is no pruritus. Biopsy of the liver shows biliary cirrhosis.

Epicrisis. Bile-duct tumors are easily overlooked in the preicteric stage. Biopsy confirmation is difficult because these tumors have a dominant desmoblastic reaction and the epithelial components are scattered and difficult to identify. Excisional surgery is sometimes possible, but there is some doubt that it has any advantage over intubation decompression. These are slowly growing cancers.

The important lesson here is that about 20% of patients with a calcified gallbladder have an associated biliary tract cancer. If cancer is not found in the gallbladder, the ductal system should be especially carefully evaluated with this statistic in mind.

Such unilateral uninfected lobar obstruction need have no associated chemical abnormalities. The diagnosis is on the film and suggested by the gallbladder pathology and the elevated alkaline phosphatase.

9. OBSTRUCTION OF THE COMMON HEPATIC DUCT CARINA

History. A 74-year-old male had undergone cholecystectomy for cholecystitis 20 years ago. He remained asymptomatic until 3 months ago, when symptoms of icterus and weakness suggested the diagnosis of hepatitis. Diarrheal stool cultures were normal. Serum bilirubin rose to 17 mg/100 ml. Hypotonic duodenography performed elsewhere was said to be normal.

Findings. No physical abnormalities were present. The liver edge was smooth and palpable on deep inspiration. Blood chemistries revealed elevated alkaline phosphatase, cholesterol, and serum bilirubin. The gastrointestinal series was normal—specifically no duodenal deformity and no grooving of the duodenum to indicate an enlarged bile duct.

Diagnosis. The diagnosis of obstructive jaundice was confirmed, the differential being a choledochal stone or biliary-pancreatic cancer. The low fecal urobiligen was an indication of complete biliary obstruction and statistically diagnostic of cancer. The normal x-ray studies favored a tumor of the bile duct. The most rewarding study from the surgical point of view would be the percutaneous transhepatic cholangiogram because it's "what's up front that counts" in considering the alternatives in bile rerouting.

FIG. 19-4. Obstruction of the hepatic duct carina. Cholangiographic pattern is characteristic of bile duct cancer. The only serious differential diagnosis—iatrogenic stricture—is ruled out by history (Fig. 5-6).

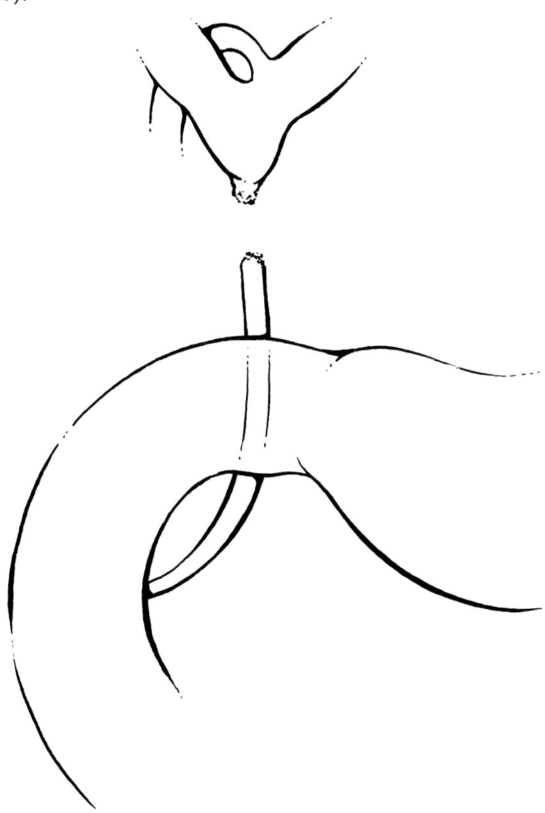

Operation. Percutaneous transhepatic cholangiogram, performed on the way to the operating room, revealed dilated intrahepatic ducts with an irregular abrupt block just distal to the carina (Fig. 19-4).

The lesion was resected to include the entire supraduodenal common bile duct and the two major hepatic ducts. Continuity was restored by hepatic Roux-Y-jejunostomy. No attempt at preresectional biopsy was made because the cholangiographic features are specific for cancer.

Result. The absence of regional lymphadenopathy or perineural invasion, and the fact that the margins were free of cancer suggested that the resection could be curative. However, the patient survived for only 15 months, during which time jaundice recurred and cholangitis and pruritis appeared.

Epicrisis. The cholangiogram is specific for the diagnosis of cancer of the bile ducts, and resectional surgery can be confidently performed without a prior biopsy. Curative resection in terms of 5-year survival free of disease is rare. It may be conjectured that a circle tube that could be readily changed could be an equally and possibly more effective way of managing the obstructive features of this cancer. Without the cholangiogram, a similar history is compatible with a calculus obstruction.

10. CYSTIC STUMP REMNANT WITH AMPULLARY CANCER

History. A 65-year-old female had cholecystectomy and choledochotomy 15 years ago. She began to complain of persistent epigastric distress, which she did not have before. Routine chemistries showed elevated bilirubin and alkaline phosphatase.

Findings. No mass was palpable. Intravenous cholangiogram showed a markedly dilated duct with a broad-based gallbladder remnant. The alkaline phosphatase was considerably elevated.

Diagnosis. Because of the dilated duct, it was assumed this was CDJS and that her symptoms were related to duct hypertension. The remnant was regarded as innocent because it was stone free.

Operation. No palpable or visible abnormalities were found except for the dilated duct. Choledochoscopy was performed as a routine. This was in the first year of my experience with the endoscope. I saw a polypoid tumor of the ampulla, which was not obstructive. A Bakes sound and a catheter could pass it. A transduodenal frozen section biopsy was reported as carcinoma. A pancreaticoduodenectomy was performed.

Result. The postoperative course was uncomplicated. The pathologist reported this as a cancer at the junction of the duct and duodenum, extending only to the submucosa. No nodes were involved.

Epicrisis. This is the earliest carcinoma of the ampulla that I have encountered. The lesion was not palpable. I wonder whether the cholangiogram would have interpreted it as papillitis. This is a striking instance of the value of biliary endoscopy as a diagnostic tool influencing the choice of surgical procedure. It also validates the concept that even though the preoperative diagnosis was wrong, a dilated common duct is an indication of past or present obstruction.

11. GALLBLADDER REMNANT WITH MULTIPLE CALCULI AND LEFT-SIDED CYSTIC DUCT

History. A 62-year-old female had a gallbladder operation 14 years ago. She was under the impression that her gallbladder had been removed. There have been recurrent bouts of colic, for which she has been treated with magnesium sulfate and "glasses full" (sic) of mineral oil. She was told that she was "liverish." When she came to the United States her family doctor obtained an oral cholecystogram. This revealed a funnel-shaped gallbladder remnant with stones and a "necklace" of stones in the greatly dilated left-sided cystic duct (Fig. 19-5).

Findings. There were no abnormal physical signs. A healed 4-in. incision was noted in the right linea semilunaris.

Diagnosis. The first procedure had been incomplete. This patient had needlessly had to endure repeated bouts of pain under an erroneous diagnosis. It would appear that the first surgeon should have known that a significant segment of diseased gallbladder was left behind and should have informed the patient about it. The segment could scarcely be considered only a cystic duct remnant.

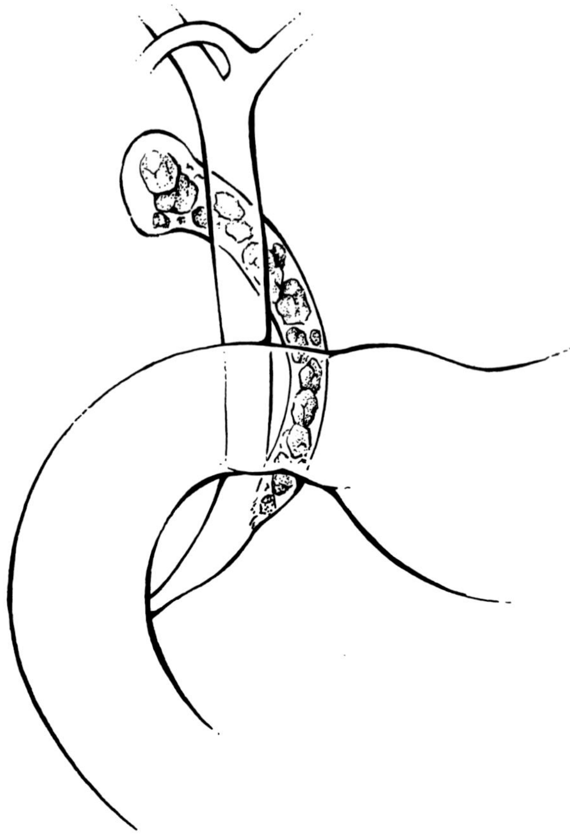

FIG. 19-5. Left-sided gallbladder remnant. The technical aspect of lithotomy in this instance can be managed via the retained ampulla of the gallbladder. It is not necessary to remove this remnant only to render it stone-free. The older literature has described doing this as a transpancreatic procedure via the posterior surface of the kocherized duodenopancreatic area, an approach that is hazardous in terms of leak and fistula.

The original procedure appears to have been only slightly more than a fundal cholecystectomy. Used in this way, cholecystostomy merits condemnation, not for being a compromise procedure, but for resulting in delayed definitive management in the severely symptomatic patient.

Operation. A subcostal incision was made and the gallbladder amputated at the right side of the common bile duct. The cystic duct was irrigated free of calculi after a small pituitary spoon was used to cradle out the accessible stones. No attempt was made to remove the now stone-free left cystic duct.

Epicrisis. One accepts the fact that the local situation in the abdomen or the general condition of the patient with gallbladder disease requires compromise procedures, such as cholecystostomy or partial amputation with intubation. However, it is later necessary to define, roentgenographically, the residual disease. Six to 12 weeks later definitive surgery should have been undertaken. I have been repeatedly seen a patient dubbed "liverish" without investigation of the anatomic status of the extrahepatic ducts having been made.

12. CALCIFICATION IN THE GALLBLADDER FOSSA SIMULATING REMNANT DISEASE

History. A 46-year-old male, an anxious patient, suffered recurrent colics after cholecystectomy 12 years ago. Blood studies and several intravenous cholangiograms were normal, the common bile duct measuring 0.8 cm. He had been treated symptomatically. The intravenous cholangiogram that was the indication for reoperation demonstrated calcified density in the right upper quadrant that had not been present previously (Fig. 8-4).

Findings. There were no abnormalities on physical examination or blood studies. The calcified mass in the right upper quadrant was interpreted as a calcified gallbladder remnant or stone.

Diagnosis. It is not clear why the mass had not been seen on any of the previous x-ray studies. The possibility of a hepatic artery aneurysm existed. There was nothing in the man's life style to implicate hydatid disease.

Operation. The may lay beneath a silk-sutured peritoneal cuff over the gallbladder fossa. It was a calcified hematoma.

Results. The symptom complex was not altered.

Epicrisis. The indication for reoperative surgery was quite clear—an extra choledochal abnormality in the symptomatic patient. There is no way of making a preoperative diagnosis of the condition.

13. LONG, INNOCENT CYSTIC DUCT REMNANT

History. A 56-year-old female had undergone cholecystectomy 15 years ago for acute cholecystitis. Recovery was uneventful. A specimen confirmed the diagnosis; there were two large cholesterol calculi. The patient subsequently developed a duodenal ulcer causing seasonal complaints. In the course of the ulcer study, an intravenous cholangiogram revealed a cystic duct remnant. Was this contributing to the dyspepsia?

Findings. Physical examination and blood studies are normal. Intravenous cholangiogram shows a normal-sized duct, emptying promptly. There are no calculi. A lateral view shows a well-opacified cystic duct remnant 4 cm long, but 3 cm of this is to the left of the common bile duct (Fig. 19-6).

Diagnosis. This duct remnant is not diseased. The distal 3 cm of the duct are in the head of the pancreas. No treatment is required for this normal segment.

Epicrisis. Left-sided cystic duct entrance is rarely apparent to the surgeon. He cannot see its course

FIG. 19-6. Innocent left cystic duct remnant. This calculus-free, normally draining duct is an anatomic entity, not a disorder likely to provoke pathogenic symptoms.

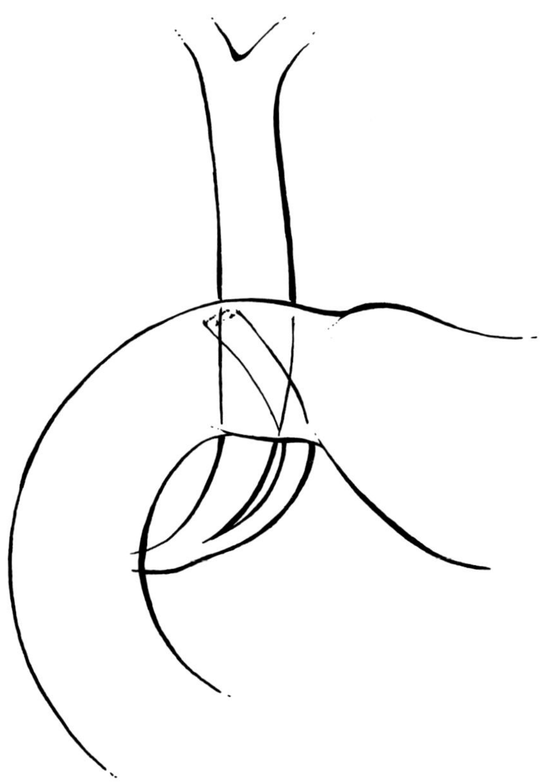

beyond the presumed entrance into the common bile duct, at which point the duct passes posteriorly. The full course of such a duct can only be appreciated on the lateral view. Such a duct can be a surgical hazard when it crosses the common bile duct anteriorly on its way to a left-sided entrance in the supravaterian segment. It is both unnecessary and hazardous to attempt removal of this remnant if it is stone-free and not dilated. The dyspepsia is related to the peptic ulcer; this is best managed medically.

14. RETAINED STONES AFTER SECONDARY CHOLEDOCHOLITHOTOMY

History. A 44-year-old male underwent cholecystectomy and choledocholithotomy 3 years ago. A second choledocholithotomy was required for a retained duct stone during the sixth postoperative week. A postoperative T-tube study is said to have been normal. The T tube was removed. The patient now presents with chills, fever, and jaundice, the second such episode in 3 months.

Findings. The man is icteric and febrile. The former cholangiograms are retrospectively viewed, showing a large stone at the hepatic carina obfuscated by an excessively dense contrast medium and the lack of a sufficient number of films (Fig. 7-5A). Incidentally noted is the progression of intrahepatic dilatation between the first and second studies.

Diagnosis. The obvious diagnosis is cholangitis due to retained stone. The size of the stone is almost 2 cm, and it is probably incarcerated in the carinal area.

Operation. The common bile duct contained infected bile with stone flakes and small pigment-stone particles. The carinal stone could not be cradled out intact. It was crushed and the fragments irrigated out. Choledochoscopy showed an ulceration at the area of calculus impaction. There were no other stones. Choledochoduodenostomy was performed.

Result. No further symptoms (8 years later).

Epicrisis. The problem was avoidable. The first intraoperative procedure was not carefully monitored. The area of proximal hepatic duct stone disease can be especially well monitored by biliary endoscopy. One must be aware of the retained stone problem in this area, where the cholangiographic duct overlap can cover over stones. The surgeon at the second operation may have been content with finding the one stone. Would a choledochoduodenostomy at that time have allowed that retained stone to pass spontaneously? It might not have been incarcerated at that time.

At all second operations for stone disease when the common bile duct is dilated, choledochoduodenostomy as a prophylactic as well as therapeutic measure should be favored over simple T-tube drainage.

15. SOLITARY RETAINED COMMON BILE DUCT STONE

History. A 72-year-old male who had severe cardiac disease with angina and two prior myocardial infarcts underwent cholecystectomy and common duct exploration. Several stones were removed. A postoperative cholangiogram revealed a retained stone. During this study and a second one 3 weeks later, he experienced a profound adverse reaction to the cholangiogram. The first time he was said to have had anaphylactic shock and second time, sepsis.

Findings. The patient had no symptoms with a clamped T tube. Review of that cholangiogram reveals a duct 1.2 cm wide with free flow into the duodenum. A 6-mm stone is seen in the suprasphincteric zone.

Diagnosis. One would prefer not to reoperate on this man. His stone is not producing symptoms and he tolerates clamping. I advised that the T-tube be removed and that nothing further be done unless he became symptomatic. The patient died 3 months later of myocardial infarction. His common duct stone had remained quiet.

Epicrisis. A large experience with spontaneous stone passage has been reported, especially Millbourne's monograph (426). This size stone (less than 7 mm) in a patient whose duct is otherwise normal is in a most favorable situation for spontaneous passage. Because of the patient's idiosyncrasy to the contrast material, I preferred this to any method requiring cholangiographic monitoring.

16. MULTIPLE RETAINED STONES IN A 1.2-CM COMMON BILE DUCT

History. A 56-year-old female underwent an uneventful cholecystectomy after a cholecystogram showed many small stones. Common duct exploration was negative, and an intraoperative cholangiogram was interpreted as normal. The postoperative cholangiogram demonstrated three stones in an ampullary saccule (Fig. 5-3).

Findings. Retrospectively, the stones were seen in the poor-quality intraoperative cholangiogram. Chemistries were normal.

Diagnosis. A repeat cholangiogram 3 weeks later confirmed the presence of stones. That they had not changed position was probably related to the saccule or quasi-diverticulum in which they lie. The same study done after another 3 weeks showed no change.

Operation. The fistulous tract is now well established. Under x-ray control employing the steering catheter and the Dormia loop, two of the stones were extracted uneventfully. The third remains. It will be observed and approached surgically only if symptoms warrant.

Epicrisis. If retained stones are diagnosed with the T tube *in situ,* the modalities that can be employed depend, in part, on the expertise and experience of personnel. Early in the course one considers the following alternatives 1) perfusion with cholic acid or heparin or other solutions (see Perfusion, under Management of Retained Stones Demonstrated by Postoperative Cholangiography, Ch. 18; my experience with such solutions has been so unsatisfactory that this is the very last resort); 2) pass a catheter to dilate the Vaterian segment; 3) wait for spontaneous passage.

In the later phase (6 weeks) one can consider closed extraction by the basket or transduodenal endoscopic sphincterotomy, dilatation, and basketing.

It is not necessary to get all stones out of all ducts, however desirable this may be from a theoretical viewpoint. The practical problem is to balance tolerance to the stone against the probability for spontaneous stone passage. In so doing one must be prepared to change the therapy as the situation alters.

17. SYMPTOMATIC TUBULAR STENOSIS OF THE TRANSPANCREATIC PORTION OF THE COMMON BILE DUCT

History. A 72-year-old male with diabetes was operated on 6 weeks ago for acute suppurative cholecystitis. A single large elliptical stone was removed from the gallbladder. The landmarks were difficult to define; so the surgeon did a cholecystostomy. The patient recovered uneventfully, but the postoperative problem was presented by the cholecystocholangiogram. There was no history of pancreatitis or alcoholism.

Findings. The opacification study revealed no calculi. There was a long tubular stenosis of the common bile duct in the area in which it coursed through the pancreas. The duct was not deviated, and the contrast material passed through readily. The proximal duct was dilated. The cholecystostomy tube was clamped and the opacification studies repeated in 3 weeks and at 10 weeks. There was no change (Fig. 19-7).

Diagnosis. The change in this segment of the common bile duct was the result of gallstone-linked pancreatitis. This duct passes through the pancreatic parenchyma and is circumferentially compressed from without by the pancreatic interstitial fibrosis. The pancreatic reaction to acute cholecystitis is reversible in the vast majority of instances and only rarely eventuates in this type of stricture. It is highly probable—the history of only one severe attack notwithstanding—that the pancreatic reaction was the result of recurrent pancreatitis, and that the acute cholecystitis was, in fact, aggravated by the tubular stenosis. Because the patient was in good condition and diabetic, elective corrective surgery was advised.

Operation. Cholecystectomy, common-duct exploration, and choledochoduodenostomy were carried out. There were no choledochal calculi. Manometry demonstrated an elevated passage pressure.

Result. The postoperative course was uneventful.

Epicrisis. When performed electively, definitive and totally corrective biliary surgery in the diabetic carries no greater risk than it does for others in the same age group. Emergency surgery

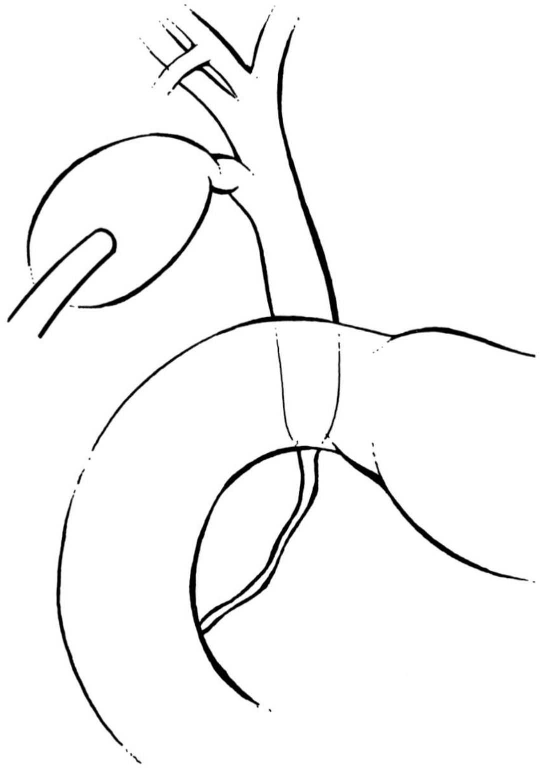

FIG. 19-7. Symptomatic tubular stenosis of the common bile duct. Manometric findings did not integrate with the rest of the clinical facts. A choledochoduodenostomy was added to the cholecystectomy because of proximal dilatation and associated vesicle disease. This dissociation of manometric findings has been encountered frequently (533).

in the elderly diabetic, over 70, for the infectious complications of gallbladder disease is the single most morbid combination of circumstances that this institution ordinarily encounters in the surgery for gallstone disease.

In the presence of the anatomic findings of proximal dilatation in relation to the tubular stenosis, and a suppurative cholecystitis, an obstructive feature is assumed. In the diabetic it is more hazardous in this circumstance to risk a recurrence by removing the cholecystostomy tube than it is to do definitive elective surgery.

18. INNOCUOUS TUBULAR STENOSIS OF THE TRANSPANCREATIC SEGMENT OF THE COMMON BILE DUCT

History. A 61-year-old male was experiencing recurrent bouts of abdominal pain, such as he had had before cholecystectomy 2 years earlier. The operation was difficult: "There was a lot of bleeding and I had to get three transfusions." Liver biopsy disclosed early cirrhosis and fatty changes. The patient was never jaundiced, is a heavy drinker, mostly on weekends, but holds a responsible position.

Findings. Liver function tests are normal except for BSP retention. No stigma of cirrhosis is apparent on physical examination. Gastrointestinal series is normal, and there are no varices. Intravenous cholangiogram shows tubular narrowing of the distal common bile duct (Fig. 19-8), but there are no stones, and the duct

FIG. 19-8. Innocuous tubular stenosis. This finding is suggested by the normal time–density factor and the absence of calculi. However, the proximal duct is dilated. If there is no pain, obstruction, or infection, then surgery need not be advised.

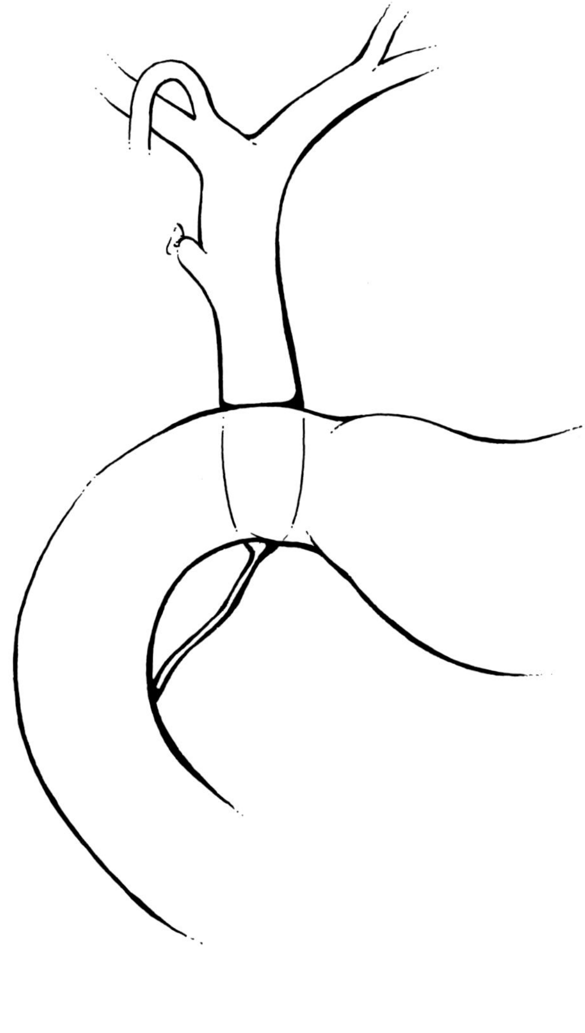

clears all the contrast material in 60 min. Percutaneous liver biopsy shows fatty changes.

Diagnosis. There is no evidence of functionally significantly biliary disease. The symptoms could be due to gastritis or pancreatitis. The stricture of this portion of the common bile duct is due to associated pancreatitis. No surgery is indicated at this time. Re-evaluate later.

Epicrisis. It is possible that the difficult first operative procedure was related to a dilated cystic vein. This vein is very rarely recognized as a distinct structure. Could this have been part of early portal hypertension?

In the MHMC experience, there is a reduced incidence (5%) of common bile duct stones in patients with established Laennec's cirrhosis. It is not possible to know whether this is pertinent to this patient. Gallstones in the cirrhotic patient are often totally silent. There is the after-the-fact consideration of whether the cholelithiasis was the source of the initial symptoms and whether cholecystectomy was indicated. One has to distinguish cholelithiasis as an anatomic fact from calculous disease as a pathogenetic entity.

19. CHOLEDOCHODUODENAL JUNCTION STENOSIS (IATROGENIC?)

History. A 46-year-old female underwent cholecystectomy and common duct exploration 3 years ago. No calculi were found in the gallbladder; the surgeon "vigorously explored the common bile duct to account for the elevated serum bilirubin." The ampulla was serially dilated to the width of a number 10 Bakes dilator. No stones were found, and the intraoperative and postoperative T-tube cholangiograms were normal.

The patient was well for about 3 months. Recently she complained of recurrent episodes of epigastric pain, more severe than formerly and longer lasting. She did not improve on a fat-free diet and bile salts.

Findings. No abnormalities were found on physical examination. An intravenous cholangiogram showed the common bile duct width to be 1.6 cm. The bile duct was still opacified at 150 min. No formed stones were detected. The previous intraoperative cholangiogram showed the common bile duct to be 0.9 cm wide.

Diagnosis. This patient had delayed flow through the choledochoduodenal junction—a roentgen diagnosis based on the prolonged time-density relationship demonstrated on the intravenous study. The duct was considerably dilated compared to earlier measurements, an indication of an organic obstructive component. The severity of symptoms warranted surgical correction.

Operation. Passage pressure was 27 cm of saline. The duct contained sludge (Fig. 19-9). A number 3 Bakes dilator could not negotiate the choledochoduodenal junction, and a choledochoduodenostomy was performed. Hepatic plexus vagectomy could not be expected to relax the fibrotic Vaterian segment.

FIG. 19-9. Choledochoduodenal junction stenosis. The diagnosis is suggested by a dilated duct with delayed transit time on the intravenous cholangiogram. At the time of operation, the obstruction is verified manometrically and by difficulty in passing a number 3 Bakes dilator through the Vaterian segment.

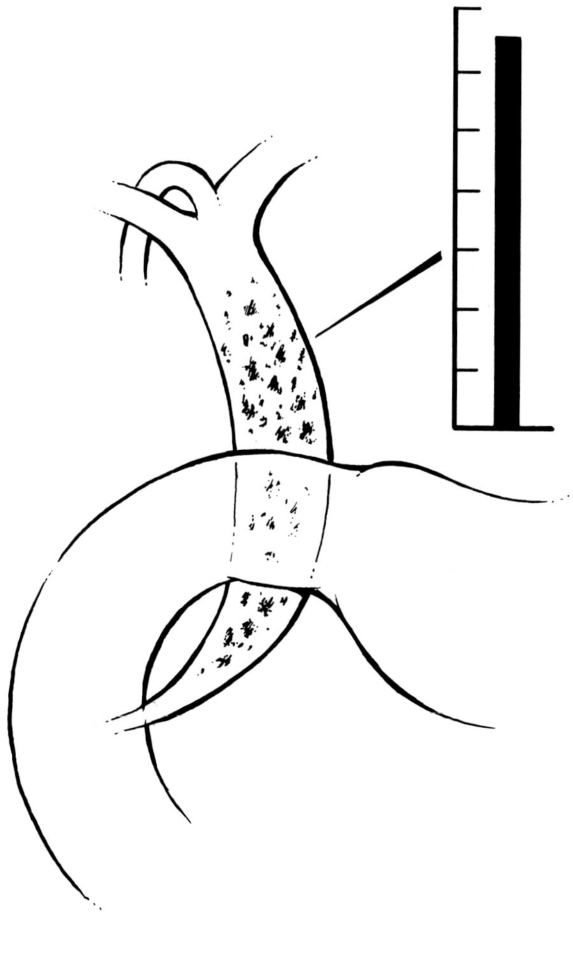

Result. The patient has no further pain but is still flatulent. She has gained considerable weight, because "I eat without fear."

Epicrisis. Because there are no stones in the duct and there was no documentation of either acute cholecystitis or acute pancreatitis, one might infer that the distal choledochal obstruction resulted from the prior surgery. There is another unprovable possibility: could this have been an example of what the Europeans so often termed papillitis in its early prefibrotic functional stage?

Did the inflammatory process go on to an obstructive CDJS because of fibrotic healing or because of operative trauma? In either instance the bypass now circumvents the obstruction. More significant is the thought that the indication for the initial operation is not clear.

20. CHOLECYSTOSTOMY WITH RETAINED GALLSTONE

History. A 64-year-old female underwent elective cholecystostomy 8 days ago. She has hypertensive cardiac disease and is in chronic congestive failure but well controlled. There is severe peripheral venous stasis with thrombophlebitic changes. At initial surgery several stones were removed from a large, distended, acutely inflamed gallbladder.

Findings. A postoperative cholecystocholangiogram, through the malecot catheter, revealed a stone in the gallbladder. The cystic duct was patent and the common duct was normal. The stone was 2 cm in diameter and unlikely to pass spontaneously through the cystic duct.

Diagnosis. Retained stone. Because of this patient's general condition, one would prefer not to do surgery at all unless the indications are pressing. However, this type of retained stone can re-initiate an outlet obstruction.

Operation. The cholecystostomy tube was removed and the tract dilated with the Hegar dilator. An infant-size sigmoidoscope was inserted and the stone visualized. It was crushed and the fragments washed out (Fig. 14-2). A cholecystogram 5 days later showed a normal extrahepatic biliary tree. A tube was removed and the patient was asymptomatic during a 6-week follow-up.

Epicrisis. Retained calculi in the gallbladder alone do not require formal reoperative laparotomy if an adequate sinus tract is present. The modalities for stone retrieval include 1) endoscopic identification and crushing, as in this instance, 2) irrigation in the prone position, 3) Dormia basket retrieval, 4) intravesical forefinger manipulation with a forceps guiding the intravesical sponge forceps, 5) continuous irrigation with one of the "dissolving agents."

In all instances the cholecystostomy tube should be reinserted after the manipulation and definitively removed only after a contrast study shows an unobstructed pathway.

21. CHOLECYSTODUODENAL FISTULA PERSISTING AFTER GALLSTONE ILEUS

History. An 84-year-old female was admitted with 3 days of abdominal pain. A pattern of intestinal obstruction and a pneumocholangiogram made the diagnosis of gallstone ileus. The surgeon performed an enterotomy with removal of a large stone from terminal ileum. He palpated another large stone in the gallbladder, and cholecystostomy was carried out, with removal of stone. The postoperative course was uneventful, but the problem now relates to the findings on the cholecystocholangiogram.

Findings. The patient is now asymptomatic. There is minimal drainage via the cholecystostomy tube, and no duodenal contents come through. The film shows a wide cholecystoduodenal fistula; the cystic duct is patent, there are no calculi, and the common duct empties.

Diagnosis. The problem is whether to surgically remove the gallbladder and close the fistula, or to leave the cholecystostomy tube in, or to remove the tube.

Epicritic. The vast majority of elderly patients tolerate this fistula without an infection or obstructive component if there are no stones in the extrahepatic system. This fistula appears to be valved, and there is no evidence for a duodenocholecystocutaneous spill. I suggested removing the cholecystostomy tube and intervening only if symptoms recur. The patient and family should be advised regarding the warning signs.

There is a much more aggressive opinion that

favors doing a primary biliary cleanout at the same time that the intestinal obstruction is managed. That approach puts at considerable risk a number of patients who do not require the operation. The greater number of elderly patients live out the fistula without further problems. Up to 1968, only 20 cases of simultaneous correction had been reported and morbidity was high. Many of these fistulas close after passing the stone.

22. PERSISTING SYMPTOMS DESPITE CHOLEDOCHODUODENOSTOMY

History. A 50-year-old female underwent cholecystectomy and common duct exploration 5 years ago. A postoperative T-tube cholangiogram revealed multiple retained stones in the duct. After the tube was removed, the patient became symptomatic. Choledocholithotomy and choledochoduodenostomy were done 4 years ago. The patient complains of epigastric pain and burning, intensifying with sleep. She has gained weight and is severely constipated, but has no fever or icterus.

Findings. A gastrointestinal series shows a hiatal hernia without reflux. The barium swallow reveals (see Fig. 18-11) a patent anastomosis between the duodenum and a large accessory hepatic duct (not the choledochus). The blood studies are normal. Esophagogastroduodenoscopy is normal.

Diagnosis. This patient is regarded as having functional complaints only because an anatomic diagnosis has not been made.

Epicrisis. In the absence of truly demonstrable biliary tract malfunction, no revisional surgery is advised. The symptoms, though distressing, and unrelieved by antiacids, choleretics, laxatives, and tranquilizers, have no, as yet, demonstrable treatable etiology. Therefore, I chose to observe and follow.

23. AMPULLARY DILATATION FOR RETAINED COMMON DUCT STONE

History. A 60-year-old female underwent an uneventful cholecystectomy for acute cholecystitis. The common duct was explored because the duct was dilated. There were no abnormal findings. No operative cholangiogram was available at 1:00 o'clock in the morning. A number 16 T tube was inserted.

Findings. The course was uneventful, and the patient tolerated T-tube clamping. Postoperative study showed a solitary retained 6-mm stone.

Operation. Rather than waiting for spontaneous passage or for basketing weeks later, the surgeon elected to withdraw the T tube and pass a red rubber catheter through the ampulla into the duodenum. The catheter was left that way for 48 hours, then pulled back into the duct, proximal to the stone. A continuous saline drip was started. A film taken 24 hours later showed no stone, and it is assumed to have passed into the duodenum.

Result. There was no bile leak, and the patient left the hospital 24 hours later.

Epicrisis. It is hard to be sure of cause and effect in this instance since spontaneous passage is likely. Catheter intubation is a simple method; and there is the advantage that it can be positioned at the same time that the diagnostic cholangiogram has demonstrated the problem.

24. MALFUNCTIONING CHOLEDOCHODUODENOSTOMY

History. A 47-year-old female underwent cholecystectomy and choledochoduodenostomy 20 years before in another country. She was well until 2 years ago. Since then, bouts of chills, fever, and jaundice every few months have been managed with antibiotics. She regards herself as invalided and worries about "my liver."

Findings. The patient is timid, subdued by her disability. There are no physical findings.

Diagnosis. Barium meal shows a choledochoduodenostomy with a 1-cm opening. The duct proximally is 1.6 cm wide and is full of stones. The liver radicles empty poorly and show evidence of serrations consistent with cholangitis. The Vaterian segment is patent.

Operation. Anastomotic stricture was found. The anastomosis was opened, the duct cleared out, and a revision done by increasing the stoma size to 3 cm. The common duct was opened to the carina and the duodenum brought well up into the hilus of the liver.

Result. The patient was well for 2 years, then lost to follow-up.

Epicrisis. The problem in this patient resolved down to an inadequate anastomosis, with proximal stasis and infection—an intolerable state that must be corrected.

The intraoperative choices are between a revision or a dismantling of the fistula with Roux-Y choledochojejunostomy. The fault did not lie in the indication for the procedure but in technical inadequacy or stricture for reasons that are not clear.

With present-day techniques, an attempt at endoscopic cleanout could have been attempted. Silvis (564) has reported on this. The duodenoscope is passed and the stasis calculi are manipulated and irrigated out. This has the limitation of not correcting the anastomotic stricturing, but it may be effective for a long period and it is certainly less likely to result in morbidity for the patient than the revisional procedure. Endoscopic surgery of the retained stone and anastomotic stricture is evolving. Its role in the management of ampullary fibrosis and the retained common duct stone is now being established (319).

25. SECONDARY OPERATION FOR A PSEUDOCALCULUS

History. A 60-year-old hypertensive, diabetic female underwent cholecystectomy and common bile duct exploration for calculous disease. The duct was 1.4 cm in width. Two large calculi were removed and a T tube inserted. A postoperative cholangiogram was interpreted as demonstrating a 0.7-cm solitary stone impacted in the suprasphincteric segment.

Diagnosis. Retained common duct stone. No repeat study was undertaken.

Operation. At a second operation no stone could be found with duct exploration and duodenostomy. The T tube was reinserted. The operative procedure went smoothly.

Result. On the third postoperative morning, the patient was found dead in bed. Autopsy demonstrated a massive acute myocardial infarct. The entire biliary tree was normal.

Epicrisis. I participated in this patient's care during my surgical residency. It is, I believe, fitting that I conclude this monograph with a consideration of this patient and the current viewpoint on management.

Because the common bile duct was significantly dilated and contained calculi, it would now be initially managed by choledochoduodenostomy rather than T-tube drainage.

The postoperative T-tube cholangiogram should have been repeated. I strongly suspect that the single film showed a phase of choledochal sphincter function of the type shown in Figure 19-10D, that there was, in fact, no retained stone, and that this was a pseudocalculus sign.

If a stone was present, then there was a reasonable chance for it to pass spontaneously. Secondary surgery was ill-advised at that time.

The lessons that revisional surgery have taught can be applied to the first operation as a total corrective procedure.

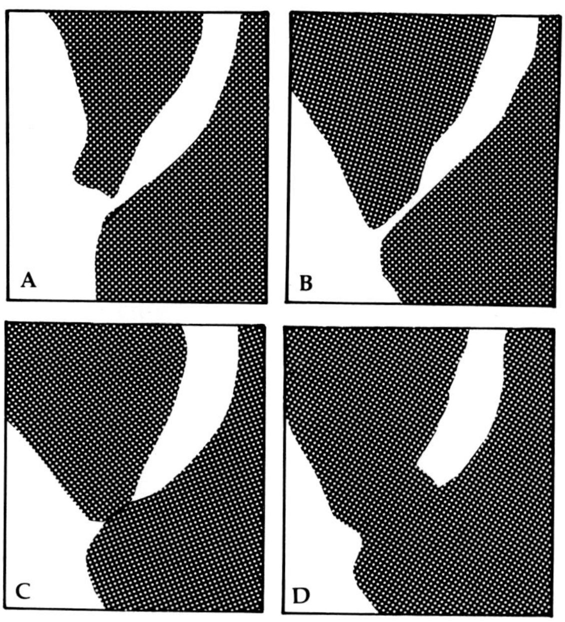

FIG. 19-10. Choledochal sphincter function as demonstrated in sequential views of the distal common duct as visualized by cine film cholangiography. **A.** Full diastolic filling. **B.** Early systolic phase. **C.** Mid systolic phase, simulating stricture or stenosis of the distal duct. **D.** Full systolic phase with a meniscus simulating a stone. This is the pseudocalculus phenomenon. All four phases are normal. This distal duct has no stone and is not strictured.

References

1. Acosta JM, Civantos F, Nardi GL, Castleman B: Fibrosis of the papilla of Vater. Surg Gynecol Obstet 124:787, 1967

2. Acosta JM, Ledesma CL: Gallstone Migration as a cause of acute pancreatitis. N Engl J Med 290: 484, 1974

3. Acosta JM, Nardi GL, Civantos F: Distal pancreatic duct inflammation. Ann Surg 172:256, 1970

4. Acosta JM, Rosario A, Nardi GL: Papillitis: Inflammatory disease of the ampulla of Vater. Arch Surg 92:354, 1966

5. Adams JT, Libertino JA, Schwartz SI: Significance of an elevated serum amylase. Surgery 63: 877, 1968

6. Adler GG: Choledochussteinbildung durch nichtresorbierbares nahtmaterial. Chirurg 11:508, 1971

7. Adlercreutz E: Corpus luteum hormone in the treatment of biliary dyskinesia and especially of the postcholecystectomy syndrome. Acta Med Scand 145:15, 1953

8. Ahlberg A: Silk ligature as a cause of choledocholithiasis after cholecystectomy. Acta Chir Scand 118:22, 1959

9. Albot G, Olivier C, Libauda H: Radiomanometric examination of the biliary ducts: experience with 418 cases. Gastroenterology 24:242, 1953

10. Alexander S, McAlpine FS: Cholecystectomy in the cardiac patient. Med Clin North Am 50:495, 1966

11. Alexander WM: The innervation of the biliary system. J Comp Neurol 72:357, 1940

12. Alonso–Lej F, Rever WB, Pessagno DJ: Congenital choledochal cyst with a report of 2 and an analysis of 94 cases (abstr). Int Surg 108:1, 1959

13. Altemeier WA, Gall EA, Culbertson WR, Inge WW: Sclerosing carcinoma of the intrahepatic (hilar) bile ducts. Surgery 60:191, 1966

14. Amdrup BM, Griffith CA: The effects of vagotomy upon biliary function in dogs. J Surg Res 10:209, 1970

15. Amdrup BM, Steinoe K, Bille–Brahe NE: An experimental study of the incidence of gastric ulcers in rabbits following truncal vagotomy, selective gastric vagotomy and highly selective gastric vagotomy. Acta Chir Scand 137:794, 1971

16. Anda B: Constipation in post-cholecystectomy syndrome. Acta Chir Scand 108:437, 1955

17. Andersen PT: Traumatic false aneurysm of the right hepatic artery: an unusual complication of cholecystectomy. Aust NZ J Surg 40:273, 1971

18. Anderson MC, Gregor WH: Papilloma of the ampulla of Vater. Am J Surg 102:865, 1961

19. Anderson MC, Mehn WH, Method HL: An evaluation of the common channel as a factor in pancreatic or biliary disease. Ann Surg 151:379, 1960

20. Anderson RP, Leand PM, Zuidema GD: Uses of the balloon-tipped catheter in biliary tract surgery. Am J Surg 117:55, 1969

21. Andresen AFR: Gastrointestinal allergy—its present status. South Med J 34:415, 1941

22. Applegate WV: Abdominal cutaneous nerve entrapment syndrome. Surgery 71:118, 1972

23. Archibald E: The experimental production of pancreatitis in animals as a result of resistance of the common duct sphincter. Surg Gynecol Obstet 28:529, 1919

24. Arianoff AA: Duodenopancreatic disorders associated with biliary diseases in the light of cholangiomanometry. Acta Gastroenterol Belg 23:188, 1960

25. Arianoff AA: Les papillo-oddites. Scalpel 25:3, 1969

26. Arianoff AA, Vielle G, DeWulf E: Réflexions sur la lithiase de la voie biliaire principale, primitive et residuelle. Acta Chir Belg 72:20, 1973

27. Arianoff AA, Vielle G, Van Reepinghen P: Considerations sur la chirurgie du sphincter d'oddi. Acta Chir Belg 67:779, 1968

28. Arner O, Hagberg S, Seldinger SI: Percutaneous transhepatic cholangiography in the diagnosis of posthepatic jaundice. Surgery 48:295, 1960

29. Babcock WW: Management of biliary diseases and their surgical complications. Pa Med 40: 604, 1937

30. Baggenstoss AH: Major duodenal papilla: variations of pathologic interest and lesions of the mucosa. Arch Pathol 26:853, 1938

31. Bainbridge FA, Dale HH: The contractile mechanism of the gallbladder and its extrinsic nervous control. J Physiol (Lond) 33:138, 1905–06

32. Bakes J: Die choledochopapilloskopie, nebst bermerkungen uber hepaticus drainage und dilation per papille. Arch Klin Chir 126:473, 1923

33. Bakes J: Zur drainagelosen gallenchirurgie und der methodischen dilatation der papille. Zentralbl Chir 2:1858, 1928

34. Ban JL, Hirose FM, Benfield JR: Foreign bodies of the biliary tract. Ann Surg 176:102, 1972

35. Barber H, Barber WH: Pancreatic heterotopia causing post-cholecystectomy symptoms and obstructive jaundice. Ann Surg 138:124, 1953

36. Barbosa JJC, Dockerty MB, Waugh JM: Pancreatic heterotopia. Review of the literature and report of 41 authenticated surgical cases, of which 25 were clinically significant. Surg Gynecol Obstet 82:527, 1946

37. Bardenheier JA III, Kaminski DL, Willman VL: Pancreatitis after biliary tract surgery. Am J Surg 116:773, 1968

38. Barge J, Marche C: The value of histologic diagnosis in patients with odditis. Ann Chir 2:321, 1966

39. Barker JR, Williams JA: The effect of cholecystectomy on oesophageal symptoms. Br J Surg 61:346, 1974

40. Bartlett MK: Retained and recurrent common duct stones. Am Surg 38:63, 1972

41. Bartlett MK, Waddell WR: Indications for common duct explorations, evaluation of 1000 cases. N Engl J Med 258:164, 1958

42. Beattie WG, Kuppusami M: Sphincteroplasty, an individualized operation: an anatomic study in autopsy material. Am J Surg 15:6, 1972

43. Beck K, Dischler W, Helms M, Kiani B, Sickinger K, Tenner R: Color Atlas of Laparoscopy. Stuttgart, Verlag, 1970

44. Beecher HK: Surgery as a placebo: a quantitative study of bias. JAMA 19:642, 1961

45. Beneventano TC, Schein CJ: The pseudocalculus sign in cholangiography. Arch Surg 98:731, 1968

46. Beneventano TC, Schein CJ: Pyloric sphincter incompetence in man—a physiologic variant. Gastroenterology 59:518, 1970

47. Bengolea AJ, Negri A: La maladie du choledoque terminal. Rev Chir Orthop 43:65, 1947

48. Benson KW: Dilatation of bile ducts and its relation to distress after cholecystectomy. Am J Dig Dis 7:1, 1940

49. Berci G: Endoscopy and radiology. In Endoscopy. New York, Appleton–Century–Crofts, 1976, p 222

50. Berci G: Laparoscopy in general surgery. In Endoscopy. New York, Appleton–Century–Crofts, 1976, p 382

51. Berci G, Morgenstern L, Shore JM, Shapiro S: A direct approach to the differential diagnosis of jaundice. Am J Surg 126:372, 1973

52. Berci G, Stevenson JK, Nyhus LM, Harkins HN, Majewska A, Smuckler E: The behavior of foreign bodies (imitated "gallstones") in the extrahepatic biliary system. Am J Surg 108:250, 1964

53. Berg J: Studien uber die function der gallenwege unter normalen und gewissen abnormen verhältnissen. Acta Chir Scand Suppl 2, 1922

54. Bergner LH: Internal biliary fistulas. Am J Gastroenterol 43:11, 1965

55. Bergvist A, Seldinger SI: Pancreatic reflux in operative cholangiography in relation to pre- and postoperative pancreatic affection. Acta Chir Scand 114:191, 1957

56. Berk JE: Post Cholecystectomy syndrome. Critical evaluation. Gastroenterology 34:1060, 1958

57. Berman LG, Dunn E, Straehley CJ: Survey of pancreatitis—Central New York Surgical Society. Gastroenterolgy 40:94, 1961.

58. Besancon F, Pironneau A, Lopes–Macedo L, Longuet YJ, Debray C: Technique nouvelle et simple d'exploration opératoire du canal choledoque: le débit-matre à flotteur perfusé sous pression constante et élevés. Arch Mal Dig 54: 59, 1965

59. Best RH: Incidence of liver stones associated with cholelithiasis and its clinical significance. Surg Gynecol Obstet 78:325, 1944

60. Beye HL: Conditions necessitating surgery following cholecystectomy: an analysis of 66 cases and a discussion of certain technical problems concerned in the removal of the gallbladder and in operations upon the common bile duct. Surg Gynecol Obstet 62:191, 1936

61. Birnstingl M: A study of pancreatography. Br J Surg 47:128, 1959

62. Bismuth H, Kuntziger H, Corlette MB: Cholangitis with acute renal failure. Ann Surg 181: 881, 1975

63. Bivens BA, Meeker WR, Weiss DL, Griffen WO: Carcinoma in situ of the gallbladder: a dilemma. South Med J 68:297, 1975

64. Blatherwick NH, Pattison AC: Acute pancreatitis complicating choledochal sphincterotomy. Am J Surg 88:129, 1954

65. Block MA, Brush EE, Ponka JL, Chepeau A: Stenosis of the sphincter of Oddi as a cause of jaundice. Arch Surg 76:88, 1958

66. Block MA, Brush BE, Ponka JL, Priest RH: The diagnosis of postcholescystectomy biliary tract stones. Arch Surg 73:694, 1956

67. Blumenberg RM, Powers SR Jr: Acute biliary pancreatitis: an experimental reappraisal of factors governing biliary reflux into the pancreas. Ann Surg 158:1058, 1963

68. Blumgart LH, Salmon MB, Cotton PB: Endoscopy and retrograde choledochopancreatography

in the diagnosis of the patient with jaundice. Surg Gynecol Obstet 138:565, 1974

69. Bode FF: Acute pancreatitis before and after biliary tract surgery. Chirurg 34:207, 1963

70. Bodvall B: Late results following cholecystectomy in 1930 cases and special studies on postoperative biliary distress. Acta Chir Scand Suppl 329:9, 1964

71. Bodvall B, Overgaard B: Cystic duct remnant after cholecystectomy: incidence studied by cholegraphy in 500 cases and significant in 102 reoperations. Ann Surg 163:382, 1966

72. Bodvall B, Overgaard B: Computer analysis of postcholecystectomy biliary tract symptoms. Surg Gynecol Obstet 124:723, 1967

73. Boecker W: Health resort therapy in gastrointestinal diseases and liver-biliary tract diseases. Internist (Berlin) 3:313, 1962

74. Boeckl O: Objectivierung der indikation zur sphincterotomie durch electromanometric. Langenbecks Arch Chir 325:1144, 1969

75. Bogoch A, Roth JLA, Bockus HL: The effects of morphine on serum amylase and lipase. Gastroenterology 26:697, 1954

76. Bohmig HJ, Fitsch A: Die bedeutung der cholangiometrie fur die intraoperative gallenwegsdiagnostik. Chirurg 37:446, 1966

77. Bohmig HJ, Fitsch A, Kux M, Stacher G: Indikationen und ergebnisse der transduodenalen sphincterotmie. Langenbecks Arch Chir 323:173, 1969

78. Bourke JB, Ritchie HD: The pressure profile of the sphincter of Oddi in man and the pig. Br J Surg 57:848, 1970

79. Bove P, De Oliveira M, Speranzini M: Intrahepatic lithiasis. Gastroenterology 44:251, 1963

80. Boyden EA: An analysis of the reaction of the human gallbladder to food. Anat Rec 40:147, 1928

81. Boyden EA: Hypertrophy of the sphincter choledochus. Surgery 10:567, 1941

82. Boyden EA: The anatomy of the choledochoduodenal junction in man. Surg Gynecol Obstet 104:641, 1957

83. Braasch JW: Segmental surgical disease of the liver. Ann Surg 168:110, 1968

84. Braasch JW, McCann JC: Normal luminal size of choledochoduodenal junction as determined by probe at choledochostomy. Surgery 62:258, 1967

85. Braasch JW, Preble HE: Unilateral hepatic duct obstruction. Ann Surg 158:17, 1963

86. Braasch JW, Whitcomb FF, Watkins E Jr, Maguire RR, Khazei A: Segmental obstruction of the bile duct. Surg Gynecol Obstet 134:915, 1972

87. Branch CD, Bailey OT, Zollinger R: Consequences of instrumental dilatation of papilla of Vater: an experimental study. Arch Surg 38:358, 1939

88. Bretino GG, Cole JW: Air contrast cholangiography: a preliminary report. Surgery 43:795, 1958

89. Brocks H: Choledoscopy versus cholangiography. Experiences of a 12 month trial. Acta Chir Scand 118:434, 1960

90. Brooks FP: Testing pancreatic function. N Engl J Med 286:300, 1972

91. Brooks PM, Cutforth R: Gallbladder disease and the heart. Med J Aust 1:340, 1973

92. Brown JO, Echenberg RJ: Mucosal reduplications associated with the ampullary portion of the major duodenal papilla in humans. Anat Rec 150:293, 1964

93. Brown MJ: The diseased cystic duct remnant. Arch Surg 79:304, 1959

94. Brown RB, Osborne DP: The reliability of palpation for common duct stones. Arch Surg 78:310, 1959

95. Brücke H: Débitmétrie et calibration de la papilla. Un procédé simple et cliniquement applicable. Rev Int Hepat 15:1009, 1965

96. Brücke H: Physikalische mesmethoden in der gallenchirurgie. Langenbecks Arch Chir 321: 334, 1968

97. Brush BE, Ponka JL, Damazo F, Whitcomb J: An evaluation of dilatation of the sphincter of Oddi. Arch Surg 706:766, 1955

98. Burden VG: Observations on the histologic and pathologic anatomy of the hepatic, cystic and common bile ducts. Ann Surg 82:584, 1925

99. Burhenne HJ: Nonoperative retained biliary tract stone extraction. A new roentgenologic technique. Am J Roentgenol Radium Ther Nucl Med 117:388, 1973

100. Burhenne HJ: Extracting retained biliary tract stones without reoperation. Contemp Surg 7: 27, 1975

101. Burhenne HJ: Complications of nonoperative extraction of retained common duct stones. Am J Surg 131:260, 1976

102. Burnett W, Gairns FW, Bacsich P: Some observations on the innervation of the extrahepatic biliary system in man. Ann Surg 159:8, 1964

103. Butsch JL: A technique for the prevention of hepatic duct disruption caused by the use of the Fogarty biliary catheter. Arch Surg 108:381, 1974

104. Butsch JL, Ali MV, Nolan JP: Serendipitous passage of a common duct stone following ampullary cannulation. Arch Surg 110:433, 1975

105. Byrne JJ, Melekatos CJ: Foreign bodies in the common duct. Arch Surg 71:91, 1955

106. Camishion RC, Goldstein F: Partial, noncalculus cystic duct obstruction (Cystic duct syndrome). Surg Clin North Am 47:1107, 1967

107. Capper WM: External choledochoduodenostomy. An evaluation of 125 cases. Br J Surg 49: 292, 1961

108. Capper WM, Butler TJ, Kilby JO, Gibson MJ: Gallstones gastric secretion and flatulent dyspepsia. Lancet 1:413, 1967

109. Caroli J: La radiomanométrie biliaire. Sem Hop Paris 22:1985, 1946

110. Caroli J: Les icteres par retention. Paris, Masson et cie, 1956

111. Caroli J, Gilles E: La radiomanométric biliaire: étude technique. Sem Hop Paris 44:1278, 1945

112. Caroli J, Gilles E: Cholecystography during pain crisis in biliary dyskinesias (especially in migraine). Arch Mal Appau Dig 40:883, 1951

113. Caroli J, Mercadier M: Les Dyskinésies Biliaires. Paris, Vigot, 1948

114. Carter RF, Saypol GM: Transabdominal cholangiography. JAMA 148:253, 1952

115. Casal MA: Cholangiografia laparoscopia y curgia des las visas biliares. Prensa Med Argent 40:1484, 1953

116. Catt PB, Hogg DF, Clunie JA, Hardie IR: Retained biliary calculi: removal by a simple nonoperative technique. Ann Surg 180:247, 1974

117. Cattell RB, Braasch JW: Secondary operations on the biliary tract. Lahey Clin Bull 6:162, 1959

118. Cattell RB, Braasch JW, Kahn F: Polypoid epithelial tumors of the bile ducts. N Engl J Med 226:57, 1962

119. Cattell RB, Colcock BP: Fibrosis of the sphincter of Oddi. Ann Surg 137:797, 1953

120. Cattell RB, Colcock BP, Pollack JL: Stenosis of sphincter of Oddi. N Engl J Med 256:429, 1957

121. Cattell RB, Colcock BP, Pollack JL: Stenosis of the sphincter of Oddi. In Surgical Practice of the Lahey Clinic. Philadelphia, W. B. Saunders, 1962, pp 595–603

122. Cattell RB, Pyrtek LJ: Premalignant lesions of the ampulla of Vater. Surg Gynecol Obstet 90: 21, 1950

123. Cattell RB, St Ville J: Amputation neuromas of the biliary tract. Arch Surg 83:242, 1961

124. Charcot JM: Thesis: Leçons sur les maladies du foie des voies filiaires et des reins. Paris, Faculté de Médecine de Paris, 1877

125. Cherrick GR, Kuehner CR, McCabe R: Megacholedochus. A condition arising from long standing biliary tract obstruction in the patient with cholecystectomy. Am J Surg 115:845, 1968

126. Chetlin SH, Elliott DW: Biliary bacteremia. Arch Surg 102:303, 1971

127. Chetlin SH, Elliott DW: Preoperative antibiotics in biliary surgery. Arch Surg 107:319, 1973

128. Childs P: Dietary fat, dyspepsia, diarrhoea and diabetes. Br J Surg 59:48, 1972

129. Chu PT: Benign neoplasm of the extrahepatic bile tract. Arch Pathol 50:84, 1950

130. Classen M, Demling L: Endoskopische sphinkerotomie der papilla Vateri und steinextraktion aus dem ductus choledochus. Dtsch Med Wochenschr 99:496, 1974

131. Classen M, Hellwig H, Rosch W: Anatomy of the pancreatic duct. A duodenoscopic radiological study. Endoscopy 5:14, 1973

132. Classen M, Schwamberger K: Reintervention an den gallenwegen internistische diagnostik. Chirurg 45:145, 1974

133. Cohn I Jr, Cotlar AM, Atik M, Lumpkin WM, Hudson TL, Werenette GJ: Bile peritonitis. Ann Surg 152:827, 1960

134. Cohn R, Hibner R: The cystic duct remnant. Am J Surg 98:296, 1959

135. Colcock BP, Perey B: Exploration of the common bile duct. Surg Gynecol Obstet 118:20, 1964

136. Cole GJ: The implications of bile in the stomach. Gut 10:864, 1969

137. Cole WH, Grove WJ: Persistence of symptoms following cholecystectomy with special reference to anomalies of the ampulla of Vater. Ann Surg 136:73, 1952

138. Cole WH, Harridge WH: Disappearance of stone shadows in postoperative cholangiograms. JAMA 164:238, 1957

139. Coley GM, Howes EL: Effects of injury to the ampulla of Vater on the biliary tract. An experimental study. Am J Surg 108:794, 1964

140. Comfort MW, Walters W: Intermittent jaundice due to neuroma of cystic and common bile ducts. Ann Surg 93:1142, 1931

141. Cooperman AM, Dickson ER, Re Mine WH: Changing concepts in the surgical treatment of gallstone ileus: a review of 15 cases with emphasis on diagnosis and treatment. Ann Surg 167:377, 1968

142. Copher GH, Illingworth CFW: Experimental study of factor of biliary stasis in production of gall stones. Surg Gynecol Obstet 46:658, 1928

143. Corbitt JD Jr, Levin JM, Walker LG Jr, Haynes CD: Relationship between biliary tract distention and the blood flow in the aorta and the right coronary and renal arteries. Am J Surg 120:14, 1970

144. Corlette MB, Bismuth H: Bibliobiliary fistula, a trap in the surgery of cholelithiasis. Arch Surg 110:384, 1975

145. Cotton PB: Cannulation of the papilla of Vater by endoscopy and retrograde cholangiopancreatography (ERCP). Gut 13:1014, 1972

146. Cotton PB, Chapman M, Whiteside CG, LeQuesne LP: Duodenoscopic papillotomy and gallstone removal. Br J Surg 63:709, 1976

147. Cowie AGA, Clark CG: The lithogenic effect of vagotomy. Br J Surg 59:365, 1972

148. Crain RC, Walsh EL; Effect of an acute chemical duodenitis on the emptying time of the gallbladder. Surg Gynecol Obstet 55:753, 1931

149. Crema A, Berte F, Benzi G, Frigo GM: The responses of the sphincterial areas of the extrahepatic biliary tract to the stimulation and parasympathetic nerves. Acta Physiol (Lat Am) 14:24, 1964

150. Crispin JS, Choi YW, Wiseman DGH, Gillespie DJ, Lind JF: A direct manometric study of the canine choledochoduodenal junction. Arch Surg 101:215, 1970

151. Crook NJ, Smith DC, McAllister RA, MacKay C: The effect of cholecystectomy on the size of the bile salt pool in the dog. Br J Surg 58: 867, 1971

152. Cullen ML, Reese HL: Myocardial circulatory changes measured by clearance of a Na–24. Effect of common duct distention on myocardial circulation. J Appl Physiol 5:281, 1952

153. Custer MD Jr, Clore JN Jr: Source of error in operative cholangiography. Arch Surg 100:664, 1970

154. Dadgar–Dehkordi I: Uber den wert der papillenplastik. Ergebnisse der nachuntersuchung der in den jahren 1956 bis 1965 operierten patienten. Bruns Beitr Klin Chir 216:256, 1968

155. Dahl–Iversen E, Sorenson H, Westengaard E: Pressure measurements in the biliary tract in patients after cholecystolithotomy and in patients with dyskinesia. Acta Chir Scand 114:181, 1958

156. Dale WA: Splanchnic block in the treatment of acute pancreatitis. Surgery 32:605, 1952

157. Dalhamn T: Biliary motility studies. Arch Intern Med 126:424, 1970

158. Dancer JT, Hawley WD, DuVal MK: The intrinsic contractile activity of the duodenum. Arch Surg 88:984, 1964

159. Dardik H, Schein CJ, Warren A, Gliedman ML: Adrenergic receptors in the canine biliary tract. Surg Gynecol Obstet 128:823, 1969

160. Dardinsky VJ: Inflammatory adenomatoid hyperplasia of the major duodenal papilla in man. Am J Pathol 7:519, 1931

161. Darnborough A, Geffen N: Drip infusion cholangiography. Br J Radiol 39:827, 1966

162. Davidson CL, Hirsch C, Angrist A: Survey of common duct stones in clinical necropsy cases. Am J Surg 78:486, 1949

163. Davis JL, Mulligan FD, Cameron JL: Septic complications following endoscopic retrograde cholangiopancreatography. Surg Gynecol Obstet 140:365, 1975

164. Degenshein GA: Choledochoduodenostomy: an 18 year study of 175 consecutive cases. Surgery 76:319, 1974

165. Degenshein GA, Hurwitz A: The techniques of side-to-side choledochoduodenostomy. Surgery 61:972, 1967

166. DelGuercio LRM: Savings through the direct approach to jaundice. Am J Surg 127:157, 1974

167. DelValle D Jr, Donovan R: Choledoco-odditis retractil cronica; concepto clinco-quirugico. Arch Argent Enferm Appar Dig 1:141, 1926

168. Del Valle D: Patologia y Chirurgica de Esfinter de Oddi. Buenos-Aires, El Ateneo, 1939

169. De Santis C, Tagliaferri G: Ampullary biopsy: A critical appraisal based on a histological study of the normal papilla of Vater. Br J Surg 55:250, 1968

170. DeWeese JA: Cholecystoscopy. NY J Med 52:2805, 1952

171. DiDio LJA, Boyden EA: The choledochoduodenal junction in the horse—a study of the musculature around the ends of the bile and pancreatic ducts in a species without a gallbladder. Anat Rec 143:61, 1962

172. Dineen R: Importance of the route of infection in experimental biliary tract obstruction. Surg Gynecol Obstet 119:1001, 1964

173. Domelloff L, Schersten T: Prognosis of early post-cholecystectomy distress. Acta Chir Scand 134:291, 1968

174. Doran FSA: The sites to which pain is referred from the common bile duct in man, and its implication for the theory of referred pain. Br J Surg 54:599, 1967

175. Doubilet H, Colp R: Resistance of the sphincter of Oddi in the human. Surg Gynecol Obstet 64:622, 1937

176. Douglas TC, Lawes RB, Mehn WH: Operating room cholangiography errors in technique and interpretation. Arch Surg 68:427, 1954

177. Dowdy GS, Olin WG, Shelton EL, Waldron GW: Benign tumors of the extrahepatic bile ducts. Arch Surg 85:503, 1962

178. Dreiling DA: The postcholecystectomy syndrome. Am J Dig Dis 7:603, 1962

179. Dreiling DA, Janowitz HD, Perrier CV: Pancreatic Inflammatory Disease. A Physiologic Approach. New York, Harper & Row, 1964

180. Drouin JP: Cholecystectomy with routine sphincteroplasty. Can J Surg 7:367, 1964

181. Dubecz S, Nagy T: Significance of liver biopsy in the treatment of cholelithiasis and symptoms after cholecystectomy. Orv Hetil 102:1791, 1961

182. Duff JH, Salvian AG, Finley R: The incidence of secondary common bile duct exploration. Surg Gynecol Obstet 139:723, 1974

183. Eaton SB Jr, Benedict KT, Ferrucci JT: Hypotonic duodenography. Radiol Clin North Am 8:125, 1970

184. Eaton SB Jr, Wirtz RD, Ten Eyck JR, Richards JC: Iatrogenic liver injury resulting from ductal instrumentation with the Fogarty biliary balloon catheter. Radiology 100:581, 1971

185. Edholm P, Jonsson G: Bile duct stones related to age and duct width. Acta Chir Scand 124:75, 1962

186. Edlund Y, Christoffersson E: Alkaline phosphatase and transaminases in serum and hepatic duct bile in patients with normal or blocked biliary flow. Acta Hepatosplenol (Stuttg), 14:230, 1967

187. Edlund Y, Jacbsson B: Section of the Sphincter of Oddi in pathological conditions of the choledocho-duodenal junction. Acta Chir Scand 114:262, 1957

188. Edlund Y, Kewenter J: Isolated hyperphosphatasemia in hepatobiliary disease. Acta Chir Scand 123:322, 1962

189. Eiseman B, Brown WH, Virabutr S, Gottesfeld S: Sphincterotomy—an evaluation of its physiologic rationale. Arch Surg 79:294, 1959

190. Ekdahl PH: On late distress following biliary tract operations. Acta Chir Scand 106:339, 1953

191. Ekeland A, Ofstad E, Stiris G: Hemobilia pseudoaneurysm in the gastroduodenal artery fol-

lowing choledochotomia. Acta Chir Scand 140: 422, 1974

192. Elfving G: Gallenblasen ohne steine. Langenbecks Arch Chir 325:572, 1969

193. Elliott DW, Williams RD, Zollinger RM: Alterations in pancreatic resistance to bile and pathogenesis of acute pancreatitis. Ann Surg 146:669, 1957

194. Elman R, McMaster PD: The physiological variations in resistance to bile flow to the intestine. J Exp Med 44:151, 1926

195. Engstrom J, Groth CG, Lundh G, Lonnqvist B: Infectious complications after surgery for biliary calculus. Acta Chir Scand 138:357, 1972

196. Falkmer S, Sjostrom B: Histological changes in the liver in diseases of the biliary tract. Gastroenterologia 91:16, 1959

197. Fegiz G, Tonelli F: Comparative results of papillostomy and choledocho-duodenostomy for lithiasis of the common bile duct. Surgery Italy 4:54, 1974

198. Ferrante WA, Maxfield WS: Comparison of diagnostic accuracy of liver scans, liver function tests and liver biopsies. South Med J 61: 1255, 1968

199. Fevery J, Tanghe W, Kerremans R, Desmet V, De Groote J: Congenital dilatation of the intrahepatic bile ducts associated with the development of amyloidosis. Gut 13:604, 1972

200. Fischer MG, Geffen A, Ozoktay S: Percutaneous transhepatic cholangiography. Am J Gastroenterol 60:557, 1973

201. Flament JB: Les Diverticules Muqueux de la Fenêtre Duodenale. Paris, Impressions, 1973

202. Florcken H: Gallenblasenregeneration mit steinrecidiv nach cholecystectomie. Dtsch Zentralbl Chir 113:604, 1912

203. Foley FE, Kilpatrick JT, Crabtree SF: Chronic recurrent pancreatitis due to injury to the duct of Santorini: a complication of subtotal gastrectomy. Ann Surg 144:87, 1956

204. Franksson C: Innervation of the common bile duct duodenal junction from a surgical point of view. Acta Chir Scand 96:163, 1947

205. Friedman GD: The relationship between coronary heart disease and gallbladder disease. A critical review. Ann Intern Med 68:222, 1968

206. Fritsch A: The effect of transecting the sphincter of Oddi on the bile flow and function of the papilla of Vater. Klin Med Wien 21:49, 1966

207. Fritsch A: Erfahrungen mit der sphincterotomie bei 634 fällen seit 1956. Langenbecks Arch Chir 325:590, 1969

208. Fritz ME, Brooks FP: Control of bile flow in the cholecystectomized dog. Am J Physiol 204: 825, 1963

209. Fuchsig P, Hartmann G: Zur kenntnis gutartiger stenosen der papilla Vateri. Wien Med Wochenschr 108:937, 1958

210. Gaensler EA, McGowan JM: Activity of some newer spasmolytic agents on the biliary tract of man. J Pharmacol Exp Ther 99:304, 1950

211. Gaisford WD: Peritoneoscopy: a valuable technic for surgeons. Am J Surg 130:671, 1975

212. Galambos A: True intrahepatic lithiasis. Am J Gastroenterol 21:54, 1954

213. Gambill EE: Pancreatitis. St Louis, CV Mosby, 1973

214. Gambill EE, Mason HL: One hour value for urinary amylase in 96 patients with pancreatitis. JAMA 186:24, 1963

215. Gardner B, Dennis CR, Patti J: Current status of heparin dissolution of gallstones. Experimental and clinical observations. Am J Surg 130:293, 1975

216. Garlock HA, Hurwitt ES: Cystic duct stump syndrome. Surgery 29, 883, 1951

217. Gerdes MM, Boyden EA: The role of emptying of the human gallbladder in pregnancy. Surg Gynecol Obstet 66:145, 1938

218. Gertz T: Om resultaterne af galdestensoperationer. København, Steen Hasselbachs, 1946

219. Gessner FB, Nykvist WE, Zinner NR: Pressure pulse reflections as a means of diagnosing obstructions in the lower urinary tract. J Biomech 4:391, 1971

220. Giermann H, Holle G: Stereoskopische und mikroskopische untersuchungen zur pathologie des schleimhautreliefs und klappenapparates der papilla Vateri. Acta Hepatosplenol 8:189, 1961

221. Gilman PK, Gibbons JC, Kaplan MS: Unusual diagnostic aspects and current management of pancreatic pseudocysts. Am Surg 40:326, 1974

222. Ginsberg AL: Very high levels of SGOT and LDH in patients with extrahepatic biliary tract obstruction. Am J Dig Dis 15:803, 1970

223. Ginzburg L, Geffen A, Friedman JH: Pseudoobstruction following postcholedochotomy cholangiography. Ann Surg 166:83, 1967

224. Glenn F: Pain in biliary tract disease. Surg Gynecol Obstet 122:495, 1966

225. Glenn F: Postcholecystectomy choledocholithiasis. Surg Gynecol Obstet 134:249, 1972

226. Glenn F, McSherry CK: Secondary abdominal operations for symptoms following biliary tract surgery. Surg Gynecol Obstet 121:979, 1965

227. Glenn F, McSherry CK: Biliary tract obstruction and duodenal diverticula. Surg Gynecol Obstet 130:829, 1970

228. Glenn F, Moody F: Acute obstructive suppurative cholangitis. Surg Gynecol Obstet 113:265, 1961

229. Gliedman ML, Bolooki H, Rosen RG: Acute pancreatitis. Curr Prob Surg, Aug, 1970

230. Glystorff H, Faber H: Choledochus changes after cholcystectomy. (Pre- and post-operative examination of 400 patients). Acta Chir Scand 125:499, 1963

231. Goinard P, Plessier G: Exploration pharmacodynamique peroperation du sphincter d'Oddi. J Chir (Paris) 78:507, 1959

232. Goor DA, Ebert PA: Anomalies of the biliary tree. Arch Surg 104:302, 1972

233. Gothlin J, Mansoor M, Tranberg KG: Combined percutaneous transhepatic cholangiography (PTC) and selective visceral angiography (SVA) in obstructive jaundice. Am J Roentgenol Radium Ther Nucl Med 117:419, 1973

234. Gots RE, Zuidema GD: Dilatation of the intrahepatic biliary ducts in a patient with a choledochal cyst. Am J Surg 119:726, 1970

235. Grace RH, Peckar VG: The value of operative cholangiography using an image intensifier and television monitor. Br J Surg 55:933, 1968

236. Grage TB, Lober PH, Imanoglu K, Wangenstein OH: Stenosis of the sphincter of Oddi: a clinical pathologic review of fifty cases. Surgery 48:304, 1960

237. Grassberger A, Seyss R: Uber veranderungen der papilla Vateri. Bruns Beitr Klin Chir 200: 446, 1960

238. Gray HK, Sharpe WS: Biliary dyskinesia: the role played by a remnant of the cystic duct. Mayo Clin Proc 19:164, 1944

239. Greissman H: Erfahrungen mit die choledochoskopie. Bruns Beitr Klin Chir 195:251, 1957

240. Griffen WO, Schaefer JW, Schindler S, Hyde G, Bryant LR: Ampullary obstruction by benign duodenal polyps. Arch Surg 97:444, 1968

241. Gunnarson E: The bile ducts of cholecystectomized patients with and without dyskinesia before and after morphine injection. Acta Radiol [Diagn] (Stockh) 45:298, 1956

242. Haff RC, Torma MJ: Oddi sphincteroplasty in the management of complicated biliary and pancreatic disease. Am J Surg 129:509, 1975

243. Haff RC, Wise L, Ballinger WF: Biliary enteric fistulas. Surg Gynecol Obstet 135:84, 1971

244. Hagerstrand I, Norden JG, Ohlsson EG: Histochemical studies of hepatic enzymes in dogs subjected to lobar bile duct obstruction. Acta Chir Scand 140:391, 1974

245. Hagstrom WM Jr, France TD, Anderson MC: A comparison of pancreatic and biliary pressures recorded simultaneously in man. Northwest Med 35:311, 1961

246. Hallberg D, Jonson G, Sadersjoo B: The icteric index and the alkaline phosphatase activity in biliary obstruction—the influence of the gallbladder. Acta Chir Scand 119:29, 1960

247. Hallenberg HG, Eikner WC, Spings C: Cholecystoscopy. Surgery 2:37, 1937

248. Halsted WS: Contributions to the surgery of the biliary passages, especially of the common bile duct. Johns Hopkins Med J 4:1, 1900

249. Ham JM, Sorby W: Measurement of stoma size following choledochoduodenostomy by transduodenal cholangiography. Br J Surg 60:940, 1973

250. Hand BH: Anatomical study of the choledochoduodenal area. Br J Surg 223:486, 1963

251. Hardy JD: Some lesions of the biliary tract. Idiopathic retroperitoneal fibrosis and other problems. Am J Surg 103:457, 1962

252. Harting K: Uber die feinere innervation der extrahepatischen gallenwege. Z Zellforsch Mikrosk Anat 12:518, 1931

253. Hayes MA, Goldenberg IS, Bishop CC: The developmental basis for bile duct anomalies. Surg Gynecol Obstet 107:447, 1958

254. Hays DM, Glenn F: Fate of the cholecystostomy patient. J Am Geriatr Soc 3:21, 1955

255. Heimburger IL, King RD; Surgery and gallstones—from helplessness to triumph. Surgery 57:325, 1965

256. Hellstrom HR, Perez–Stable EC: Retroperitoneal fibrosis with disseminated vasculitis and intrahepatic sclerosing cholangitis. Am J Med 40:184, 1966

257. Hendrickson WF: Study of the musculature of the entire extrahepatic biliary system, including that of the duodenal portion of the common bile duct and of the sphincter. Johns Hopkins Med J 9/10:221, 1898

258. Herzog KH: Indikation and technik der choledochoduodenostomie. Chirurg 37:486, 1966

259. Hess W: Die primare stenosierende papillitis. Helv Chir Acta 21:433, 1954

260. Hess W: Operative Cholangiographic Tecknik Diagnostik Praxis. Stuttgart, Georg Thieme Verlag, 1955

261. Hess W: Cholangiographische befunde beim beschwerden nach cholecystektomie. Langenbecks Arch Chir 282:856, 1955

262. Hess W: Die Erkrangungen der Gallenwege und des Pankreas. Stuttgart, George Thieme Verlag, 1961

263. Hess W: Die schlecht functionierende choledochoduodenostomie. Ber Proc Surg Int Coll 14: 545, 1965

264. Hess W: Diagnosis of papillitis and stenosis. Dtsch Med Wochenschr 90:2289, 1965

265. Hicken NF, McAllister AJ, Call DW: the problem of hepatolithiasis. A study of thirty five personal cases. Am Surg 19:695, 1953

266. Hicken NF, McAllister AJ, Call DW: Residual choledochal stones: etiology and complications in 110 cases. Arch Surg 68:643, 1954

267. Hicken NF, McAllister AJ, Franz BJ, Crowder E: Does the removal of the gallbladder produce functional changes of the sphincter of Oddi and the choledochus? Am Surg 17:598, 1951

268. Hicken NF, White LB, Coray OB: Incomplete removal of the cystic duct as a factor in producing postcholecystectomy complications. Surgery 21:309, 1947

269. Hill HA: Functional disorders of the extrahepatic biliary system: biliary dyssynergia or dyskinesia. Radiology 29:261, 1937

270. Hill MJ, McColl I: Ultrasonic detection of choledochlithiasis. Nature (Lond) 190:627, 1961

271. Hinchey EJ, Couper CE: Acute obstructive suppurative cholangitis. Am J Surg 117:62, 1969

272. Hodes PJ, Pendergrass EP, Winston NJ: Pancreatic, ductal and Vaterian neoplasms: their roentgen manifestations. Radiology 62:1, 1954

273. Hoff RC, Torma MJ: Oddi sphincterplasty in the management of complicated biliary and pancreatic disease. Am J Surg 129:509, 1975

274. Hoffman E: Acute pancreatitis due to a Peri–Vaterine. Arch Surg 78:177, 1959

275. Hofmann AF, Thistle JL: Chenodeoxycholic acid: the Mayo Clinic experience. Hosp Prac 41, Aug, 1974

276. Hofmeister V: Die methodische dilatation der papilla duodeni und die choledochoduodenaldrainage. Zentralbl Chir 40:5, 1913

277. Holle G: Die bauprinzipien der Vater'schen papille und ihre funktionelle bedeutung unter normalen und krankhaften bedeutung. Ger Med Mon, April, 1960, 648

278. Hollinshead WH: The lower part of the common bile duct: a review. Surg Clin North Am 37:939, 157

279. Hopton D, White TT: Effect of hepatic and celiac vagal stimulation on common bile-duct pressure. Am J Dig Dis 16:1095, 1971

280. Howard JM, Jordan GL Jr: Relapsing pancreatitis secondary to choledochlithiasis. Arch Surg 73:960, 1956

281. Huang T, Bass JA, Williams RD: The significance of biliary pressure in cholangitis. Arch Surg 98:629, 1969

282. Huchzermeyer H, Seidenabel KH, Eickmeier C, Burgmann W: Zum problem der choledochusdilatation bei gallenblasenerkrankungen und nach cholezystektomie. Munch Med Wochenschr 115:1831, 1973

283. Hughes ESR: Recurrent and residual stones in the common bile duct. Br J Surg 43:198, 1955

284. Hughes L, LoCurcio SB, Edmunds R, Finby N: The common duct after cholecystectomy. JAMA 197:247, 1966

285. Hunt T: Cholagogues and choleretics. Practitioner 206:51, 1971

286. Hunter FM, Akdamar K, Sparks RD, Reed RJ, Braun CL: Congenital dilatation of the intrahepatic bile ducts. Am J Med 40:188, 1966

287. Hurvitz SA, Averbook BD, Hurvitz RJ: Pancreatitis with biliary disease. Arch Surg 86:664, 1963

288. Ibach JR, Hume HA, Erb WH: Cholecystectomy in the aged. Surg Gynecol Obstet 126:523, 1968

289. Ikeda S, Okada Y: Classification of choledochoduodenal fistula diagnosed by duodenal fiberscopy and its etiological significance. Gastroenterology 69:130, 1975

290. Illiescu G: Vagotomia selective hepatica. Chirurgia (Bucur) 22:981, 1973

291. Imamoglu K, Perry JF, Wangensteen OH: Experimental production of gallstones by incomplete stricture of the terminal common bile duct. Surgery 42:623, 1957

292. Ingelfinger FJ: Digestive disease as a national problem. Gastroenterology 55:102, 1968

293. Iser JH, Dowling H, Mok HYL, Bell GD: Chenodeoxycholic acid treatment of gallstones. N Engl J Med 293:378, 1975

294. Ishioka T: Electromyographic study of the choledochoduodenal junction and duodenal wall muscle. Tohoku J Exp Med 70:73, 1959

295. Ivy AC: Motor dysfunction of the biliary tract. An analytical and critical consideration. Am J Roentgenol 57:1, 1947

296. Jacobi M, Zuckerman IC, Kogut B: Studies on human biliary physiology effect of food factors and orally administered bile on rate and quantity of bile secretion. Am J Dig Dis 6:270, 1939

297. Jacobsson B: Determination of pressure in the common bile duct at and after operation. Acta Chir Scand 113:483, 1957

298. Jacobsson B: The morphology of the choledochoduodenal junction and the functional properties of the extra-hepatic biliary ducts in cholecystectomized patients. Rev Int Hepat 15: 939, 1965

299. Jacobsson B, Kjellander J, Rosengren B: Cholangiovenous reflux: an experimental study. Acta Chir Scand 123:316, 1962

300. Jacobsson B, Lanner LO, Radberg C: The dynamics of the choledochoduodenal junction studied by cineroentgenography during pressure recording. Acta Chir Scand 113:488, 1957

301. Jacobsson B, Lanner LO, Radberg C: The dynamic variability of the choledochopancreaticoduodenal junction. A roentgen cinematographic investigation. Acta Radiol [Diagn] (Stockh) 52: 269, 1959

302. Jansen W: Intraduodenal cyst containing bile and stones: report of a case with recurrent pancreatitis. Gastroenterology 58:397, 1970

303. Jelinek R: Komplikationen and todesursachen nach der sphincterotomie. Langenbecks Arch Klin Chir 325:594, 1969

304. Jennings WK, Ortega LR, Braslow L: Relationship of postcholecystectomy disturbances to bacterial sensitivity. Surg Gynecol Obstet 95: 439, 1952

305. Joannides M: The mechanics of eructation. A hitherto undescribed function of the diaphragm. J Thorac Cardiovasc Surg 380:1932–1933

306. Johnson AG: Pyloric function and gall-stone dyspepsia. Br J Surg 59:449, 1972

307. Johnson AG: Cholecystectomy and gallstone dyspepsia. Ann R Coll Surg Engl 56:69, 1975

308. Johnson AG, Rains AJH: Choledochoduodenostomy: a reappraisal of its indications based on a study of 64 patients. Br J Surg 59:277, 1972

309. Johnson G Jr, Glenn F: Multiple liver abscesses following biliary tract surgery. Ann Surg 140: 227, 1958

310. Jones AA, Smith LL: A reappraisal of sphincteroplasty (not sphincterotomy). Surgery 71: 565, 1972

311. Jonsson G: Relative diagnostic significance of bilirubin and phosphatase values in the postcholecystectomy syndrome. Acta Chir Scand 115:299, 1958

312. Joseph WL, Fonkalsrud EW, Longmire WP: Cystic dilatation of common bile duct in adults. Arch Surg 91:468, 1965

313. Judd ES, Burden VG: Internal biliary fistula. Ann Surg 81:305, 1925

314. Kaden VG, Howard JM, Doubleday LC: Cholecystographic studies during and immediately following acute pancreatitis. Surgery 38:1082, 1955

315. Kaiser E: Postoperative veraenderungenden normalen und des pathologischen choledochus. Helv Chir Acta 5:25, 1958

316. Kaiser E: Das postcholecystektomie syndrom. J Int Coll Surg 31:80, 1959

317. Kantor JL, Marks JA: A study of intestinal flatulence. Ann Intern Med 3:403, 1929

318. Kasugai T, Kuno N, Kobayashi S, Hattori K: Endoscopic pancreatocholangiography. Gastroenterology 63:217, 1972

319. Kawai K, Nakajima M, Kimoto K, Sugawara K, Fukumoto K: Endoscopic sphincterotomy of the ampulla of Vater. Endoscopy 7:30, 1975

320. Keclik M, Fric P, Smat V, Friedberger V: Chronic pancreatitis and choledochoduodenal anastomosis. Gut 9:311, 1968

321. Keclik M, Kolominsky J: Spa treatment of cholelithiasis. Practitioner 201:474, 1968

322. Kehr H: Die Praxis der Gallenwege Chirurgie, Vol 1, 2. Munchen, Lehmann, 1913

323. Keighley MRB, Lister DM, Jacobs SI, Giles GR: Hazards of surgical treatment due to microorganisms in the bile. Surgery 75:578, 1974

324. Kern E: Operationstaktik der gallenwegsrevision. Langenbecks Arch Klin Chir 313:264, 1965

325. Kirk J: Observations on the histology of the choledochoduodenal junction and papilla duodeni, with particular reference to the ampulla of Vater and sphincter of Oddi. J Anat 78:118, 1944

326. Kirsteins A, Govostis MC, Van Prohaska J: Benign tumors of the ampulla of Vater. Arch Surg 67:708, 1953

327. Kjaergaard S: Choledocho-duodenostomy in postoperative dyskinesia. Acta Chir Scand 104: 87, 1952

328. Klatskin G: Adenocarcinoma of the hepatic duct at its bifurcation within the porta hepatis. An unusual tumor with distinctive clinical and pathological features. Am Med 38:241, 1965

329. Koch H, Glassen M, Schaffner O: Endoscopic papillotomy. Scand J Gastroenterol 10:441, 1975

330. Koch RL, Gorder JL: Bile-blood fistula: a complication of percutaneous transhepatic cholangiography. Radiology 93:67, 1969

331. Kocher T: Cholelithothripsie bei choledochusverschluss mit volliger genesung. Basel, Cor–Bl f schweiz Aerzte, 8:577, 1878

332. Kocher T: Ein fall von choledochoduodenosto nia interna wegen gallensteines. Korrespondenz-blatt fur Arzte 7:193, 1895

333. Kocher T: Textbook of Operative Surgery, Vol. 2, 3rd ed. New York, Macmillan, 1911

334. Kock NG, Kewenter J, Jacobsson B: The influence of the motor activity of the duodenum on the pressure in the common bile duct. Ann Surg 160:950, 1964

335. Kourias B: Reintervention an den ableitenden gallenwegen diagnostik, indikation, operative methodik. Chirurg 39:283, 1968

336. Kourias B, Papacharalampous NX: Die chronische pankreatitis als begleiterkrankung des gallensteinleidens. Chirurg 37:11, 1966

337. Kourias B, Tierris EJ: Transduodenal sphincterotomy with strict indications. Am J Surg 112: 426, 1966

338. Kourias B, Tobler A: Das postcholecystektomie syndrom. Chirurg 30:398, 1959

339. Kreilkamp BL, Boyden EA: Variability in the composition of the sphincter of Oddi. A possible factor in the pathologic physiology of the biliary tract. Anat Rec 76:485, 1940

340. Kune GA: Gallstones in diverticula of lower common bile duct. Gut 6:95, 1965

341. LaCalle JP: Transduodenal sphincterotomy. Contemp Surg 7:51, 1975

342. Lagerlof H: Choledochal denervation in biliary dyskinesia. Acta Chir Scand 95:297, 1947

343. Lahana DA, Bonorris GG, Schoenfield LJ: Gallstone dissolution in vitro by bile acids, heparin and quaternary amines. Surg Gynecol Obstet 138:683, 1974

344. Lahey FH: Exposure of the gallbladder and bile ducts. Surg Gynecol Obstet 75:445, 1942

345. Lansford C, Mehta S, Kern F: The treatment of retained stones in the common bile duct with sodium cholate infusion. Gut 15:48, 1974

346. Larmi TKI: Surgical treatment of the postcholecystectomy syndrome. Ann Chir Genecol Fenn 52:Suppl 126, 1963

347. Larmi TKI: Hemobilia associated with cholecystitis, post-cholecystectomy conditions and trauma: review of 12 cases. Surgery 60:547, 1966

348. Larmi TKI, Mokka R, Kemppainen P, Seppala A: A critical analysis of the cystic duct remnant. Surg Gynecol Obstet 141:48, 1975

349. Larmi T, Silvennoinen E: Rate of formation of common bile duct stones from nonabsorable silkworm gut. Acta Chir Scand 134:82, 1968

350. Lasser RB, Bond JH, Levitt MD: The role of intestinal gas in functional abdominal pain. N Engl J Med 293:524, 1975

351. Laubersheimer A: Cholecystoscopy following cholecystostomy: report of procedure and twelve cases. West J Surg 48:357, 1940

352. Laursen T, Schmidt A: Increase in serum–GPT and serum–LDH after administration of morphine to patients suffering from bile duct dyskinesia. Scand J Clin Lab Invest 18 (90–93): 175, 1966

353. Layne JA, Bergh GS: Experimental study of pain in the human biliary tract induced by spasm of sphincter of Oddi. Surg Gynecol Obstet 70:18, 1940

354. Lempke RE: Sphincter of Oddi and gallbladder function. II. The effect of sphincterotomy upon sphincter resistance. Ann Surg 158:9, 1963

355. LeQuesne LP, Whiteside CG, Hand BH: The common bile duct after cholecystectomy. Br Med J 1:329, 1959

356. Leslie D: Endoscopy of the bile duct: an evaluation. Aust NZ J Surg 44:340, 1974

357. Levine T: Chronic Cholecystitis. Its Pathology and the Role of Vascular Factors in its Pathogenesis. Jerusalem, Israel Universities Press, 1975

358. Levitt MD: Intestinal gas. Postgrad Med 57:77, 1975

359. Lichtenstein ME, Nicosia AJ: The clinical significance of accessory hepato-biliary ducts. Ann Surg 141:120, 1955

360. Liden K, Lindgremy M: Cholangiographic examinations. Acta Radiol [Diagn] (Stockh) 38:1, 1952

361. Light W: Extraction of residual biliary calculi in the x-ray department. J Can Assoc Radiol 24:209, 1973

362. Lin T: Actions of gastrointestinal hormones and related peptides on the motor function of the biliary tract. Gastroenterology 69:1006, 1975

363. Lindenauer SM, Lavanway JM: Surgical management of congenital choledochal cyst. Surgery 65:972, 1969

364. Lindner J, Lautenschlager HJ: Die laparoskopische differtialdiagnose des intraund extrahepatischen Verschlusssyndroms. Leber Magen Darm 4:319, 1974

365. Lindskog BI: Evaluation of operative cholangiography in gallstone surgery with special reference to residual stones. Lund, 1970

366. Lloyd GAS: The "Four-day telepaque test" in the investigation of the postcholecystectomy syndrome. Br J Radiol 33:522, 1960

367. Loeweneck H, Bruckner W, Rux I: Vagotomie und choledochusinnervation. Chirurg 44:126, 1973

368. Longmire WP: Tumors of the extrahepatic biliary radicals. Curr Probl Cancer 1:5, 1976

369. Longmire WP, Mandiola SA, Gordon HE: Congenital cystic disease of the liver and biliary system. Ann Surg 174:711, 1971

370. Longmire WP, Rangel PM: Difficult problems encountered in the management of biliary obstruction due to stones and other benign conditions. Adv Surg 4:105, 1970

371. Longmire WP, Tompkins RK: Lesions of the segmental and lobar hepatic ducts. Ann Surg 182:478, 1975

372. Longo MF, Hodgson JR, Ferris DO: Size of the common bile duct following cholecystectomy. Ann Surg 165:250, 1967

373. Lubbers EJC: Sphincterotomy. Arch Chir Neerl 20:15, 1968

374. Ludwick JR: Observations on the smooth muscle and contractile activity of the common bile duct. Ann Surg 164:1041, 1966

375. Ludwick JR, Bass P: Contractile and electric activity of the extrahepatic biliary tract and duodenum. Surg Gynecol Obstet 124:536, 1967

376. Lumsden K, Holden WS: The act of vomiting in man. Gut 10:173, 1969

377. Lutkens U: Aufbau and funktion der extrahepatischen gallenwege. Leipzig, Vogel, 1926

378. Luttwak E, Schwartz A: Jaundice due to obstruction of common duct by aberrant artery. Ann Surg 153:134, 1961

379. Lytle WJ: The common bile duct groove in the pancreas. Br J Surg 47:209, 1959

380. MacDonald D: A two way T–tube for continuous postoperative perfusion of biliary tree. Can Med Assoc J 62:481, 1950

381. Madden JL: Primary and secondary common duct stones. Surg Gynecol Obstet 130:1091, 1970

382. Madden JL, Chun JY, Kandalaft S, Parekh M: Choledochoduodenostomy. An unjustly maligned surgical procedure? Am J Surg 119:45, 1970

383. Maddocks AC, Hilson GR, Taylor R: The bacteriology of the obstructed biliary tree. Ann R Coll Surg Engl 52:316, 1973

384. Magarey CJ: Removal of retained bile duct calculus without operation. Br J Surg 56:312, 1969

385. Mahour GH, Wakim K, Ferris DO: The common bile duct in man: its diameter and circumference. Ann Surg 165:415, 1967

386. Mahour GH, Wakim KG, Soule EH, Ferris DO: Structure of the common bile duct in man: presence or absence of smooth muscle. Ann Surg 166:91, 1967

387. Maingot R: Stenosis of the sphincter of Oddi. In Smith R, Sherlock S: Surgery of the Gall-Bladder and Bile Ducts. Washington, Butterworth, 1964, pp 177–196

388. Maki T, Sato T, Matsushiro T: A reappraisal of surgical treatment for intrahepatic gallstones. Ann Surg 175:155, 1972

389. Maki T, Sato T, Yamaguchi I, Sato T: Treatment of intrahepatic gallstones. Arch Surg 88:260, 1964

390. Malagelada JR, Go VLW, Summerskill WHJ, Gamble WS: Bile acid secretion and biliary bile acid composition altered by cholecystectomy. Am J Dig Dis 18:455, 1973

391. Mallet–Guy P: La maladie du sphincter d'Oddi. Lyon Chir 40:553, 1945

392. Mallet–Guy P: Value of peroperative manometric and roentgenographic examination in the diagnosis of pathologic changes and functional disturbances of the biliary tract. Surg Gynecol Obstet 94:385, 1952

393. Mallet–Guy P: Pathogenese, symtomatologie und therapie pathologischer veranderungen der

papilla Vateri. Dtsch Med Wochenschr 16:652, 1960

394. Mallet-Guy P: Der platz der choledochoduodenostomie in der behandlung des postcholecystektomiesyndroms. Langenbecks Arch Chir 325: 400, 1969

395. Mallet-Guy P, Duffield RJ: Peroperative manometry and radiology in biliary tract disorders. Br J Surg 44:183, 1956

396. Mallet-Guy P, JeanJean R, Feroldi J: La maladie du sphincter d'Oddi. Hypertonie oddienne, oddite sténosante. Lyon Chir 40:553, 1945

397. Mallet-Guy P, Kestens PJ, Gignoux M, Murat J: Syndrome Post-Cholecystectomie. Paris, Masson, 1970

398. Manier JW: Diet in gastrointestinal diseases. Med Clin North Am 54:1357, 1970

400. Manier JW, Cohen WN, Printen KJ: Dysfunction of the sphincter of Oddi in a postcholecystectomy patient. Am J Gastroenterol 62:148, 1974

401. Marshall RD: Transduodenal ampullaplasty in the surgery of the common bile duct. Aust NZ J Surg 23:160, 1954

402. Marteinsson BTH, Musgrove JE: Heterotopic bone formation in abdominal incisions. Am J Surg 130:23, 1975

403. Mattig H: Die verbreitung der radiomanometrie im 25 jahr ihres bestehens. Zentrabl Chir 26: 899, 1968

404. Mattig H: Beurteilung von abflusstorungen der gallenwege mit hilfe der peroperativen debitmetrie. Zentrabl Chir 94:715, 1969

405. Mazzariello R: Removal of residual biliary tract calculi without reoperation. Surgery 67: 566, 1970

406. Mazzariello R: Review of 220 cases of residual biliary tract calculi treated without reoperation. Surgery 73:299, 1973

407. McBurney C: Removal of biliary calculi from the common duct by the duodenal route. Ann Surg 28:481, 1898

408. McCarthy JD: Radiomanometry during biliary operations. Arch Surg 100:424, 1970

409. McClenahan JL, Evans JA, Braunstein PW: Intravenous cholangiography in the postcholecystectomy syndrome. JAMA 159:1353, 1955

410. McDougall RM, Walker K, Thurston OG: Prolonged secretion of lithogenic bile after cholecystectomy. Ann Surg 182:150, 1975

411. McFarland JO, Currin J: Cholecystokinin and the cystic duct syndrome. Am J Gastroenterol 52:515, 1969

412. McGowan JM, Butsch WL, Walters W; Pressure in the common bile duct of man: its relation to pain following cholecystectomy. JAMA 106:2227, 1936

413. McGowan JM, Knepper PA, Walters W, Snell AM: The relation of spasm of the second portion of the duodenum to biliary colic. Surg Gynecol Obstet 66:979, 1938

414. McHenry MC, Martin WJ: Bacteremic shock due to gram-negative enteric bacilli. Mayo Clin Proc 37:162, 1962

415. McIver MA: An instrument for visualizing the interior of the common duct at operation. Preliminary Note. Surgery 9:112, 1941

416. McKenzie G: Extravasation of bile after operations on the biliary tract. Aust NZ J Surg 24: 181, 1955

417. McManus JE: The early history of surgery for common duct stones. N Engl J Med 254:17, 1956

418. McMaster PD, Elman R: On the expulsion of bile by the gall bladder and a reciprocal relationship with the sphincter activity. J Exp Med 44:173, 1926

419. McPhedran NT, Ainslie JDT, McCrae WH, Blundell PE, Trimble AS: Fibrosis of the ampulla of Vater. Arch Surg 83:146, 1961

420. McSwain B, Herrington L, Edwards WH, Sawyer JL, Cole WR: Intrahepatic cholangitic hepatitis. Its surgical significance. Ann Surg 147:805, 1958

421. Meier AL, Schweingruber B, Meinardus K: Indikation and Resultate der Choledochoduodenostomie. Helv Chir Acta 26:516, 1959

422. Meltzer SJ: The disturbance of the law of contrary innervation as a pathogenetic factor in the disease of the bile ducts and the gallbladder. Am J Med Sci 153:469, 1917

423. Mercadier M: Aetiology and morbid anatomy of chronic pancreatitis: analysis of 163 cases. Bibl Gastroenterol 7:1, 1965

424. Metzger AL, Vlahcevic ZR, Bell CC Jr, Gregory DH, Small L: Effect of cholecystectomy on bile acid metabolism. N Engl J Med 289:1213, 1973

425. Meyhoff HH: Sphincterotomy treatment for biliary tract stones. Acta Chir Scand 141:645, 1975

426. Millbourn E: Klinische studien uber die choledocholithiasis. Acta Chir Scand 86; Suppl 65, 1941

427. Millbourn E: On re-operation for choledocholithiasis. Acta Chir Scand 99:285, 1949

428. Molnar W, Stockum AE: Relief of obstructive jaundice through percutaneous transhepatic catheter—a new therapeutic method. Am J Roentgenol Radium Ther Nucl Med 122:356, 1974

429. Monge JJ: Secondary exploration of the biliary tract. Am J Surg 111:673, 1966

430. Morton CB: Post-cholecystectomy symptoms from cystic duct remnants. Ann Surg 139:679, 1954

431. Mossberg S, Bloom A, Berkowitz J, Ross G: Serum enzyme activities following morphine. Arch Intern Med 109: 105, 1962

432. Moynihan GGA: Gallstones and Their Surgical Treatment, 2nd ed. Philadelphia, WB Saunders, 1905

433. Mujahed Z, Glenn F, Evans JA: Communicating cavernous ectasia of the intrahepatic ducts. (Caroli's disease). Am J Roentgenol Radium Ther Nucl Med 113:21, 1971

434. Myers RN, Haupt GJ, Birkhead NC, Deaver JM: Cinefluorographic observations of common bile duct physiology. Ann Surg 156:442, 1962

435. Nahrwold DL, Grossman MI: Effect of cholecystectomy on bile flow and composition in response to food. Am J Surg 119:30, 1970

436. Nakayama F, van der Linden W: Role of gallbladder in gallstone formation. Acta Chir Scand 139:45, 1974

437. Nana A, Toader C, Soltuz V, Neumann E, Nana M: The electrical biopotentials of the sphincter territories within the biliary pathways. Gastroenterologia 100:182, 1963

438. Nardi GL, Acosta JM: Papillitis as a cause of pancreatitis and abdominal pain: role of evocative test, operative pancreatography and histologic evaluation. Ann Surg 167:611, 1966

439. Nardi GL, Lyon DC, Sheiner HJ, Bartlett MK: Solitary occult retention cysts of the pancreas. N Engl J Med 280:11, 1969

440. Nash TP: The behaviour of the sphincter of Oddi in health and disease. Aust NZ J Surg 31–32:40, 1961–63

441. Naunyn B: A Treatise on Cholelithiasis (translated by AE Garrod). London, The New Sydenham Society, 1896. HK Lewis, 197 pp.

442. Nebel OT: Manometric evaluation of the papilla of Vater. Gastrointest Endosc 21:126, 1975

443. Nicholas P, Rinaudo PA, Conn HO: Increased incidence of cholelithiasis in Laennec's cirrhosis. Gastroenterology 63:112, 1972

444. Niedner FF: Uber die ostiumstenose der papilla Vateri. Fortschr Roentgenstr 103:147, 1965

445. Nillson S, Stattin S: Gallbladder emptying during the normal menstrual cycle. Acta Chir Scand 133:648, 1967

446. Nishimura A, Den N, Sato H, Takeda B: Exfoliative cytology of the biliary tract with the use of saline irrigation under choledochoscopic control. Ann Surg 178:594, 1973

447. Nora PF, Dorazio RA, Kirshenbaum G, Shore JM, Wilson SD, Tompkins RK: Operative choledochoscopy: results of a prospective study in several institutions. Am J Surgery 133:105, 1977

448. Nuboer JF: Die altersveranderungen der extrahepatischen gallenwege. Frankfurt Z Pathol 42: 292, 1931

449. Nuboer JF: Studien uber des extra hepatic gal-enweges-system. Frankfurt Z Pathol 41:198, 1931

450. Ochsner AJ: Further observations on the anatomy of the duodenum. Am J Med Sci 132: 1–8, 1906

451. Oddi R: D'une disposition á sphincter speciale de l'ouverture du canal choledoque. Arch Ital Biol 8:317, 1887

452. Ohlsson EG, Aronsen KF: Carcinoma of the gallbladder. Acta Chir Scand 140:475, 1974

453. Ominsky SH: Intravenous cholangiogram contrast medium reflux into pancreatic ducts in a patient with acute pancreatitis. Radiology 111: 97, 1974

454. Ong GB: A study of recurrent pyogenic cholangitis. Arch Surg 84:199, 1962

455. Ono K, Watanabe N, Suzuki K, Tsuchida H, Sugiyama V, Abo M: Bile flow mechanism in man. Arch Surg 96:869, 1968

456. Op den Orth JO: A radiologically demonstrated fistula between the common bile duct and the right renal pelvis. Radiol Clin Biol 38:402, 1969

457. Opie EL: The etiology of acute hemorrhagic pancreatitis. Johns Hopkins Med J 121, 1, 2, 3, 182, 1901

458. Orr KB: External choledochoduodenostomy for retained common duct stone: reappraisal of an old technique. Med J Aust 2:1027, 1966

459. Parry EW, Hallenbeck GA, Grindlay PW: Pressure in the pancreatic and common ducts. Arch Surg 70:757, 1955

460. Partington PF: Sphincterotomy for stenosis of the sphincter of Oddi. Surg Gynecol Obstet 123:282, 1966

461. Paulino A, Paulino F: Pancreatic ductal reflux. Am J Dig Dis 8:166, 1963

462. Paulino F, Cavalcanti A: Biopsy of the ampulla of Vater for demonstration of organic stenosis. Surgery 48:698, 1960

463. Paulino F, Cavalcanti A: Anatomy and pathology of the distal common duct; special reference to stenosing odditis. Am J Dig Dis 5:697, 1960

464. Paulino F, Roselli A: Stenosis of sphincter of Oddi. Surgery 54:865, 1963

465. Pemberton LB, Manax WG: Complications after vertical and transverse incisions for cholecystectomy. Surg Gynecol Obstet 132:892, 1971

466. Pereira–Lima J, Pereira–Lima LM, Nestowski M, Cuervo C: Anomalous locations of the papilla of Vater. Am J Surg 128:71, 1974

467. Pfeffermann R, Floman Y, Rozin RR: Ascariasis of the biliary system. Arch Surg 105:118, 1972

468. Pikula JV, Dunphy JE: Some effects of stenosis of the terminal common bile duct on the biliary tract and liver: an experimental study. N Engl J Med 260:315, 1959

469. Pinotti HW, DeSousa OM, Parolari JB, Conte VP, Raia A, Netto AC: The dynamics of the main biliary duct and the mechanism of the biliopancreatic reflux. Am J Dig Dis 12:878, 1967

470. Pinotti HW, Tacla M, Pontes JF, Bettarello A: Juxta–Ampullar duodenal diverticula as cause of bilio-pancreatic disease. Digestion 4:353, 1971

471. Pirola RC, Davis AE: Effects of ethyl alcohol on sphincteric resistance at the choledocho-duodenal junction in man. Gut 9:557, 1968

472. Pirola RC, Davis AE: Effects of intravenous alcohol on motility of the duodenum and of the sphincter of Oddi. Australas Ann Med 19:1, 1970

473. Polk HC Jr: Carcinoma and the calcified gallbladder. Gastroenterology 50:582, 1966

474. Pollack EL, Tabrisky J: The aberrant divisional bile duct: a surgical hazard. Surgery 73:234, 1973

475. Pomare EW, Heaton KW: The effect of cholecystectomy on bile salt metabolism. Gut 14:753, 1973

476. Poppel MH, Jacobson HG, Smith RV: The Roentgen Aspects of the Papilla and Ampulla of Vater. Springfield, Charles C Thomas, 1953

477. Potter JC, Mann FC: Pressure changes in the biliary tract. Am J Med Sci 171:202, 1926

478. Poulsen H, Christoffersen P: Histological changes in liver biopsies from patients with surgical bile duct disorders. Acta Pathol Microbiol Scand [A] 78:571, 1970

479. Preshaw RM, Knouf RJ: The effect of sham feeding on the secretion and motility of canine duodenal pouches. Gastroenterology 51:193, 1966

480. Preston DJ: Transduodenal ampullo-duodenostomy for treatment of common bile duct obstructions without a T tube drain. Surg Gynecol Obstet 100:499, 1955

481. Pribram BOC: Postcholecystectomy syndromes. JAMA 142:1262, 1950

482. Price WH: Gall-bladder dyspepsia. Br Med J 2:138, 1963

483. Prudhomme P, Niloff P, Skoryna SC, Webster DR: Experimental studies on fibrosis of sphincter of Oddi and on sphincterotomy. Can J Surg 8:201, 1965

484. Puestow CB: Choledochus after cholecystectomy. Surg Gynecol Obstet 67:82, 1938

485. Quattlebaum JK, Quattlebaum JK Jr: Malignant obstruction of the major hepatic ducts. Ann Surg 161:876, 1965

486. Quintana EV, Labat R: Ectopic drainage of the common bile duct. Ann Surg 180:119, 1974

487. Raines DR, Van Heertum RL, Johnson LJ: Intrahepatic hematoma: a complication of percutaneous liver biopsy. Gastroenterology 67:284, 1974

488. Raskin HF, Wenger J, Sklar M, Pleticka S, Yarema W: The diagnosis of cancer of the pancreas, biliary tract and duodenum by combined cytologic and secretory methods. Gastroenterology 34:996, 1958

489. Ratchke L: Steinrezidiv und gallenwegsanastomsen Stuttgart, Ferdinand Enke, 1956

490. Ray BS, Neill CL: Abdominal visceral sensation in man. Ann Surg 126:709, 1947

491. Raymer JB, Tarpinian DA, Meyers SG: Symptoms following cholecystectomy. Am J Dig Dis 5:55, 1960

492. Rehfuss ME, Nelson GM: The Medical Treatment of Gallbladder Disease. Philadelphia, WB Saunders, 1935

493. Reich H: Choledochal denervation. New procedure for relief of biliary dyskinesia. Surg Gynecol Obstet 71:39, 1940

494. Reiss, R, Pikielny S: The clinical significance of the diameter of the common bile duct in cholecystectomized patients. Isr J Med Sci 7:1070, 1971

495. Re Mine WH: Biliary enteric fistulas: natural history and management. Adv Surg 7:69, 1973

496. Reynolds BM: Immediate effects of instrumental dilatation of the ampulla of Vater. Ann Surg 164:271, 1966

497. Reynolds BM, Dargan EL: Acute obstructive cholangitis, a distinct clinical syndrome. Ann Surg 150, 299, 1959

498. Rhind JA, Watson L: Gallstone dyspepsia. Br Med J 1:32, 1968

499. Riddell DH, Kirtley JA: Stenosis of the sphincter of Oddi. Transduodenal sphincterotomy and some other surgical aspects. Ann Surg 149:773, 1959

500. Riedel B: Die pathogenese, diagnose und behandlung des gallensteinleidens. Jena, Verlag Von Gustav Fischer, 1903

501. Ritter U: Untersuchungen zur retrograden insuffizienz der papilla Vateri. Z Gastroenterol 1:36, 1963

502. Ritter U: Zur pathophysiologie des postcholecystektomiesyndroms. Gastroenterologia 107:73, 1967

503. Robson MC, Bogart JN, Heggers JP: An endogenous source for wound infections based on quantitative bacteriology of the biliary tract. Surgery 86:471, 1970

504. Roeckerath W: Der nachweis der papilla minor duodeni in Rontgenbild und ihre differentialdiagnostische bedeutung. Fortschr Roentgenstr 75:479, 1952

505. Rosato EF, Oram–Smith JC, Reber HA, Czernobilsky B, Rosato FE: Papillary integrity as a factor in pancreatic reflux. Am J Surg 121:13, 1971

506. Rose JD: Biliary vesicular stasis. Lancet 1:1356, 1958

507. Rose JD: The problems of biliousness. Newcastle Med J 30:69, 1968

508. Rosen RG, Garret M, Aka E: Cytologic diagnosis of pancreatic cancer by ductal aspiration. Ann Surg 167:427, 1968

509. Rosenberg J, Matzner M: Neuroma in dilated stump of cystic duct preoperative visualization by intravenous cholangiography. Am J Gastroenterol 29:471, 1957

510. Ross FP, Dunphy JE: Studies in acute cholecystitis. II. Cholecystostomy. Indications and technic. N Engl J Med 242:359, 1950

511. Ross RJ, Pudvan WR: Peptic ulcers and gallbladder disease. Radiology 95:119, 1970

512. Rousselot L, Sanchez–Ubeda R, Giannelli S: Choledochoenterostomy in chronic relapsing pancreatitis: a study of five cases with prolonged follow up observation. New Engl J Med 250:267, 1954

513. Roux M, LeCanuet R, Vayre P: Estimation of the functional value of the main biliary tract by the peroperative radiomanometric study of the biliary output. J Chir (Paris) 89:587, 1965

514. Roux M, Rettori R, Debray C, LeCanuet R,

Laumonier R: Diagnosis of chronic odditis. J Int Coll Surg 32:599, 1959

515. Royer H, Solari AV: Cholangiography performed with the help of periteonoscopy. Gastroenterology 8:586, 1947

516. Rundle FF, Perry D, Cass M, Oddie TH: Rise in serum bilirubin with biliary obstruction and its decline curve after operative relief. Surgery 43:555, 1958

517. Safrancy L: Duodenoscopic sphincterotomy and gallstone removal. Gastroenterology 72:338, 1977

518. Saharia PC, Cameron JL: Clinical management of acute cholangitis. Surg Gynecol Obstet 142: 369, 1976

519. Saik RP, Greenburg AG, Farris JM, Peski GW: Spectrum of cholangitis. Am J Surg 130:143, 1975

520. Salembier Y: Removal of intrahepatic bile duct stones. Int Surg 60:149, 1975

521. Salik JO, Siegel CI, Mendeloff AI: Biliary duodenal dynamics in man. Radiology 106:1, 1973

522. Saltzstein EC, Subbarao V, Evani SV, Mann RW: Routine operative cholangiography. Arch Surg 107:289, 1973

523. Sandblom P: Hemobilia (Biliary tract hemorrhage). History, Pathology, Diagnosis, Treatment. Springfield, Ill, CC Thomas, 1972

524. Sanders RL: Indications for and value of choledochoduodenostomy. Ann Surg 123:847, 1946

525. Sasse F: Ueber choledocho-duodenostomie. Arch Klin Chir 100:969, 1913

526. Sasson L: Dissolution and flushing technics for removal of retained common duct stone. Am J Gastroenterol 51:394, 1969

527. Schein CJ: Biliary endoscopy: an appraisal of its value in biliary lithiasis. Surgery 65:1004, 1969

528. Schein CJ: Acute Cholecystitis. New York, Harper & Row, 1972

529. Schein CJ, Allen LB, Hurwitt ES: Biopsy of the common bile duct in acute cholecystitis. Arch Surg 83:835, 1961

530. Schein CJ, Beneventano TC: Choledochoduodenal junction stenosis in the postcholecystectomy syndrome. Surgery 64:1039, 1968

531. Schein CJ, Beneventano TC: Choledochal dynamics in man. Surg Gynec Obstet 126:591, 1968

532. Schein CJ, Beneventano TC: Biliary manometry: its role in clinical surgery. Surgery 67:255, 1970

533. Schein CJ, Beneventano TC, Rosen RG, Dardik HM, Gliedman ML: Hepatic plexus vagectomy as an adjunct to cholecystectomy. Surg Gynecol Obstet 128:241, 1969

534. Schein CJ, El Tawil V, Dardik H, Beneventano TC: Common duct dynamics in man. Am J Surg 119:261, 1970

535. Schein CJ, Hurwitt ES: A safe technique for the difficult cholecystectomy, utilizing intravesical manipulations. Surg Gynecol Obstet 102:113, 1956

536. Schein CJ, Hurwitt ES, Herskovitz A: Andoscopy of the bile ducts; sound, color, 16 mm. motion picture. In Motion Picture Library of the American College of Surgeons, produced in April 1961, presented at meeting of the American College of Surgeons, Oct, 1961

537. Schein CJ, Shapiro N, Gliedman ML: Choledochoduodenostomy: as an adjunct to choledocholithotomy: Surg Gynecol Obstet. In press

538. Schein CJ, Stern WZ, Hurwitt ES, Jacobson HG: Cholangiography and biliary endoscopy as complementary methods of evaluating the bile ducts. Am J Roentgenol Radium Ther Nucl Med 89:864, 1963

539. Schein CJ, Stern WZ, Jacobson HG: The Common Bile Duct. Operative Cholangiography, Biliary Endoscopy and Choledocholithotomy. Springfield, Ill, CC Thomas, 1966

540. Schoenfield LJ: Clinical aspects of the chenodeoxycholic acid trial. Hosp Prac Aug, 1974, 53

541. Schoenfield LJ, Coyne MJ: Cholesterol gallstones, 1975. Viewpoints Dig Dis 7:1, 1975

542. Schreiber H: Der muskelapparat des duodenalen choledochusendes (Papilla Vateri) beim menschen. Langenbecks Arch Klin Chir 206:211, 1944

543. Schultz NJ, Sanders RJ: Evaluation of pancreatic biopsy. Ann Surg 158:1053, 1963

544. Schwarz SI: Primary sclerosing cholangitis. A disease revisited. Surg Clin North Am 53:1161, 1973

545. Schwegler RA, Boyden EA: The development of the pars intestinalis of the common bile duct in the human fetus with special reference to the origin of the ampulla of Vater and the sphincter of Oddi. II. The early development of the musculus proprius. Anat Rec 68:17, 1937

546. Scott GW, Smallwood RE, Rowland S: Flow through the bile duct after cholecystectomy. Surg Gynecol Obstet 140:912, 1975

547. Sedlack RE, Hodgson JR, Butt HR, Stobie GHC, Judd ES: Gas in the biliary tract. General and experimental observations. Gastroenterology 41:551, 1961

548. Seel DJ, Yang J, Lee KY: Inflammatory hemobilia. Surgery 66:821, 1969

549. Selberg W: Das morphologische substrat der sogen. Papillitis stenosans cholangica. Zentralbl Allg Pathol 96:551, 1957

550. Semb BKH, Norderval Y, Halvorsen JF: The non-operative removal of retained common duct stones after biliary surgery. Acta Chir Scand 140:469, 1974

551. Sewell JH, Sewell RL: The incompetent sphincter of Oddi. Am J Surg 101:390, 1961

552. Shaffer EA, Braasch JW, Small DM: Bile composition at and after surgery in normal persons and patients with gallstones—influence of cholecystectomy. N Engl J Med 287:1317, 1972

553. Shafiroff GP, Hinton JW: Surgical anatomy of the choledochal nerves. Arch Surg 60:944, 1950

554. Shehadi WH: Urography and cholangiography

not contraindicated by history of allergy. JAMA 218:1836, 1971

555. Sherlock S, Scheuer PJ: The presentation and diagnosis of 100 patients with primary biliary cirrhosis. N Engl J Med 289:674, 1973

556. Shingelton WH, Anlyan WG, Hart D: Effects of vagotomy, splanchnicectomy and celiac ganglionectomy on experimentally produced spasm of sphincter of Oddi in animals. Ann Surg 135: 721, 1952

557. Shingleton WW, Gamburg D: Stenosis of the sphincter of Oddi. Am J Surg 119:35, 1970

558. Shore JM, Berci G: Operative management of calculi in the hepatic ducts. Am J Surg 119: 625, 1970

559. Shore JM, Berci G, Morgenstern L: The value of biliary endoscopy. Surg Gynecol Obstet 140: 601, 1975

560. Shore JM, Morgenstern L, Berci G: An improved rigid choledochoscope. Am J Surg 122:567, 1971

561. Shore JM, Silverman A, Siegel M, Bakal M: Direct observations of the canine sphincter of Oddi. Ann Surg 174:264, 1971

562. Sigler L, Sahler CO: Silk: the nidus of a common bile duct calculus. Surgery 65:276, 1969

563. Silvennoinen E, Asp K: Clinical observations on complications from nonabsorbable suture material on gallbladder surgery. Acta Chir Scand 132:587, 1966

564. Silvis SE, Rohrmann C, Vennes JA: Diagnostic criteria for the evaluation of endoscopic pancreatograms. Gastrointest Endosc 20:51, 1973

565. Sivak MV Jr, Sullivan BH Jr: Endoscopic retrograde cholangiopancreatography (RCP). Cleve Clin Q 41:93, 1974

566. Skinner DB, Belsey RHR, Hendrix TR, Zuidema GD: Gastroesophageal Reflux and Hiatal Hernia. Boston, Little, Brown, 1972

567. Small DM: The formation of gallstones. Adv Intern Med 16:243, 1970

568. Smith RB, Conklin EF, Porter MR: A five year study of choledocholithiasis. Surg Gynecol Obstet 116:731, 1963

569. Sorby WA, Ham JM: A new method for roentgenologic assessment of the stoma after choledochoduodenostomy. Surg Gynecol Obstet 135:438, 1972

570. Spjut HJ, Ramos AJ: An evaluation of biopsy-frozen section of the ampullary region and pancreas: a report of 68 consecutive patients. Ann Surg 146:923, 1957

571. Sprayregen S, Messinger NH: Angiography of the jaundiced patient with emphasis upon the angiographic appearance of biliary dilatation. Am J Roentgenol Radium Ther Nucl Med 122: 335, 1974

572. Staffen A, Staudacher M: Der "symptomlose" choledochusstein. Chirurg 41:377, 1970

573. Stafford ES, Isaacs JP: Stone in the left hepatic duct causing jaundice. Ann Surg 147:812, 1958

574. Stauber R: Leber parenchym und gallsteinkrankheit. Wien Med Wochenschr 112:677, 1962

575. Stauber R: Registrierung der muskelaktivität an der Vaterschen papille und deren bedeutung für die intraoperative diagnostik. Langenbecks Arch Klin Chir 325:1139, 1969

576. Stein AA: The surgically resected gallbladder. A morphologic evolution. Arch Surg 82:556, 1961

577. Stein D: The diagnosis of jaundice by the mini-laparotomy open transhepatic cholangiogram. Ann Surg 181:386, 1975

578. Stiller H, Eisenreich F: Second operations on the extrabiliary system; choledochoduodenostomy versus sphincter cutting operation. (Wiederholungseingriffe an den Gallenwegen). Langenbecks Arch Chir 325:386, 1969

579. Strasberg SM, Dorn BC, Redinger RN, Small DM, Egdahl RH: Effects of alteration of biliary pressure on bile composition—a method for study. V. Primate biliary physiology. Gastroenterology 63:357, 1971

580. Sullivan FJ, Eaton SB Jr, Ferrucci JT Jr, Dreyfuss JR, Sloan RW: Cholangiographic manifestations of acute biliary colic. N Engl J Med 288: 33, 1973

581. Sutton JP, Sachatello CR: The confluence stone: a hazardous complication of biliary tract disease. Am J Surg 113:719, 1967

582. Szeleczky G, Megyeri L: Beitrage zur morphologie der gegend des sphincter Oddi. Langenbecks Arch Klin Chir 305:139, 1964

583. Szelczky G, Megyeri L: Angaben zur frage der gutartigen paillenstenose. Acta Chir Acad Sci Hung 11:23, 1970

584. Tanturi CA, Ivy AC: On the existence of secretory nerves in the vagi for, and the reflex excitation and inhibition of, bile secretion. Am J Physiol 121:270, 1938

585. Thomas E, Grant AK, Holford D, Ringwood AW, Magarey JR: Bacterial flora in the duodenum of patients after biliary fenestration. Br J Surg 60:107, 1973

586. Thompson JA, Howard JM, Vowles DU: Acute pancreatitis following choledochotomy. Surg Gynecol Obstet 105:706, 1957

587. Tierney JM, Carter JF, Van Goidsenhoven GE: Screening for pancreatic disease. Ann Intern Med 58:229, 1963

588. Toland CG: Foreign bodies in the biliary tract. Ann Surg 99:904, 1933

589. Trapnell J: The operative diagnosis of carcinoma of the pancreas. Br J Surg 58:849, 1971

590. Trier JS: Per oral cannulation of pancreatic and bile ducts. Gastroenterology 60:470, 1971

591. Trommold JP, Seabrook BB: Benign fibrosis of the sphincter of Oddi. West J Surg Obstet Gynecol 58:89, 1950

592. Trotman BW, Petrella EJ, Soloway RD, Sanchez HM, Morris TA, Miller WT: Evaluation of radiographic lucency or opaqueness of gallstones as a means of identifying cholesterol or pigment stones. Gastroenterology 68:1563, 1975

593. Tumen HJ: What is the "postcholecystectomy syndrome?" Am J Dig Dis 2:289, 1957

594. Turner GG: The surgery of the gall-bladder and bile ducts. (Lettsomian Lectures). London, Transcript Medical Society, Vol. 62:238, 1939

595. Tylen U, Hoevels J, Vang J: Percutaneous transhepatic cholangiography with external drainage of obstructive biliary lesions. Surg Obstet Gynecol 144:13, 1977

596. Ustach TJ, Tobon F, Hambrecht T, Bass DD, Scjister MM: Electrophysiological aspects of human sphincter function. J Clin Invest 49:41, 1970

597. Vajcner A, Grossling S, Nicoloff DM: Physiologic evaluation of sphincteroplasty. Surgery 62:589, 1967

598. Valberg LS, Jabbari M, Kerr JW, Curtis AC, Ramchard S, Prentice RSA: Biliary pain in young women in the absence of gallstones. Gastroenterology 60:1020, 1971

599. Van der Linden W: Hemobilia: a case with recurrent jaundice cured by removal of a blood clot from the common bile duct. Acta Chir Scand 141:445, 1975

600. Van der Linden W, Norman A: Composition of human hepatic bile. Acta Chir Scand 133:313, 1967.

601. Van Houten FX, Lewicki AM: Cystic duct remnant duodenal fistula. Radiology 107:75, 1973

602. Villemin F: Recherches d'anatomie comparée sur le duodénum de l'homme et des mammiferes. Sa signification morphologique et fonctionnelle. Arch Morphol Gen Exp 3:1, 1922

603. Vos A: Duodenal ulceration after diversion of bile. Digestion 6:227, 1972

604. Wakim KG, Mahour GH: Pathophysiologic consequences of cholecystectomy. Surg Gynecol Obstet 133:113, 1971

605. Walters W: Spasm of the common duct producing pain after sphincterotomy. Arch Surg 72:547, 1956

606. Walters W: Postcholecystectomy dyskinesia with pancreatic sphincteritis and choledochlithiasis as causes. JAMA 160:425, 1956

607. Walz UM: Die transduodenale sphincterotomie. Langenbecks Arch Klin Chir 323:1, 1968

608. Warren A, Beneventano TC, Schein CJ: The influence of extra biliary peritonitis on cholecystography. Am J Surg 116:872, 1968

609. Warren KW, Athanassiades S, Monge JI: Primary sclerosing cholangitis. A study of forty two cases. Am J Surg 111:23, 1966

610. Warren KW, McDonald WM: Facts and fiction regarding strictures of the extrahepatic bile ducts. Ann Surg 159:996, 1964

611. Warshaw AL, Schapiro RG, Ferrucci JJ, Galdabini JJ: Persistent obstructive jaundice, cholangitis, and biliary cirrhosis due to common bile duct stenosis in chronic pancreatitis. Gastroenterology 70:562, 1976

612. Watts DR, Lorenzo GA, Beal JM: Congenital dilatation of the intrahepatic biliary ducts. Arch Surg 108:592, 1974

613. Watt J McK, Dunphy JE: The role of the common bile duct in biliary dynamics. Surg Gynecol Obstet 122:1207, 1966

614. Waugh JM, Johnson EV, Cain JC: Choledocholithiasis. JAMA 154:734, 1954

615. Way LW, Admirand WH, Dunphy JE: Management of choledocholithiasis. Ann Surg 176: 347, 1972

616. Webb WR, DeGuzman VC, Hoopes JE, Doyle RA: Experimental evaluation of sphincteroplasty with and without long arm T tubes. Surg Gynecol Obstet 119:1, 1964

617. Webb WR, Hoopes JE, DeGuzman VC, Doyle RA: Sphincterotomy and sphincteroplasty. An experimental evaluation. Surg Forum 14:94, 1963

618. Weber F: Zur frage der choledochusweite nach transduodenaler papillotomie. Wien Klin Wochenschr 9:1, 1969

619. Weiner S, Gramatica L, Voegle LD, Hauman RL, Anderson MC: Role of the lymphatic system in the pathogenesis of inflammatory disease of the biliary tract and pancreas. Am J Surg 119:55, 1970

620. Weinstein BR, Korn RJ, Zimmerman HJ: Obstructive jaundice as a complication of pancreatitis. Ann Intern Med 58:245, 1963

621. Weitz G: 3194 operationen wegen cholelithiasis in 15 jahren. Langenbecks Arch Klin Chir 312: 139, 1965

622. Welch CE: Choledochotomy. Surg Gynecol Obstet 102:495, 1956

623. Wenckert A, Robertson B: The natural course of gallstone disease. Gastroenterology 50:376, 1966

624. Wendth AJ, Cross VF, Moriarty DJ, Vitale P, Lopez F, Samson RVS: Hypotonic duodenography. Radiology 108:274, 1973

625. Wenzl M, Lorbeck W: Fremdkorper im choledochus als ursache von postcholecystektomiebeschwerden. Wien Klin Wochenschr 66:451, 1954

626. Westphal K: Muskelfunction, nervensystem and pathologies der gallenwege. II. Experimentelle untersuchungen uber die nervoise beeinflussung der bewgungsvorgange der gallenwege. Z Klin Med 96:52, 1923

627. Whelton MJ, Petrelli M, George P, Young WB, Sherlock S: Carcinoma at the junction of the main hepatic ducts. Q J Med 38:211, 1969

628. White C: Sampling in medical research. Br Med J 2:1284, 1953

629. White TT: Indications for sphincteroplasty as opposed to choledochoduodenostomy. Am J Surg 126:165, 1973

630. White TT, Waisman H, Hopton D, Kavlie H: Radiomanometry, flow rates, and cholangiography in the evaluation of common bile duct disease. Am J Surg 123:73, 1972

631. Whiting EG, Nusynowitz ML: Radioactive rose bengal testing in the differential diagnosis of jaundice. Surg Gynecol Obstet 127:732, 1968

632. Whitman EJ, Buie LA, Huizenga KA, Waugh JM: Cystic artery—cystic duct fistula: an un-

usual cause of gastrointestinal hemorrhage: report of case. Mayo Clin Proc 35:55, 1960

633. Wiechel KL: Percutaneous transhepatic cholangiography. Acta Chir Scand [Suppl] 330:1, 1964

634. Wildegans H: Die Operative Gallengansendoskopie. Munchen, Urban & Schwarzenberg, 1960

635. Williams RD: Postcholecystectomy bilious state. JAMA 208:541, 1969

636. Williams RD, Fish JC, Williams DD: The significance of biliary pressure. Arch Surg 95:374, 1967

637. Winchester DP, Seed RW, Bergan JJ, Conn J: Jaundice, hemobilia and hemoperitoneum consequences of rupture of hepatic artery aneurysm. Am J Surg 120:385, 1970

638. Wise RE: Intravenous Cholangiography. Springfield, Ill, CC Thomas, 1962

639. Wolfman NT, Short WF: T-tube cholangiography with barium after reaction to iodinated contrast medium. JAMA 232:523, 1975

640. Womack NA, Crider RL: Persistence of symptoms following cholecystectomy. Ann Surg 126: 31, 1947

641. Wormsley KG: Tests of pancreatic function. Scand J Gastroenterol 5:1, 1970

642. Wyatt AP, Belzer FO, Dunphy JE: Malfunction without constriction of the common bile duct. Am J Surg 113:592, 1967

643. Zawisch–Ossenitz C: Histologische untersuchungen zur frage der kinstilichen dehnung der papilla Vateri. Zentrabl Chir 30:1868, 1928

644. Zeff RH, Pfeffer RB, Adams PX, Rouff M: Reoperation for amputation neuroma of the cystic duct. Am J Surg 131:369, 1976

645. Zer M, Chaimoff C, Dinstsman M, Glanz I: Cystic dilation of intrahepatic bile ducts. Arch Surg 106:225, 1973

646. Zimmermann G, Laszcz M, Boeckl O: Zur wahl des zeitpunktes der intervallcholezystektomie bei cholelithiasis mit begleit pankreatitis. Munch Med Wochenschr 115:1837, 1973

647. Zimmon DS, Breslaw J, Kessler RE: Endoscopy with endoscopy cholangiopancreatography. The combination as a primary diagnostic procedure. JAMA 233:447, 1975

648. Zimmon DS, Falkenstein DB, Kessler RE: Endoscopic removal of biliary stones and sludge: preliminary experience. Gastroenterology 68: 1052, 1975

Monographs in Biliary Surgery

I included in *Acute Cholecystitis*, published in 1972, a specific section referring to pertinent monographs related to that subject. Several criteria served as the indication for inclusion: that I knew the text and could read or understand it, that it be so available as to be physically present in my library, and that I found it useful. Obviously eclecticism is the author's privilege.

I have expanded that initial list of 55 monographs to 85. The premise is that the surgery for postcholecystectomy complaints touches on virtually the entire diagnostic and therapeutic armamentarium of biliary-pancreatic disorders. I have excluded text books and nonmonographic material. The aim is to have access to in-depth reference material. Age has not withered some of the material, nor custom invalided its utility. There is something new and something old. They have been of value to me.

CLASSICS

M–1. Thudichum JLW: A Treatise on Gallstones: Their Chemistry, Pathology and Treatment. London, Churchill, 1863, 315 pp

This is one of the oldest monographs in English on the biliary tract. A facsimile of the text is obtainable from University Microfilms, in Ann Arbor, Michigan. The author, a German chemist, suggested a two-stage cholecystotomy, the gallbladder being stitched to the abdominal wall in the first stage and opened in the second, and then removing the stones with a lithotrite.

M–2. Naunyn BA: Treatise on Cholelithiasis (translated by AE Garrod). London, New Sydenham Society, 1896, 197 pp

Naunyn was Professor of Medicine in Strassburg. He postulated that an inflammatory "lithogenic catarrah" initiated the formation of gallstones, its nidus being derived from mucous membrane cholesterol. This viewpoint regarded pigment stones as originating in the liver. The second half of the treatise deals with the entire panorama of clinical disorders. The descriptions of the symptomatology and all of the known complications of the entity indicate how far he was able to go in diagnosis without the use of extensive laboratory aids. The case details are a model of the now-declining art of elaborate descriptive clinical observations based on pathologic-anatomic correlations.

M–3. Moynihan GGA: Gallstones and Their Surgical Treatment, 2nd ed. Philadelphia, WB Saunders, 1905, 458 pp

This was a surgical classic in its time because each operation was a daring giant step forward. Moynihan describes the patient's history in intimate detail, the precedents and procedural variants of other surgeons, and then his own attitudes, experiences, and results.

M–4. Bland–Sutton J: Gallstones and Diseases of the Bile Ducts. New York, Wood, 1907, 233 pp

The text is especially interesting because it is the compendium of a series of lectures delivered to the house staff of The Middlesex Hospital in London. The etiological factors which were unexplained more than 60 years ago, have still not been clarified. Many aspects of the case presentations remain pertinent.

M–5 Lutkens U: Aufbau und Funktion der Extrahepatischen Gallenwege. Vogel, 1926, 205 pp

This was written at the time of the active Freiburg Şchool of Medicine with its interest in biliary pathology directed by Aschoff, and the clinical studies of Naunyn. The text is dedicated to Naunyn. On the basis of operative and postmortem material studied in 1923, the author presents a detailed study of the pathology of the extrahepatic biliary passages. The viewpoint is to correlate morphology with function. Lutkens redefines a gross, microscopic, and functioning sphincter at the cholecystocholedochal junction which he calls the "collum-cysticus" sphincter. He held that disorders in this area may be a primary factor in the genesis of gallbladder disease.

SURGICAL SYSTEMS

M–6. KEHR H: Die Praxis der Gallenwege Chirurgie, Vol 1, 404 pp, 2, 661 pp. Munchen, Lehmann, 1913

This is the most comprehensive, detailed, and best illustrated monograph on the surgery of the biliary passages. Some of its illustrated surgical procedures were initiated by Kehr. The presentation is done in the elaborate detail often found in the German publications. The numerous color illustrations are another example of the personal expertise which has gone into the making of this book. This is one of the outstanding monographs in all surgery by one who limited his practice to biliary problems.

M–7. WALTERS W, SNELL AM: Diseases of the Gallbladder and Bile Ducts. Philadelphia, WE Saunders, 1940, 645 pp

The Mayo Clinic attitudes and experiences of that time are presented in this volume.

M–8. PUESTOW CB: Surgery of the Biliary Tract, Pancreas and Spleen. Chicago, Year Book Medical, 1953

Clearly done drawings illustrating operative techniques. The opposing page is a concise description of the procedure. Simplistic, especially good as an introductory text.

M–9. BEHREND M: Diseases of the Gallbladder and Allied Structures: Diagnosis and Treatment. Philadelphia, Davis, 1947, 290 pp

This is a short text of general methods.

M–10. BRUCKE H: Die Eingriffe am Gallensystem. Versuch Einer Neuen Darstellung. Bonn, Wilhelm Maudrich, 1956, 167 pp

A short but detailed and strongly opinionated monograph devoted to the practical aspects of the surgery of the biliary tract. It is obviously the product of a seasoned hand and rich experience. It voices a critical attitude toward the physiologic validity and practical significance of procedures directed at the assumed functional disorders of the biliary tract.

M–11. RATHCKE L: Steinrezidiv und Gallenwegsanastomosen. Stuttgart, Ferdinand Enke, 1956, 145 pp

This book, based on the author's personal experience, emphasizes the satisfactory role in both short- and long-term evaluation, of choledochoduodenostomy as a way of avoiding the problem of the residual or recurrent stone. In a personal communication in 1965, Professor Rathcke of Ludwigsburg wrote that the routine use of cholangiography and choledochoscopy has greatly decreased his indication for this procedure.

M–12. Lahey Clinic Number of the Surgical Clinics of North America. Symposium on the Surgery of the Biliary Tract, Liver, Pancreas, and Spleen. Philadelphia, WE Saunders, June, 1958

Pages 611 to 815 by several authors, deal with this Clinic's surgical practice relative to the technical aspects of surgery of the biliary tract and related areas.

M–13. ROUX M, DEBRAY C, LECANUET R, LAUMONIER R: Pathologie Chirurgicale des Voies Biliaires Extra-Hepatique. Paris, Masson et Cie, 1961, 345 pp

This volume is especially valuable for its cholangiograms of unusual problems and the technical aspects of their surgical management.

M–14. SMITH R, SHERLOCK S: Surgery of the Gallbladder and Bile Ducts. London, Butterworth, 1964, 378 pp

An outstanding text on all clinical aspects of biliary problems. It is well illustrated and authoritative. The emphasis is on surgical problems, their diagnosis, and the alternatives in their management. Maingot and DeQuesne have also contributed surgical sections.

M–15. HESS W: Surgery of the Biliary Passages and Pancreas. Princeton, Van Nostrand, 1965, 638 pp

This is the English translation of the original text entitled *Die Erkrankungen der Gallenwege und des Pankreas* as published by George Thieme in Stuttgart, in 1961. This is a comprehensive, detailed monograph on all aspects of biliary pancreatic disease. There has been no other modern, single-authored volume that compares with its encyclopedic references, numerous clear illustrations, and details of an extensive experience based on the surgical material at the University of Basel. The section on radiomanometry (cholangiomanometry), represents the most intensive original published clinical experience with this modality. The text compares with Kehr's magnum opus.

M–16. SCHEIN CJ, JACOBSON HG, STERN WZ: The Common Bile Duct. Operative Cholangiography, Biliary Endoscopy and Choledocholithotomy. Springfield, Ill, CC Thomas, 1966, 290 pp

M–17. PATEL J, LEGEL L: Nouveau Traité de Technique Chirurgicale. Paris, Masson et Cie, 1968

An excellent monograph in terms of illustrations of operative technique related to the liver factors in biliary surgery. In French, but the illustrative material is self-explanatory.

M–18. KUNE A: Current Practice of Biliary Surgery. Boston, Little, Brown, 1972

The author derived his viewpoints from experience at the Lahey Clinic in Boston and the Royal Melbourne Hospital. There is a basic text encompassing all biliary surgery. The line drawings are simple and declarative. The reference section is extensive and the textual arrangement makes for facile reading. It is not intended as an extensive, in-depth consideration.

M–19. WHITE TT, HARRISON RC: Reoperations on the biliary tract. In Reoperative Gastro-intestinal Surgery. Boston, Little, Brown, 1973, pp. 100–243

A personal viewpoint on the subject, well referenced and in detail.

M–20. ORLOFF MJ: Surgery of the biliary tree. Surg Clin North Am 53:961, 1973

A review of attitudes toward the still current problems by authorities in the particular area.

MEDICAL ASPECTS

M–21. LYON BBV: Nonsurgical Drainage of Gall Tract: A Treatise Concerned with the Diagnosis and Treatment of Certain Diseases of the Biliary and Allied Systems, in their Relation to Gastroenterology and General Clinical Medicine. Philadelphia, Lea & Febiger, 1923, 640 pp

The author presents an extensive ambulatory patient experience in the treatment of biliary disorders by duodenal tube drainage. The text presents the rationales, technique, and results of this procedure. The microscopy of the biliary sediment is especially well illustrated.

M–22. Rehfuss ME, Nelson GE: The Medical Treatment of Gallbladder Disease. Philadelphia, WF Saunders, 1935, 465 pp

This text originated from Jefferson Medical College. It summarizes the nonsurgical approach to biliary dysfunction in the preantibiotic era. The authors recognize the definitive role of surgery for the inflammatory component, and advise it. Otherwise their medical regime places emphasis on diet, cholegogues, choleretics, and especially on the control of concomittant focal infection and the spastic constipated colon. Good bowel hygiene often alleviates biliary symptoms. The role of duodenal intubation, vaccine therapy, and spa hydrotherapy now appear remote but the authors consider their therapeutic efficacy apart from the often tenuous physiological considerations.

M–23. Weiss S: Clinical Lectures on the Gallbladder and Bile Duct. Chicago, Year Book, Medical, 1944, 504 pp

This book is written from the viewpoint of a gastroenterologist and what problems defeat him enough to advise the use of surgery.

M–24. Popper H, Schaffner F: Liver Structure and Function. New York, McGraw-Hill, 1952, 777 pp

An in-depth reference text to the pathology and clinical physiology of the liver and its appendages. The bibliographic references number 3735

M–25. Arianoff AA: Les Cholecystoses. Bruxelles, Editions Arscia SA, 1966

An inclusive consideration of the subject; important in this regard because wittingly or not, this was the indication for the many initial operative procedures.

GENERAL TEXTS

M–26. Graham EA, Cole WH, Colpher GH, Moore S: Diseases of the Gallbladder and Bile Ducts. Philadelphia, Lea & Febiger, 1928, 477 pp

A presentation of the anatomy, physiology, and clinical disorders of the biliary tract. There is a section on the history of cholecystography and an evaluation of its diagnostic efficacy by the founders of the procedure. It is interesting that some of the illustrations are modified from Kehr. It was the "compleat" book in English in its time.

M–27. Carter RF, Greene CH, Twiss JR: The Diagnosis and Management of Disease of the Biliary Tract. Philadelphia, Lea & Febiger, 1939, 432 pp

M–28. Sterling JA: The Biliary Tract. Baltimore, Williams & Wilkins, 1955, 424 pp

A comprehensive survey of the medical and surgical problems including differential diagnosis. There are adequate line drawings and a comprehensive bibliography. There is an original presentation of some aspects of the anatomy of the Vaterian segment.

M–29. Millbourn: Klinische Studien Über die Choledocholithiasis. Acta Chir Scand [Suppl] 86, Suppl 65, 1941

A statistical study dealing with spontaneous passage of stones and the early and late results of operative and non-operative management.

M–30. Rains AJH: Gallstones, Causes and Treatment. Springfield, ILL, CC Thomas, 1964, 188 pp

Professor Rains writes from the University of London at Charing Cross Hospital. This is a succinct and highly personalized presentation. The first major section deals with the classic controversies on the origins of gallstones and the more recent thinking along clinical and metabolic lines. The second half is a terse presentation of the clinical problems.

M–31. Taylor EW: The Biliary System. A Symposium of the NATO Advanced Study Institute. Philadelphia, Davis, 1965, 712 pp

These are the papers of a meeting held in London representing contemporary American, English, and French viewpoints on: *1*) structural and functional relationships of the liver, biliary system, and hepatic-lymphatic system; *2*) metabolism and function of bile acids and salts; *3*) bilirubin metabolism; *4*) gallbladder function and control of bile secretion; *5*) excretion of hormones and antibiotics in bile; *6*) mechanisms of bile secretion; *7*) bromsulphalein (B.S.P.) tests of bile function; and *8*) clinical aspects of the biliary system.

M–32. Bouchier IAD (ed): Disease of the Biliary Tract. Clinics in Gastroenterology, Vol 2. Philadelphia, WB Saunders, 1973

British viewpoint, clinically oriented considers all factors from epidemiology to tumors. An excellent section on postcholecystectomy syndromes by Bodvall from Gothenburg.

M–33. Najarian JS, Delaney JP (eds): Surgery of the Liver, Pancreas and Biliary Tract. New York, Stratton Intercontinental Medical Book Corp, 1975

These are the papers presented at a University of Minnesota Department of Surgery symposium. Its value lies not only in the presentation of current status (basketing for stone, operative endoscopic extraction, laboratory aids in jaundice, etc.) but for the direct transcript of the panel discussions by the authorities on their own subjects. The presentations are informally succinct and particularized.

M–34. Longmire WP: Tumors of the extrahepatic biliary radicals. Curr Probl Cancer 1:5, 1976

An in depth consideration of the diagnosis, course and management of this increasingly common problem. A masterly presentation.

RADIOLOGY

M–35. Frimann–Dahl J: Roentgen Examinations in Acute Abdominal Diseases, 2nd ed. Springfield, Ill, CC Thomas, 1960, 518 pp

Only a short section is devoted to acute cholecystitis, but the concept of the plain-film differential diagnosis is elaborated with numerous illustrative roentgenograms.

M–36. Hess W: Operative Cholangiographie. Tecknik, Diagnostik, Praxis. Stuttgart, George Thieme, 1955, 201 pp

A profusely illustrated work on the technique of manometric cholangiography. The illustrations bear on all aspects of technique and interpretation required to make the intraoperative diagnosis.

M–37. Mirizzi PH: (1) Lithiase de la Voie Biliaire Principale. Paris, Masson et Cie, 1957. (2) Chirurgie du Système du Canal Hepatique. Lésions Bénignes. Paris, Masson et Cie, 1962, 203 pp

Monographs in French, written by the innovator of operative cholangiography. Some of the examples are unique and bizarre. The text includes complicated diagnostic problems and their solution.

M–38. Poppel MH, Jacobson HG, Smith RW: The Roentgen Aspects of the Papilla and Ampulla of Vater. Springfield, Ill, CC Thomas, 1953, 195 pp

This is a roentgen morphologic study of the Vaterian segment as evaluated by barium study of the upper gastrointestinal tract. The roentgen anatomy is altered by intrinsic as well as extrinsic diseases in the duodenum, pancreas and biliary tract. Standards for the normal are established.

M–39. Wise RE: Intravenous Cholangiography. Springfield, Ill, CC Thomas, 1962, 130 pp

This is the summary of the extensive experience of the Lahey Clinic. The indications for the study are broad and the complications were infrequent. The x-rays constitute a veritable atlas.

M–40. Wise RE (ed): Symposium on the Biliary System in the Radiologic Clinics of North America. Philadelphia, WB Saunders, 1966, pp 453–632

A multiauthored text dealing with the pharmacology, roentgen physiology, and interpretation of the oral and intravenous cholecysto-cholangiogram.

M–41. Shehadi W: Clinical Radiology of the Biliary Tract. New York, McGraw-Hill, 1963, 305 pp

This is a general text of biliary roentgenography with a generous number of illustrations.

M–42. Hepp J, Hernandez C, Moreaux J, Bismuth H: L'Artériographie dans les Afféctions Chirurgicales du Foie, du Pancreas et de la Rate. Paris, Masson et Cie, 1968

Valuable for the roentgen vascular anatomy of the pancreas and liver. The roentgen reproductions are excellent.

OPERATIVE CHOLANGIOGRAPHY

M–43. Schulenburg CAR: Operative Cholangiography. London, Butterworth, 1966, 261 pp

Operative cholangiography presented in an English text, based on experiences originating in South Africa. The techniques are given in detail including the positioning of the operating table for the cassette. Each cholangiogram is accompanied by a line drawing that emphasizes the salient features. Cautions in interpretations are interposed.

M–44. Magoldi P: Atlas Cholangiografico. Tecnica de la Cholangiografia Operatoria. Buenos Aires, Lopez & Etchegoyan, 1957, 251 pp

This volume contains 100 cholangiograms each multilingually interpreted in Spanish, French, and English.

M–45. Mirizzi PO: Chirurgie du Système du Canal Hépatique. Lésions Bénignes. Paris, Masson et Cie, 1962

M–46. Mirizzi PO: Lithiase de la Voie Biliaire Principale. Paris, Masson et Cie, 1957

A veritable atlas of unusual cholangiograms. Especially interesting for the personal surgical techniques of the founder of cholangiography. Copiously illustrated.

M–47. Creagh RE: Radiomanometric Cholangio-Pancreatography. Vol 18, No. 8, 1965

This is a well done review and presentation of the subject in a soft cover, 63 page document which originates from a surgical staff meeting held at the Veterans Administration Center in Des Moines, Iowa on February 12, 1965.

M–48. Kourias B, Stucke K: Atlas der per-und postoperativen Cholangiographie. Stuttgart, George Thieme, 1967, 207 pp

The book contains over 240 well-reproduced, illustrative cholangiograms with their pertinent case histories derived from the authors' enormous experience in Athens and Wurzburg.

M–49. Mallet–Guy P, Jeanjean R, Marion P: La chirurgie biliaire sous control manométrique et radiologique per-operatoire. Paris, Masson et Cie, 1947, 137 pp

The early experience of these authors is presented in great illustrative detail. The method and techniques are used as a physiologic tool to evaluate the "dyskinesias" of the biliary system.

ATLASES

M–50. Bickham WS: Operative Surgery, Vol IV. Philadelphia, WR Saunders, 1924, pp 437–609

A description, with accompanying drawings, of the techniques described by other surgeons. The author has collected them in one volume. Many of the procedures have long since been discarded. Some of the illustrations have been redrawn from the original publications, but the styles of the original artists are preserved in redrawn figures. It is an encyclopedic compilation without attempting a critical evaluation.

M–51. Glenn F: Atlas of Biliary Tract Surgery. New York, Macmillan, 1963, 145 pp

Glenn's atlas consists of pages of line drawings with accompanying explanatory text on the opposite side. The format is that of the popular Cutler and Zollinger *Atlas of Surgical Operations.* There is accompanying discussion of the details of the clinical and technical problems.

M–52. Dogliotti AM, Fogliati B: La Chirurgia della Vie Biliare. Turino, Minerva, 1958, 216 pp

Dogliotti's and Fogliati's text contains many color illustrations. The simplified drawings make the procedures look less formidable than they are in fact.

PANCREAS

M–53. Cattell RB, Warren RW: Surgery of the Pancreas. Philadelphia, WB Saunders, 1953, 374 pp

This is a comprehensive presentation of surgical techniques and attitudes and results from the Lahey Clinic.

M–54. Blumenthal AT, Probstein JG: Pancreatitis: A Clinical Pathologic Correlation. Springfield, Ill, CC Thomas, 1959, 379 pp

M–55. Dreiling DA, Janowitz JD, Perrier CV: Pancreatic Inflammatory Disease. A Physiologic Approach. New York, Hoeber, 1964, 238 pp

A collected review of the entire published experience with an extensive bibliography and reference to their own postmortem material in the first instance and to the extensive physiological studies on pancreatic excretory function and secretin testing in the second.

M–56. Howard JM, Jordan GL Jr: Surgical Diseases of the Pancreas. Philadelphia, JB Lippincott, 1960, 607 pp

In addition to the major experiences of the two authors there is a statistical tabulation of pertinent data from many other publications. The charted and tabulated summaries from the general literature constitute a comprehensive statistical review of virtually all of the important problems in this area.

M–57. Gliedman ML, Bolooki H, Rosen RG: Acute Pancreatitis. Curr Probl Surg. Year Book, Chicago, August 1970

An extensive clinical experience at a municipal hospital. The emphasis is on the management of the peritoneal and renal complications.

CHEMISTRY

M–58. Sabotka C: Physiological Chemistry of the Bile. Baltimore, Williams & Wilkins, 1937, 202 pp

M–59. Horrall OIT: Bile: Its Toxicity and Relation to Disease. Chicago, University of Chicago Press, 1938, 434 pp

M–60. Gray CH: The Bile Pigments. New York, Wiley, 1953, 142 pp

M–61. Haslewood GAD: Bile Salts. London, Methuen, 1967, 116 pp

The first two texts were comprehensive for their time and contain a wealth of information and plethora of references which have probably not been brought sufficiently into contemporary clinical focus. The third and fourth books incorporate modern methods in steroid chemistry and chromatography. Haslewood's documentation of the species specificity of bile acids may be a clue to the genesis of calculi in man.

PATHOLOGY

M–62. Aschoff L, Bacmeister A: Die Cholelithiasis. Jena, Fisher, 1909, 113 pp

M–63. Aschoff L: Lectures on Pathology. New York, Hoeber, 1924, 362 pp

Aschoff's studies on the pathology of the gallbladder were derived primarily from surgical specimens. The examination often revealed a cholesterol stone impacted in the ampulla and behind this a number of faceted stones. The author postulated that the cholesterol stones occur aseptically as a result of stasis and metabolic increase in bile cholesterol. As this stone produces obstruction, infection occurs and secondary stones form. This classification of stones in relation to stasis, metabolic factors, and infection remains the classic way of identifying them. The unnumbered last half of the volume contains colored drawings of the gross and microscopic pathologic variants of the diseased gallbladder.

M–64. Franz VK: Tumors of the Pancreas. Washington DC, Armed Forces Institute of Pathology, 1959

Especially valuable for its photo micrographs.

M–65. Cameron R, Hou PC: Biliary Cirrhosis. Edinburgh, Oliver & Boyd, 1962

The classification and pathology of the varieties of biliary cirrhosis including that resulting from extrahepatic obstruction.

M–66. Edmondson HA: Tumors of the Gallbladder and Extrahepatic Bile Ducts. Washington DC, Armed Forces Institute of Pathology, 1967, 167 pp., containing 151 figures, some in color

This is the most detailed and authorative presentation of the microscopic aspect of tumors in this area. It conforms to the high standards of the Armed Forces Institute of Pathology fascicles. One section also considers the normal anatomy and hyperplastic pathology as well as the pathogenesis of the intramural sinuses associated with chronic inflammation. The photomicroscopy is superb and represents a contemporary extension of Aschoff and Baumeister's monograph on the pathology of inflammatory disorders of the area.

M–67. Edmondson HA: Tumors of the Liver and Intrahepatic Bile Ducts. Washington DC, Armed Forces Institute of Pathology, 1967

An atlas of gross and microscopic pathology with descriptive data. A unique collection and presentation, especially of the rarer disorders.

M–68. Levine T: Chronic Cholecystitis. Its Pathology and the Role of Vascular Factors in its Pathogenesis. New York, John Wiley & Sons, 1975

This is the report of a Russian pathologist on the detailed morphologic changes encountered in chronic cholecystitis as well as changes associated with aging alone.

ENDOSCOPY

M–69. Wildegans H: Die Operative Gallengangsendoskopie. Munchen, Urban & Schwarzenberg, 1960, 105 pp

This is the only monograph limited to choledoscopy. The author developed the major clinical aspects of biliary endoscopy including the presently employed rigid instrument. He reports on an extensive experience. Endoscopic views are particularly well reproduced.

M–70. Beck K, Dischler W, Helms M, Kiani B, Sickinger K, Tenner R: Color Atlas of Laparoscopy. Stuttgart, Verlag, 1968

Especially valuable for the large colored endoscopic photographs of the liver and gallbladder. Original in German.

M–71. Berci G (ed): Endoscopy. New York, Appleton–Century–Crofts, 1976

The text considers the entire field of endoscopy. It is valuable in this specific context because of the sections on instrumentation (including care) and choledochoscopy and peritoneoscopy. The colored photographs are a valuable diagnostic aid. The chapter on endoscopy and radiology details intraoperative image intensification cholangiography.

ANATOMY

M–72. Netter, FH: Liver, Biliary Tract and Pancreas, 2nd ed. Edited by Oppenheim E. Summit, NJ, Ciba Pharmaceutical Co, 1964, 199 pp

These are the best colored drawings of biliary anatomy and pathology. They are in the tradition established by the artists who illustrated Sabotta's *Anatomy* and Kehr's textbook. The accompanying text is contributed by Bodansky, Clifton, Kozoll, Popper, Sborov, and Pack.

M–73. Michels NA: Blood Supply and Anatomy of the Upper Abdominal Organs. Philadelphia, JB Lippincott, 1955, 581 pp

A detailed anatomy of the biliary area is included. These are colored diagrammatic illustrations, from dissected specimens, of the usual, unusual, accessory, and aberrant vessels to the area. An encyclopediac collection of variants is graphically presented in trichome diagrams that become completely and readily comprehensible when the initial impression of seeming complexity is overcome.

M–74. Otto K: Die Gefasse der Gallenblase. Morphologic und Klinik. Berlin, Walter de Gruyter, 1973

A monographic consideration based on 106 injection studies. There were 33 cadaver studies. Now of interest principally for the venous studies *in vivo*. Hepatic and superior mesenteric arteriography have illuminated this area far beyond what corrosion studies can accomplish.

M–75. Kyosola K: Structure and innervation of the choledochoduodenal junction. Ann Chir Gynaecol Fenn [Suppl] 192: 1976

This is a micro anatomical and electron microscopic examination of the feline, canine and human Vaterian segment. The data is from the University of Helsinki.

POSTCHOLECYSTECTOMY SYNDROMES

M–76. Horgan E: Reconstruction of the Biliary Tract. A Review of all the Methods that Have Been Employed. New York, Macmillan, 1932, 201 pp

Much of this is now of only historic interest. There are 77 good line drawings of the surgical reconstructive procedures and 201 references to primary sources. The evolution of biliary surgery is indicated not only by the decreased need for such reconstructions, but also by the standardization of the technical methods now employed. It tersely represents one man's ingenuity to repair another's bizarre errors. Some of the illustrated procedures are now employed in the reconstructive surgery of other areas.

M–77. Redell G: Operative anastomoses between biliary and gastrointestinal tracts. A review of earlier literature and a clinical study of 809 Swedish cases. Acta Chir Scand Vol 84, Suppl 59, 1940

A huge early monograph of 371 pages with numerous line drawings illustrating the methods. Includes 1117 references. The case presentations are explicit in regard to details, methods and results.

M–78. Van der Linden W: Some biological traits in female gallstone-disease patients. Acta Chir Scand Suppl 269, Stockholm 1961

There has been little change in more than one-and-one-half decades in the still pertinent considerations regarding body build, parity, and serum cholesterol and social background.

M–79. Adolfsson G: Circulating and respiratory function in relation to physical activity in female patients before and after cholecystectomy. Acta Chir Scand Suppl 401, 1969

The role of preoperative physical training, intercostal block and early ambulation on the end result.

M–80. Mallet–Guy P, Kesten PJ, Gignoux M, Murat J: Syndrome Post-Cholécystectomie. Paris, Masson et Cie, 1970

A viewpoint regarding 407 patients with secondary operations offering satisfactory results in 90 percent. The choice of procedures is based on the cholangiomanometric demonstration of hypotonia or hypertonia of the biliary system. The treatment was by splanchnicetomy or choledocho-duodenostomy. A prejudiced experience based on highly personalized criteria.

M–81. Bodvall B: Late results following cholecystectomy in 1930 cases and special studies on postoperative biliary distress. Acta Chir Scand Suppl 329, 1964

This is an in-detail analysis of the problem detailing the significant statistical variables including age, sex, type of gallbladder disease and the type of distress. A realistic light on some until now indistinctly defined factors. A sort of bottom line monograph on a delicate subject.

SPECIAL AREAS

M–82. LIEDBERG N: Klinische Studien Uber die Akute Cholecystitis. Acta Chir Scand Suppl 47, 1937, pp 1–274; 1–182

There are numerous Scandinavian monographs on the biliary tract. They have usually appeared as supplements to the *Acta Chirurgica Scandinavica* rather than as separately published hard-cover volumes. Some of these are referred to in the references. This one is included because it is the monograph completely devoted to acute cholecystitis. The first section is a review of the pathology, clinical course, and management. The second section is a detailed case history of each of the patients included in the study. The results analyze the accomplishments and failures in therapy.

M–83. HARLEY HRS: Subphrenic Abscess. Oxford, Blackwell Scientific Publications, 1955

The symptoms, diagnosis, and management of this postoperative problem as reflected in this experience with 188 patients. The data originates from the United Cardiff Hospitals.

M–84. SANDBLOM P: Hemobilia. History, Pathology, Diagnosis, Treatment. Springfield, Ill, CC Thomas, 1972

The only monograph on this uncommon disorder of the liver and gallbladder. Detailing the history of its recognition and the evaluation of its management as indicated by case studies.

M–85. FLAMENT JB: Les Diverticules Muqueux de la Fenêtre Duodenale. Paris, Impressions, 1973

A radiographic and line drawing monograph on the biliary-pancreatic-significance of the paravaterian diverticulum. It's one viewpoint.

INDEX

The letters t and f following a page number indicate table and figure respectively.